D1605482

Dupuytren's Disease

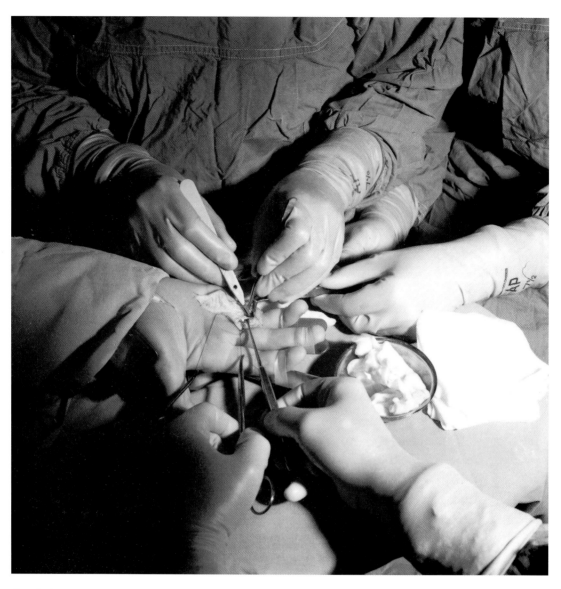

Surgical team operating on Dupuytren's disease

Dupuytren's Disease

Raoul Tubiana MD, FRCSEd (Hon)
Associate Professor, Faculty of Medicine, and
past President, Institut de la Main, Paris

Caroline Leclercq MD
Hand Surgeon, Institut de la Main, Paris

Lawrence C Hurst MD
Professor and Chairman, and Chief of Hand Surgery,
Department of Orthopaedics, SUNY at Stony Brook

Marie A Badalamente PhD
Professor, Department of Orthopaedics, SUNY at Stony Brook

Evelyn J Mackin PT
Executive Director, Hand Rehabilitation Foundation, Philadelphia

With contributions by Jean-Jacques Comtet
and Terri M Skirven

With illustrations by Léon Dorn

MARTIN DUNITZ

© Martin Dunitz Ltd 2000

First published in the United Kingdom in 2000 by
Martin Dunitz Ltd
The Livery House
7–9 Pratt Street
London NW1 0AE

Tel: +44 (0)20 7482 2202
Fax: +44 (0)20 7267 0159
E-mail: info@mdunitz.globalnet.co.uk
Website: http://www.dunitz.co.uk

A CIP catalogue record for this book is available from the British Library

ISBN 1–85317–475–0

Distributed in the United States by:
Blackwell Science Inc.
Commerce Place, 350 Main Street
Malden MA 02148, USA
Tel: 1 800 215 1000

Distributed in Canada by:
Login Brothers Book Company
324 Salteaux Crescent
Winnipeg, Manitoba R3J 3T2
Canada
Tel: 1 204 224 4068

Distributed in Brazil by:
Ernesto Reichmann Distribuidora de Livros, Ltda
Rua Coronel Marques 335
03440–000 São Paulo–SP
Brazil

Composition by Scribe Design, Gillingham, Kent
Printed and bound in China by Imago

Contents

Contributors

Raoul Tubiana
Associate Professor, Faculty of Medicine, and past President, Institut de la Main, Centre Orthopédique Jouvenet, 75016 Paris, France

Caroline Leclercq
Hand Surgeon, Institut de la Main, Centre Orthopédique Jouvenet, 75016 Paris, France

Lawrence C Hurst
Professor and Chairman, and Chief of Hand Surgery, Department of Orthopaedics, Health Science Center, State University of New York at Stony Brook, Stony Brook, NY 11794, USA

Marie A Badalamente
Professor, Department of Orthopaedics, Health Science Center, State University of New York at Stony Brook, Stony Brook, NY 11794, USA

Evelyn J Mackin
Executive Director, Hand Rehabilitation Foundation, Philadelphia, PA 19107, USA

Jean-Jacques Comtet
Professor, Polyclinique Orthopédique de Lyon, Clinique du Parc, 69006 Lyon, France

Terri M Skirven
Director of Hand Therapy, Hand Rehabilitation Foundation, Philadelphia, PA 19107, USA

Acknowledgments

Developing this book on Dupuytren's disease has been a stimulating experience as there are so many aspects to be considered. This would not have been possible without a multidisciplinary collaboration of researchers, surgeons, and therapists.

I would first like to thank the co-authors of this book: Caroline Leclercq, Marie Badalamente, Lawrence Hurst, and Evelyn Mackin; I am particularly grateful to Dr Hurst who has corrected most of the text.

In addition to the authors, I wish to extend my thanks to the contributors and others: Jean-Jacques Comtet (who has allowed us to publish his excellent study on reflex sympathetic dystrophy), Guy Foucher (who has created a new fasciotomy technique – the needle fasciotomy; he has modified the original hazardous technique and he gives his first results here); A Messina (who has been the pioneer of the preoperative elongation technique; he has sent us the encouraging results of this salvage procedure); Y Djermag (who uses a smaller fixator for longitudinal traction and has demonstrated the efficiency of this technique); François Iselin and A Logan, J Armstrong, and J Huerren (who have kindly sent us the results of their dermofasciectomies); and Terri Skirven (who has collaborated with Evelyn Mackin in the chapter on hand therapy).

I hope that these combined efforts have produced a book that reflects the current knowledge of Dupuytren's disease.

I would also like to extend my thanks to all my friends with whom, in the past, I have worked on this subject. Their names are frequently quoted in this book: JIP James, C Nezelof, Jacques Michon, Jean-Michel Thomine, Hervé de Frenne, Barry Simmons, and of course John Hueston.

I am also particularly grateful to Léon Dorn who, for so many years, has enriched my books with his superb illustrations, and to the editorial staff at Martin Dunitz Ltd, Robert Peden and Mike Meakin, for their constant assistance.

Raoul Tubiana

Permissions

Although every effort has been made to ensure that copyright material has been reproduced with the permission of the copyright holder, the publisher apologizes for any omission. For permissions acknowledgment in any future edition of this book, please contact the publisher.

Many illustrations have been reproduced from Tubiana R, Gilbert A, Masquelet AC (1999) *An Atlas of Surgical Techniques of the Hand and Wrist*. Martin Dunitz, London/Lippincott–Raven, Philadelphia, and from Tubiana R, Thomine J-M, Mackin E (1996) *Examination of the Hand and Wrist*, 2nd edn. Martin Dunitz, London/Mosby–Year Book, Inc., St Louis.

The following, or their adaptations, are reproduced by kind permission of the copyright holders:

Alioto RJ, Rosier RN, Burton RI et al. (1994) Comparative effects of growth factors on fibroblasts of Dupuytren's tissue and normal plantar fascia. *J Hand Surg* **19A**: 442–52 (Figure 4.4);

Blair WF (1996) *Techniques in Hand Surgery*. Williams and Wilkins, Baltimore; from the chapter by Hurst (Figure 6.34);

Bourgery JM, Jacob NA (1832) *Traité complet de l'anatomie de l'homme comprenant la médecine opératoire*. CA Delauney, Paris (Figures 2.1, 6.8, 6.10 and 6.61);

Bruner JM (1970) The dynamics of Dupuytren's disease. *Hand* **2**: 172–77 (Figure 5.12);

Djermag Y (1999) *Traitement des formes sévères de la maladie de Dupuytren par distracteur articulaire progressif*. Communication à l'Académie Nationale de Chirurgie le 5 mai 1999 (Figures 7.6–7.8);

Eicher E, Moberg G (1970) Möglichkeiten zur Vermeidung von Amputationen bei schwerer Dupuytren'scher Kontraktur. *Handchirurgie* **2**: 56–60 (Figure 7.2);

Hueston JT, Tubiana R (1974) *Dupuytren's Disease*. Churchill Livingstone, Edinburgh (Figure 2.5); also, from the 2nd edn (1985), from the chapter by Littler (Figures 5.28 and 6.48); McGregor (Figure 6.11);

Hurst LC, Badalamente MA (1999) Non-operative treatment of Dupuytren's disease. *Hand Clin* **15**: 97–107 (Figures 6.1–6.3);

Ling RSM (1963) The genetic factor in Dupuytren's disease. *J Bone Joint Surg* **45B**: 709–18 (Figure 3.1);

McFarlane R, McGrouther D, Flint M (1990) *Dupuytren's Disease. Biology and Treatment*, Vol. 5. Churchill Livingstone, Edinburgh (Figures 4.1–4.3 and Table 4.1); also, from the chapter by Hurst and Badalamente (Figures 5.31 and 5.32);

McGrouther DA (1982) The microanatomy of Dupuytren's contracture. *Hand* **13**: 215–36 (Figure 2.24);

Messina A (1989) La TEC (Tecnica estensione continua) nel morbo di Dupuytren grave. Dall'amputazione alla ricostruzione. *Riv Chir Mano* **26**: 253–56 (Figures 7.4 and 7.5);

Milford L (1968) *Retaining Ligaments of the Digits of the Hand*. WB Saunders, Philadelphia (Figures 2.2, 2.4, 2.19 and 2.20);

Museu Nacional d'Art de Catalunya, Barcelona, Spain (Figure 1.1);

Thomine J-M (1965) Conjonctif d'enveloppe des doigts et squelette fibreux des commissures interdigitales. *Ann Chirurg Plast* **3**: 194–203 (Figures 2.14 and 2.17);

Tubiana R, Hueston JT (1986) *La Maladie de Dupuytren*, 3rd edn. L'Expansion Scientifique Française, Paris; from the chapter by Allieu and Tessier (Figures 6.63 and 6.64);

Walsh M (1984) Relationship of hand edema to upper extremity position and water temperature during whirlpool. *J Hand Surg* **9A**: 609 (Figure 9.2).

The majority of the entries in the 'References and further reading prior to 1942' have been reproduced from the 'Bibliografia' in Ferrarini M (1941) *La malattia del Dupuytren*, 409–38. Nistri–Lischi Editori, Pisa.

Many other entries in the 'References and further reading prior to 1942' have been reproduced from Elliot D (1999) Pre-1900 literature on Dupuytren's disease. *Hand Clin* **15**: 175–81.

Preface

This book traces the history, which is relatively recent, of Dupuytren's disease. In fact, the first medical descriptions of this disease only appeared in the 17th century and the first attempt at treatment was at the end of the 18th century. Until now, no medical treatment has proved effective. Surgical treatment was first directed towards the correction of deformities by performing increasingly extended procedures: aponeurotomies, then aponeurectomies. In the presence of more numerous and severe intra- and postoperative complications, the surgeon's efforts were then redirected towards the prevention of such complications. More recently, surgical intervention has also aimed to prevent recurrence.

At present, two surgical tendencies have developed; these appear divergent but are in fact complementary. When, for example, the surgeon is primarily seeking to correct deformity in the case of slowly evolving disease in the elderly patient, the current tendency is to perform only limited procedures. On the contrary, if there is a risk of early recurrence, skin grafts are more frequently carried out; this is mostly in relatively young patients presenting with rapid evolution of the disease.

Now, at the start of the 21st century, we still do not know the origin of this disease, and its treatment remains essentially palliative. What will happen during this century? One can only assume that the nature of this mysterious disease will be elucidated and that its current treatment will become medical. Scientific research, which has substantially increased in recent decades, has provided considerable advances in the fields of anatomy, anatomico-pathology, genetics, epidemiology, cellular biology, and biochemistry.

The progress in our knowledge of the nature of collagen in Dupuytren's disease, in particular, has permitted two of the authors of this book to embark on the use of local injections of Clostridial collagenase, resulting in the lysis of the collagen cord and so allowing its rupture. The results of this method have been spectacular according to both the authors and the patients. Can one therefore say that surgery will be totally abandoned? This will depend on the results of current clinical research, which will define the limits of medical treatment by eventual contraindications, by its efficacy in the presence of long-standing joint contractures and by its preventative effect on recurrence.

It appears that we are now close to solving a problem that has impassioned generations of researchers and surgeons.

Raoul Tubiana

1

History

Raoul Tubiana

HISTORY OF DUPUYTREN'S DISEASE AND OF ITS TREATMENT

Dupuytren's contracture appears to be a relatively new disease. Medical historians have not identified any condition of the hand resembling Dupuytren's disease in the medical writings of the Greeks and Romans. Even in Northern Europe, where Dupuytren's disease is now so common, there was no mention of it 'in the fragmented Anglo-Saxon of early Gaelic medical literature, nor in that of Scandinavia in the 13th and 14th Centuries. When life expectancy was short, by comparison with today, the incidence of this disease of late middle and old age may have been small and the disease considered comparatively trivial.' (Elliot, 1988a).

Yet, on the Isle of Skye in the Western Isles of Scotland, an area colonized by the Norsemen, a progressive contracture of the little finger has been known for centuries among bagpipe players in the Scottish College of Bagpiping run by the MacCrimmons (the MacCrimmons' Curse).

Whaley and Elliot (1993) identified four miracle cures set in Orkney and Iceland in the 12th and 13th Centuries and recorded in the sagas of the earls of Orkney and the bishops of Iceland, in which the condition of the hand that was healed bore a resemblance to Dupuytren's contracture.

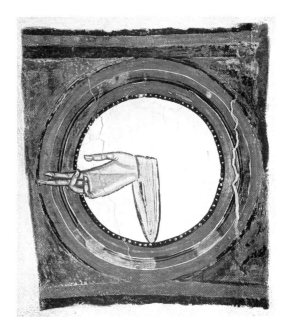

Figure 1.1 The raised hand of benediction of Sant Climent de Taüll (© Museu Nacional d'Art de Catalunya (Barcelona), reproduced with permission).

What is the relationship between the raised hand of benediction (Figure 1.1) or of legality (Figure 1.2) and Dupuytren's disease? Redfern (1986), in a correspondence newsletter of the American Society for Surgery of the Hand, supports the theory that its origin is much

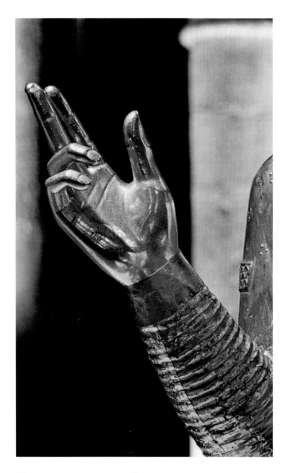

Figure 1.2 The hand of legality.

older than Christianity, and probably represents the superimposition of a Roman gesture, from earlier times, on the Christian Church.

The earliest medical description of this deformity is found in the writings of Felix Plater of Basel in 1614. In the third volume of his *Observationum* he described the case of a stone-mason with ulnar fingers contracture and the inexorable progress of this condition despite splinting and emoluments, drawing into the palm of the hand the ring and little fingers. However, he did not attempt an explanation of its cause.

Henry Cline

Henry Cline, from London, was the first to recognize the role of the palmar aponeurosis. In 1777, he dissected two cadaveric hands with this contracture of the fingers and recorded in his notebook kept at the library of St Thomas' Hospital Medical School in London (Cline, 1777):

> Fingers in the palm of the hand without any alteration in the muscles and tendons. This has been seen in dissecting two subjects, in one all the fingers were contracted, but when cutting through the fascia, they were immediately extended. In the other, the ring finger only was contracted, which was found to arise from a thickening and shortening of that portion of ligament that is inserted into that finger. It appeared from the last case, that the fascia is not blinded with the thecae of the fingers, but inserted into the phalanges distinctly, by the side of it.

Astley Cooper

Cline was Astley Cooper's teacher and the latter was invited after an apprenticeship of 5 years to share Cline's lectures. Cooper's celebrity eclipsed that of his mentor. Cooper mentioned in a brief note in 1822 in his *Treatise on Dislocations and Fractures of the Joints* (Cooper, 1822):

> The fingers are sometimes contracted by a chronic inflammation of the thecae (flexor tendon sheaths) and aponeurosis of the palm of the hand, from excessive action of the hand, in the use of the hammer, the oar ... etc, etc. When the thecae is contracted, nothing should be attempted for the patient's relief, as no operation or other means will succeed; but when the aponeurosis is the cause of the contraction, and the contracted band is narrow, it may be with advantage divided by a pointed bistory, introduced

through a very small wound in the tegument. The finger is then extended, and a splint is applied to preserve it in the straight position.

Confusion existed in France at that time as to whether flexor tendons, flexor tendon sheaths or palmar fascia were responsible for the finger's contracture. Alexis Boyer, personal surgeon to Napoleon, in his *Traité des Maladies Chirurgicales* written in 1826, attributed the contraction of the fingers to a drying and stiffening of the flexor tendons and the overlying skin, a condition called '*crispatura tendinum*', and Boyer warned surgeons strongly against dividing the flexor tendons (Boyer, 1826).

Dr Mailly, one of Boyer's pupils, was consulted by a wine-merchant, ML, in 1831 about such a contracture of the fingers. He wisely referred the patient to Dupuytren, the famous chief surgeon of the Hôtel-Dieu. Dupuytren performed his first palmar fasciotomy on this patient.

Guillaume Dupuytren

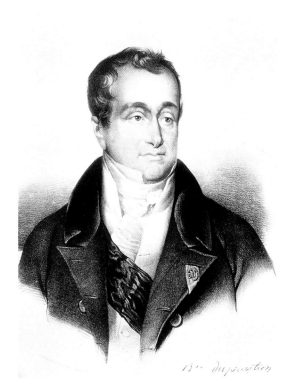

Figure 1.3. Baron Guillaume Dupuytren (1777–1835).

Guillaume Dupuytren (Figure 1.3) was born in Pierre-Buffière near Limoges in 1777. There had previously been several surgeons in the Dupuytren family. In 1719, a surgeon Michel Dupuytren lived at Pierre-Buffière, running the tobacco shop at the same time. François Dupuytren, grandfather of Guillaume, drowned while returning from visiting a sick patient. Two brothers of François, Leonard and Jacques, were also surgeons so that it is not surprising that Guillaume selected surgery, although Guillaume's own father was a lawyer. Guillaume was sent to Paris for his schooling in a Jesuit institution named after its founder, Jean de la Marche. It was during this period, from the dawn of the Revolution in 1789 through the bloody Reign of Terror in 1793–94, that young Dupuytren was a student in Paris. The changes that the Revolution wrought were to affect deeply the shape of his

life. Now the road to success was open to the talented, without distinction of birth or fortune.

Once at home again in 1794, Guillaume wanted to join the army. His father, however, insisted that, in the family tradition, Guillaume become a surgeon. As a first step in his training, he was enrolled in the medical-surgical courses in Limoges, but after a few months, Dupuytren set out for Paris, where he remained for the rest of his life.

Dupuytren's medical studies coincided with the period of Directoire, from 1795 to 1799. The Terror was over, there was money to be made in manufacture and commerce, glory to be grasped in the battlefields. This was also a period of dissipation and pleasure, but Dupuytren had given his life over completely to his studies of anatomy, experimental physiology and pathological anatomy. He became *Chef des travaux anatomiques* (Director of Anatomical Studies) in the Medical School in 1801 and the Council of the Ecole de Médecine formally requested that he be exempt from the obligatory military duty.

The reign of Napoleon (1801–14) had been for Dupuytren a period of tough 'open competition'; each post won gave rise to bitter rivalry. The Revolution had released a flood of energy and in this brilliant era of French medicine, the rising young men were Bichat, Broussais, Larrey, Roux, Laennec: all formidable rivals for Dupuytren.

Dupuytren became, at just under 25 years of age, *Chirurgien de deuxième classe* at the Hôtel-Dieu in 1802. The Hôtel-Dieu was the most important hospital in Paris. The chief surgeon was Phillippe-Joseph Pelletan, with whom Dupuytren had unceasing conflicts, which reduced his surgical activity. He continued his own researches and animal experimentation at the school of veterinary medicine at Maisons-Alfort (which still exists). Here, Dupuytren worked closely with Alexis Dupuy for many years. Dupuytren proved that the spleen could safely be removed and he published, with Dupuy, reports on the nervous, cardiac, circulatory, and cerebral systems and on the role of the nerves in respiration. In 1812 he was Professor of Operative Medicine at the Faculté de Médecine of Paris.

In 1815, Pelletan was 68 years old and wanted to 'organize' his succession at the Hôtel-Dieu. He put forward his son Gabriel, who had been a surgeon in the Imperial Guard, for the appointment as clinical assistant, but with the passing of the Napoleonic era Pelletan's position was weakened. In September 1815, the Minister of the Interior of Louis XVIII asked the Conseil des Hôpitaux to submit a list of five candidates for the post of *Chirurgien en chef* at the Hôtel-Dieu. Dupuytren's name was third on the list, after Boyer and Dubois, his elders by some 20 years. These two were passed over because of their close relationship with

Napoleon, and Guillaume Dupuytren became *Chirurgien en chef* at the Hôtel-Dieu at just under 38 years of age. For 20 years he retained a place of pre-eminence in the medical history of his time, sometimes called the Age of Dupuytren. This period corresponds with the restoration of the monarchy in France after the Revolution, and the Empire, with the return of the brother of Louis XVI, King Louis XVIII. Dupuytren had been named surgeon of King Louis XVIII in 1823 and the king conferred on him the hereditary title of baron. The king died in 1824 and was succeeded by his younger brother, Charles X; thus Dupuytren immediately became chief surgeon of the new king.

Dupuytren was admired as a brilliant surgeon and a great teacher but his ambition and his aggressiveness had aroused many envies and enemies, hence the malicious tone of so many contemporary writings. For Lisfranc, Dupuytren was 'the brigand of the Hôtel-Dieu'; for Percy 'the greatest of surgeons and the least of men'. However, so high was Dupuytren's status that his obituary in the London *Lancet* expressed the general view: 'Regarding surgery in the true sense, we hesitate not to place the late Baron Dupuytren at the head of European surgery' (*The Lancet*, 21 February 1835).

Dupuytren's powers of diagnosis were legendary and the list of his innovations is too long for enumeration. For example, in the field of orthopedics, he described in 1822 the congenital dislocation of the hip, which he distinguished from accidental dislocations. He gave the original description of fractures of the lower end of the fibula for which he devised a splint. He described a distortion of the wrist, now called Madelung's deformity. He was also the first to perform a resection of the lower jaw, and the first to excise the neck of the uterus for cancer. He described post-traumatic shock. In his thesis on 'lithotomy' (1812) he gave an anatomical description of the perineal region, layer by layer, which is still a classic. He reported a considerable number of self-mutilations of the genitalia and took account of their determining factors: 'self-punishment, guilt, jealousy, remorse, expiation, any of these may be responsible.'

In 1832 he gave his classification of burns arranged in six categories based upon the depth of the burn. He even noticed the presence of ulceration of the gastrointestinal tract in severely burned patients 10 years before Curling, to whom that insight is now credited. For Garrison (in 1966) his most enduring title to modern fame is in the field of surgical pathology and perhaps above all for his diagnosis and treatment of contracture of the fingers (Garrison, 1966), the subject of this book.

Hannah Barsky (1984) wrote a comprehensive portrait of Dupuytren in which she describes his daily activity when he was chief surgeon at the Hôtel-Dieu, which is summarized here:

For twenty years, day in, day out, the Dupuytren program was all but unvaried. When Marjolin became Dupuytren's adjunct surgeon, Dupuytren told him he was expected to act as substitute when the chief was out of the town or ill, but added 'I warn you that I am never away and never ill'. There was for Dupuytren no holiday, no vacation. Even Christmas found him at his post.

His hospital arrival came no later than six o'clock in the morning. His arrival would be signaled by the ringing of a bell. Ward round began promptly and might take as long as three hours. Dupuytren proceeded from bed to bed (the four wards of his service held 264 beds).

The daily ward rounds were followed by the daily lectures. Seated in his high-backed green armchair behind a table, he would address as many as five hundred auditors, not only hospital personnel, doctors and students, but professional colleagues and laymen from Paris, from France, from the world beyond. Dupuytren began his clinical lectures in a low voice, which would force his auditors to pay close attention, 'His voice was soft and smooth, with not only a clarity of thought but a clarity of diction, which made him, even for foreigners, so easy to follow'.

Other well-documented biographies of Dupuytren have been written by Cruveilhier (1841) and Mondor (1945).

The *Leçons Orales* (Dupuytren, 1832) recorded by his associates and promptly translated abroad attest to the method, content, and style of these model clinical lectures.

The hour's lecture over, operations began. Dupuytren valued deliberation over brilliance, safety over sleight of hand. Surgery was an extension, a demonstration of clinical lectures. In 1818, 2363 patients were admitted to Dupuytren's service and 764 major operations performed, ranging from strangulated hernias, skull fractures, mastectomies, amputations of the upper and lower jaw, artificial anus and malignant tumors, as well as a series of orthopedic and ophthalmological procedures.

His operative records were extraordinarily good. With so many eye witness accounts as we have of his operations, no error escaped the record. One failure, said Cruveilhier (1841), afflicted Dupuytren more than 20 successes delighted him. It was only his failures to which he was sensitive.

After the operations came the outpatient clinic for free consultations: 'For the cold Dupuytren, whom others saw on occasion, was not seen by these indigent patients. All those who worked with him and all who visited his clinics agreed that he showed toward these humble outpatients the same attentiveness and care he showed to the rich and famous who came to him for private consultations.'

In all, 5–6 hours had been devoted to the Hôtel-Dieu service. The rest of the day would be filled with operations on private patients, medical school duties, supervision of the laboratory, clinical research, and private consultations. Dupuytren's professional day was not yet over with the departure of the last private patient. There was always a return visit to the Hôtel-Dieu from 6–7 o'clock to see, once again, the patients on whom he had operated that day and the new admissions. And after that, there was a social life.

On 5 December 1831, at the Hôtel-Dieu, Dupuytren described the permanent contracture of the fingers. This lecture was reported verbatim in the *Journal Universel et Hebdomadaire de Médecine et de Chirurgie Pratique* by his assistants, Paillard and Marx (Dupuytren, 1831).

Dupuytren himself wrote very little apart from a huge collection of observations. The lecture notes, religiously recorded by his assistants, Brière de Boismont, Paillard and Marx, were published in the *Leçons Orales de Clinique Chirurgicale faites à l'Hôtel-Dieu de Paris par Monsieur le Baron Dupuytren*. They began in 1832 and filled five volumes. Dupuytren died in November 1835. 'La rétraction permanente des doigts', when it was published as the first article of the first edition of the *Leçons Orales* in 1832, was considered a completely unknown pathology. Later, Dupuytren's assistants and Dupuytren himself discovered that this condition had already been mentioned by Astley Cooper, and the 'Leçon sur la rétraction permanente des doigts' was relegated to article XI of Volume 4 of the second edition, which appeared in 1839, after Dupuytren's death.

Extracts of this article, in more detail than the first edition, are reported here.

> Contracture of the fingers, mainly of the ring finger, said Mr Dupuytren, had until now been of nearly unknown etiology. When we consider the multiple causes involved, the number of treatments used, and the numerous hypotheses of its origin, it is not surprising that it was considered incurable. Authors who had an interest in contracture of the fingers had given only incomplete information.
>
> Dupuytren, who had observed between 30 and 40 cases of this kind, quotes a host of diverse opinions on the cause of retraction of the ring finger. 'A few years ago, it was thought that contraction of the ring finger was dependent on a degeneration of the tendons of the flexor muscles.' Such was the state of medical knowledge relating to the disease that when a

man afflicted with it happened to die, Mr Dupuytren, who had been watching him for a long time, was informed of it and he managed to ensure this remarkable specimen was not lost to medical art. As soon as he had the arm at his disposal ... he proceeded with the dissection. The skin having been removed from the whole area of the palm and the palmar surface of the fingers, the folds or wrinkling which it formerly presented disappeared entirely ... The dissection was continued; the professor displayed the palmar fascia and noticed that it was taut, contracted and shortened; from its distal part there were cords which went to the side of the finger ... But it remained to find the exact spot affected; he cut the promulgation's passing to the sides of the fingers: immediately the contraction ceased, the finger came back to a position of semi-flexion, the least effort brought the phalanges back to complete extension. The tendons were all still intact, the sheath had not been opened at all, he could detect no change on the joint surfaces, no deterioration in the lateral ligaments, no ankylosis; the synovial sheaths and cartilages, the joint synovium, had not suffered any deterioration either. It was consequently natural to conclude that the starting point of the condition was in the exaggerated tension of the aponeurosis ... It was therefore only a question of finding the opportunity of applying the theory to new facts. The opportunity did not take long to come.

On 12 June 1831, Dupuytren operated on the right hand of ML, the wine merchant who suffered from a progressive contraction of the ring and little fingers.

> ... The ring finger and the little finger were completely bent and lying on the palm of the hand. The hand of the patient being securely fastened, Monsieur Dupuytren began by making a transverse incision one inch long, opposite the metacarpophalangeal joint of the ring finger. The scalpel cut first the skin and then the palmar aponeurosis, with an audible cracking. The incision completed, one could see the

finger becoming straight again and it could be stretched out nearly as easily as in its natural state. Wanting to save the patient the pain of another incision, Monsieur Dupuytren, tried to extend the division of the aponeurosis by sliding the scalpel transversely deep to the skin towards the ulnar side of the hand, in order to release the little finger, but this was in vain. Consequently he decided to make a fresh transverse incision opposite the proximal interphalangeal joint of the little finger and thus detached the end from the palm of the hand; but the rest of the finger remained obstinately fixed to this part ... Finally a third and last incision was made transversely, opposite the middle of the proximal phalanx itself, and immediately the little finger could be stretched.

This case was complicated by suppuration, a rather common event at that time.

On the 2nd August, ML wore the traction splint only at night and already his joints were beginning to acquire a degree of suppleness, showing that the function of the flexor tendon had remained intact, and that in a short time the movements of the fingers would be re-established to their natural state ...

On Monday 5 December Dupuytren operated successfully on another patient, a coachman, who for several years had seen his ring finger draw up towards the palm of his hand. In finishing the lesson the Professor added, 'it is necessary that you realize that all the cases are not exactly the same and that all methods are not applicable to them, and that even the best of us can be deceived and even dishonored by the wrong application of them. Such would be, for example, the application of this method to the retraction of the fingers caused by rheumatism, gout, whitlow etc.'

At 68 years of age, he developed pleurisy and died in a few days, while Cruveilhier, Bouillaud and Broussais were debating whether to drain his empyema. In Dupuytren's opinion it was 'better to die of the disease than of the operation.' On the day of his funeral, colleagues and scholars came from all over the country. His mortal remains were carried to the Père Lachaise cemetery by his students who would not delegate this last duty to anyone else.

Jean-Gaspard Goyrand

Jean-Gaspard Goyrand, from Aix en Provence, a little more than a year later challenged Dupuytren's view on this condition (Goyrand, 1833, 1835). Goyrand went to Paris in 1824 at the age of 21 years and spent four years largely under Dupuytren at the Hôtel-Dieu (Latil and Hueston, 1992). After graduating in 1828, Goyrand returned to Aix and prepared careful dissections of hands with contracture of the fingers and claimed in April 1834 at the Académie Royale de Médecine that Dupuytren was in error on three points. First, his dissections showed bands flexing fingers and the thumb, beyond the normally accepted limits of the palmar aponeurosis. Secondly, that a longitudinal incision allowed better healing and even some fascial excision. Thirdly, that the condition was more hereditary than occupational in origin.

He was back at the Académie de Médecine the next year, soon after the death of Dupuytren, and presented an experimental excision of a transverse segment of palmar aponeurosis followed by direct suture of the defect. Only the metacarpophalangeal (MP) joints were flexed but not the interphalangeal (IP) joints. He stated that the 'predigital bands', which flexed the fingers, were formed from the 'fibro-cellular subcutaneous tissue' of the fingers. Sanson and Breschet (Sanson, 1834; Sanson and Breschet, 1834), both Dupuytren's assistants, were asked to examine Goyrand's work. Sanson complimented Goyrand of the need for fasciectomies in the fingers and agreed that the disease was not always limited to the palmar aponeurosis. He proposed a theory of compromise. The new formations described by Goyrand were, in fact, not new, but a proliferation of fibrocellular tissues that were present in the normal hand. The cases presented by Goyrand were

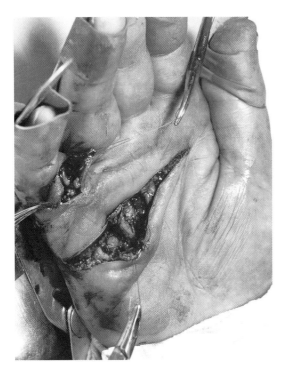

Figure 1.4 McIndoe approach for palmar and digital fasciectomy.

caused by thickening and contracture of these rudimentary fibrocellular extensions from the palmar aponeurosis extended into the fingers. One hundred and sixty years later, the debate over the actual site of the pathologic lesion continues.

THE PRESENT DAY

During the 19th Century and until the Second World War, surgeons considered mostly the palmar lesions. Correction of proximal interphalangeal (PIP) joint contracture was rarely mentioned.

Development of plastic surgery and then of hand surgery allowed surgeons to treat digital lesions. Sir Archibald McIndoe (McIndoe and Beare, 1958) performed a technique of extensive palmar fasciectomy by transverse palmar

incision associated with the excision of digital lesion by Z plasty (Figure 1.4). This was the procedure of choice used by most surgeons in the years following the war.

In 1950, the French Orthopaedic Society chose the topic of Dupuytren's disease for its annual report, and the author was designated to research and present the subject. Tradition at that time was to give this work to the youngest member of the Society. The author asked permission to work on this project with JIP James, at that time assistant to Sir Herbert Sedon, who, like the author, developed an interest in hand surgery.

The study (James and Tubiana, 1952) on both sides of the Channel highlighted the high incidence of complications after extended fasciectomies, especially when they were not performed by hand surgeons (who were rare at that time). This was due mainly to hematomas or skin necrosis. Surgeons realized that the aim of surgical treatment was not only to correct the deformity, but also to avoid complications due to surgery. In 1955, the author published a series of 100 cases of fasciectomies for Dupuytren's disease (Tubiana, 1955). Since that time, he has operated each week on one or more hands affected by this disease. This experience has allowed him to follow the evolution of the different surgical techniques over the last five decades. In the author's practice, extensive palmar fasciectomy with transverse palmar incisions, which required a vast subcutaneous undermining, were abandoned and a limited fasciectomy with a digitopalmar approach was advocated (Tubiana, 1964).

McCash (1964) reported his open palm technique, which eliminated the hematomas at the price of slow healing of the transverse palmar incision. With the development of hand surgery, the risk of complications decreased but the incidence of recurrences and extension of the disease remained (Tubiana and Leclercq, 1985). Surgeons have been slow to realize that recurrences depend less on the extent of the excision of the diseased tissue than on the rate of activity of the disease particular to each patient. The observation that recurrence did not occur beneath a skin graft led Hueston to describe a new procedure: the dermofasciectomy; however, the progression of the disease remains unchanged in the surrounding tissues.

The ultimate aim of treatment would be to prevent the proliferation of fibrous tissue and to obtain its regression without any surgical procedure. This remains an important unsolved problem, just as the origin of this affliction is still unknown. Given the considerable development of research in pathological anatomy, genetics, histopathology, cell biology and biochemistry, illustrated in the following sections, let us hope that, in the not too distant future, Dupuytren's disease will not require surgical treatment.

The history of the science of hand surgery, anatomical researches on Dupuytren's disease and its treatment may be found in the relevant chapters.

Many surgeons and scientists have been fascinated by this mysterious disease and have contributed to advances in the knowledge of Dupuytren's disease. Some of them have devoted their entire professional life to this disease. This is the case with Robert McFarlane.

Robert McFarlane

Robert Mcfarlane has, for three decades, published many important papers on the anatomy, epidemiology, and surgery of Dupuytren's disease and an excellent book (McFarlane et al., 1990).

This was also the case with John Turner Hueston who made original and significant contributions to all fields of Dupuytren's disease (Figure 1.5).

John Hueston

John Hueston was born in Kew, near Melbourne, Australia, in 1926 and graduated in 1948. He volunteered in 1952 in the Australian army as surgical specialist to serve in Japan and in Korea where he gained great experience in the management of trauma and burns. He continued his plastic surgical studies with Sir Archibald McIndoe in England, where the author met him in 1953. McIndoe's practice at the Queen Victoria Hospital at East Grinstead was at that time the mecca of plastic surgery. A few years before, in 1946, the author had met a young Swedish surgeon there, Tord Skoog, who was to become famous, carrying out a follow-up investigation on patients who had had a fasciectomy at the Plastic Surgery Unit of the Queen Victoria Hospital. Skoog's thesis, published in 1948, gave the first detailed account of McIndoe's operative technique in Dupuytren's disease (Skoog, 1948). Later, Skoog made many valuable refinements to this procedure.

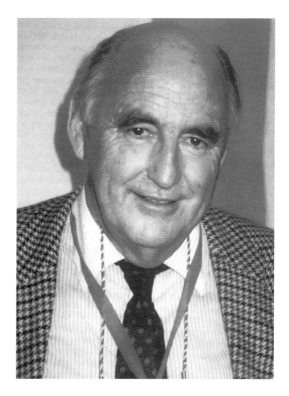

Figure 1.5 John Turner Hueston (1926–93).

Hueston, like McIndoe, was Australasian (McIndoe was born in New Zealand) and had the same buoyant personality and flair for surgical technique. Sir Archibald became his role model and, like him, Hueston became interested in Dupuytren's disease. He returned to Melbourne in 1954 as a partner to Sir Benjamin Rank and Allan Wakefield. He was asked by his mentors to edit the third edition of their book *Surgery of Repair as Applied to Hand Surgery*.

Hueston found, at the Repatriation General Hospital, hundreds of ex-servicemen with Dupuytren's disease and set up a special Dupuytren's disease clinic with operating sessions for six patients each week. This intense experience, and a similar number of operations for Dupuytren's disease each week in private practice, gave Hueston an outstanding personal experience of this condition. He published, in 1963, a brilliant and very original little book, *Dupuytren's Contracture* in which he not only set out his surgical experience of the disease, but also showed the existence of a genetic predisposition and the influence of certain factors that favor the formation of the disease that he grouped under the term 'diathesis'. He also formulated, with the pathologist MacCallum, a theory on the extra-aponeurotic starting-point of the lesions. I was impressed by this unorthodox approach and invited Hueston to join the GEM (Groupe d'Etude de la Main). Hueston came to Paris every year for the GEM meeting. The author visited him twice in Melbourne where he was Chief of Plastic Surgery at the Royal Melbourne Hospital. We co-edited two books on Dupuytren's disease, one in French (Tubiana and Hueston, 1986) and one in English (Hueston and Tubiana, 1985), in which he put forward his views on prevention of recurrences by the use of skin grafts. Hueston wrote about 70 papers on Dupuytren's disease and was also invited to publish many chapters in contributed books (Hueston, 1977, 1981, 1982, 1998). In his final lecture, in May 1992 at the Paris International Congress of Hand Surgery, he concluded, 'I have a dream, that one day

Dupuytren's disease will be treated without surgery.'

Independent, sometimes to an irritating degree, Hueston 'amputated' his surgical career at its peak and started a new life outside medicine, rather than fading away as a spectator in his old arena. He had a wide interest in art and culture, English literature and French history. He became a Bachelor of Arts in 1982. He retired to a small village in the Luberon in Provence early in 1987 where he took time to read and think. When asked why he did not write about his very full life, he insisted that he was still 'too busy living'. However, he continued his study of Dupuytren's condition and was extremely attracted by the life and work of French 19th Century medical pioneers: Dupuytren, of course, but also Goyrand, from Aix, and the neurologist Duchenne, from Boulogne. He was integrated into the local community, which awarded him the title of Honorary Citizen of Aix. He died in 1993 and rests in the grave he had already chosen in the small cemetery behind his home at Saint Saturnin d'Apt in the Luberon.

References

Barsky HK (1984) *Guillaume Dupuytren – A Surgeon in His Place and Time*. Vantage Press, New York.

Boyer A (1826) *Traité des Maladies Chirurgicales*, Vol. II. Migneret, Paris.

Cline H (1777) *Notes on Pathology and Surgery*, Manuscript 28:185. St Thomas' Hospital Library, London.

Cooper A (1822) On dislocations of the fingers and toes – dislocation from contraction of the tendon. In: Cooper A, *A Treatise on Dislocations and Fractures of the Joints*. Longman, Hurst, Rees, Orme, Brown & Cox, London.

Cruveilhier J (1841) *Vie de Dupuytren*. Béchet et Labé, Paris.

Dupuytren G (1831) De la rétraction des doigts par suite d'une affection de l'aponévrose palmaire par MM. les docteurs Paillard et Marx. *Journal Universel et Hebdomadaire de Médecine et de Chirurgie Pratiques et des Institutions Médicales*, Paris. Reprinted in *Medical*

Classics 1939–1940, Vol. 4. Royal Society of Medicine, London.

Dupuytren G (1832) *Leçons Orales de Clinique Chirurgicale faites à l'Hôtel-Dieu*. Baillière, Paris.

Dupuytren G (1834) Permanent retraction of the fingers, produced by an affection of the palmar fascia. *Lancet* **ii**: 222–25.

Elliot D (1988a) The early history of the contracture of the palmar fascia. Part 1: The origin of the disease: the curse of the MacCrimmons: the hand of benediction: Cline's contracture. *J Hand Surg [Br]* **13**: 246–53.

Elliot D (1988b) The early history of contracture of the palmar fascia. Part 2: The Revolution in Paris: Guillaume Dupuytren. *J Hand Surg [Br]* **13**: 372–78.

Elliot D (1999) The early history of Dupuytren's disease. *Hand Clin* **15**: 1–19.

Garrison FH (1966) *An Introduction to the History of Medicine*, 4th edn. WB Saunders, Philadelphia.

Goyrand G (1833) Nouvelles recherches sur la rétraction permanente des doigts. *Mem Acad Med* **3**: 489.

Goyrand G (1835) De la rétraction permanente des doigts. *Gazette Med Paris* **3**: 481–86.

Hueston JT (1963) *Dupuytren's Contracture*. E and S Livingstone, Edinburgh.

Hueston JT (1977) Dupuytren's contracture. In: Converse JM, ed., *Reconstructive Plastic Surgery*, 2nd edn, 3403–27. WB Saunders, Philadelphia.

Hueston JT (1981) Historical profiles: Guillaume Dupuytren. In: Tubiana R, ed., *The Hand*, Vol. 1. WB Saunders, Philadelphia.

Hueston JT (1982) Dupuytren's contracture. In: Flynn JE, ed., *Hand Surgery*, 3rd edn, 797–822. Williams & Wilkins, Baltimore.

Hueston JT (1998) Current views on etiology and pathogenesis. In: Tubiana R, ed., *The Hand*, Vol. 5. WB Saunders, Philadelphia.

Hueston JT, Tubiana R (1974) *Dupuytren's Disease*. Churchill Livingstone, Edinburgh.

Hueston JT, Tubiana R (1985) *Dupuytren's Disease*, 2nd edn. Churchill Livingstone, Edinburgh.

James JIP, Tubiana R (1952) La maladie de Dupuytren. *Rev Chir Orthop* **38**: 352–406.

Latil F, Hueston JT (1992) JCB Goyrand (1802–1866): Chirurgien et Académicien Aixois. *Ann Chir Plast Esthet* **37**: 574–78.

McCash CR (1964) The open palm technique in Dupuytren's contracture. *Br J Plastic Surg* **17**:271–80.

McFarlane RM, McGrouther DA, Flint MH (1990) *Dupuytren's Disease. Biology and Treatment*. Churchill Livingstone, Edinburgh.

McIndoe AH, Beare RLB (1958) The surgical management of Dupuytren's contracture. *Am J Surg* **95**: 197.

Mondor H (1945) *Dupuytren*, 2nd edn. Gallimard, Paris.

Plater F (1614) *Observationes in Hominis Affectibus*, Vol. 3. König and Brandmyller, Basel.

Redfern AB (1986) Corresp newsl of *Am Soc Surg Hand* 71.

Sanson JL (1834) Rapport sur le mémoire de Goyrand. *Mem Acad R Med* **4**: 497–500.

Sanson JL, Breschet G (1834) Rapport sur le mémoire de Goyrand. *Gaz Med Paris* **2**: 219.

Skoog T (1948) Dupuytren's contraction with special reference to aetiology and improved surgical treatment. *Acta Chirurg Scand* **96** (suppl 139):1.

Tubiana R (1955) Prognosis and treatment of Dupuytren's contracture. *J Bone Joint Surg* **37A**: 1155–68.

Tubiana R (1964) Le traitement sélectif de la maladie de Dupuytren. *Rev Chirurg Orthoped* **50**: 311–33.

Tubiana R (1967) *Maladie de Dupuytren*. L'Expansion Scientifique Française, Paris.

Tubiana R, Hueston JT (1972) *La Maladie de Dupuytren*, 2nd edn. L'Expansion Scientifique Française, Paris.

Tubiana R, Hueston JT (1986) *La Maladie de Dupuytren*, 3rd edn. L'Expansion Scientifique Française, Paris.

Tubiana R, Leclercq C (1985) Recurrent Dupuytren's disease. In: Hueston JT, Tubiana R, eds, *Dupuytren's Disease*, 2nd edn. Churchill Livingstone, Edinburgh.

Whaley DC, Elliot D (1993) Dupuytren's disease: a legacy of the North. *J Hand Surg [Br]* **18**: 363–67.

Anatomy

Raoul Tubiana

INTRODUCTION

What is the relationship between palmar aponeurosis and Dupuytren's disease?

The problem seemed to be solved by Dupuytren's operative findings and cadaver dissections: the fingers' deformities were caused by palmar fascia contracture. Nevertheless, as early as 1833, Goyrand disagreed with this assertion. He demonstrated the existence of fibrous bands superficial to the palmar fascia, which extended towards the fingers and were responsible for the interphalangeal (IP) joints' contracture (Goyrand, 1833). He performed an experimental transverse partial resection of the palmar fascia, followed by suture of the fascia. This resulted in a flexion of the metacarpophalangeal (MP) joints without affecting the proximal interphalangeal (PIP) joints. Goyrand (1834) concluded that Dupuytren's theory, which incriminated only the palmar fascia, was incorrect. He considered the disease to be localized to the plane superficial to the palmar fascia. This theory was strongly supported later in Australia: MacCallum and Hueston (1962) believed the disease arose in subdermal tissue between the skin and the fascia.

Here we must pay attention to the discrepancies between various authors in terminology.

In 1956, Landsmeer stated, in relation to the dorsal fasciae of the hand:

> All descriptions of the fasciae sooner or later run into difficulties in nomenclature between writers in French and English. There are two main differences: in English the subcutaneous layer composed of fatty tissue is invariably named the superficial fascia, while the French anatomists only distinguish the subcutaneous tissue (*tissu sous-cutané*).
>
> The second difficulty is due to the fact that the French use the word aponeurosis (aponévrose) for what the English call the deep fascia. In English the word aponeurosis is usually reserved for a layer which has a tendinous origin or connection.

For Hueston, who denied the aponeurotic origin of Dupuytren's disease, the process appears in the subcutaneous layer. Gosset (1972) challenged this theory:

> If the lesions are independent new-formations, unrelated to the recognized anatomical elements, their excision will be haphazard and will be concentrated on avoiding neurovascular structures. If, on the contrary, the lesions develop in a well-defined anatomical structure, e.g. the digitopalmar aponeurosis, their excision will be carried out in a systematic,

orderly way. There will be no unexpected anomalies, and only the uninitiated will have unpleasant surprises.

We must see first how much can be learned from microscopical examination. In this respect the works of Meyerding [1941], and those of Nezelof and Tubiana [1958] are precise and essentially in agreement. These authors have shown that two very different types of lesions are encountered in Dupuytren's disease.

In some areas, one finds fibroblastic activity, mitoses, little collagen, and a disorderly arrangement with wavy or concentric patterns. In others, there is a paucity of cells, dense collagen arranged in parallel fibers and forming actual retractile bands.

One may accept the theory, proposed by a number of authors, that the first type of lesion represents the early, progressive stage of the disease, while the other represents a late, stabilized stage. As this theory has never yet been confirmed, we feel free to suggest an alternative one; the cellular, nodular lesion and the collagen bands are two forms of the same disease occurring in different structures.

The cellular, collagenous forms are very retractile, and are the ones responsible for flexion of the metacarpo-phalangeal and interphalangeal joints. They lead to the formation of fibrous bands over which the skin of the palm remains thin, supple and mobile, except for a few millimeters proximal and distal to the flexion creases.

The nodular forms of Dupuytren's disease are quite different. Histologically, they present as a dense tissue, rich in cells and showing no organization. The picture is the same in the palmar and digital nodules, in the knuckle pads and in the plantar nodules of Ledderhose. In the hand, the round or oval-shaped nodules adhere closely to the skin, which becomes callous over the lesions. These are pretendinous and are usually found in areas where the fatty tissue is thick, between the interphalangeal creases, between the proximal IP and the MP creases, and only rarely proximal to this.

In our experience, as we shall see later, the nodules usually form in areas where no aponeurotic structure would be found in the normal hand. They are but slightly retractile. If after the removal of a large phalangeal nodule the finger still does not achieve complete extension, it is essential to look elsewhere (and we shall see where) for a band, the severing of which, will ensure a good result. Depending on the cases, any combination of these two distinct forms may be encountered.

We believe that the bands and nodules do not represent two different stages in the course of the disease, but rather two distinct forms, which originate in different tissues. When the disease develops in a well-defined sheet of aponeurosis, the lesion takes the form of dense, contracted fibrous bands, with abundant collagen and a paucity of cells. When it affects the adipose tissue, and spares the aponeurosis, the nodular form prevails. The fat disappears, the cellular fibrosis invades the deep layer of the skin and spreads inwards towards the underlying aponeurosis. In other words, we believe that the two forms, which differ macroscopically (nodules or bands) and histologically, represent lesions in different tissues: in the fatty tissue for the nodules, and in the aponeurosis for the bands.

We agree with Hueston's view that the nodular lesion is independent of the aponeurosis. It shows a preference for the pretendinous zones where there is no aponeurosis, at the base of the phalanx, distal to the first interphalangeal crease, or the area between the proximal digital crease and the MP joint. Much less frequently, a nodule may be found in the palm, proximal to the distal palmar crease, between the skin and aponeurosis. Its adhesion to the aponeurosis is only secondary and comes from intimate contact with that structure.

When, however, the disease attacks the aponeurosis, retractile bands are formed. These take their origin from the true aponeurosis and always follow a well-defined course.

It is true that the proportions of the two types of lesions in one case may vary. There are essentially nodular forms, essentially retractile forms, and mixed forms with both nodules and retractile bands. Surgically, the essential step is the excision of these bands, which are responsible for flexion of the fingers. This excision is performed according to a technique based on the normal anatomy of the palmodigital aponeuroses.

This is why we think it is important to consider the anatomy of these structures.

Gosset's view that nodules and cords occur independently is a theory of compromise supported by Strickland and Leibovic (1991). These hypotheses were, however, refuted by Hueston (1991): 'The nodule appears on the anterior aspect of the palmar aponeurosis, never on its posterior aspect... This raises the question of why only one aspect of the aponeurosis and not the other is involved primarily.'

In any case, knowledge of normal anatomy of the palmar aponeurosis, which is the network for the diseased fibrous proliferation, seems necessary for a safe fasciectomy, whatever the origin of the pathological process.

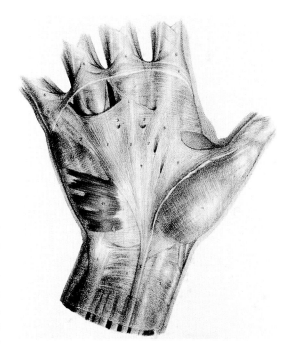

Figure 2.1. The general anatomy of the midpalmar aponeurosis with longitudinal and transverse fibers, in particular the natatory ligament with its distal extensions in the fingers forming 'gothic arches' in the interdigital skinfold. (Reproduced with permission from Bourgery and Jacob, 1832.)

HISTORY OF THE PALMAR FASCIA ANATOMICAL RESEARCH

Much anatomical research on the subject of the palmar fascia and its relevance in Dupuytren's disease has been performed. A wide search of this literature and extensive review have been provided by Graham Stack in his book, *The Palmar Fascia* (1973). Anatomical research on this subject may be divided in two periods: traditional dissections and contemporary research.

Period of traditional dissections

The midpalmar fascia seems to have been first identified by Giovanni Cannanus of Ferrara (Italy) in his study *Musculorum Humani Corporis – Picturata Dissecto* (1543) in which he shows the palmaris longus (PL) muscle and its prolongation through the midpalmar fascia to the digits (Zancolli and Cozzi, 1992). The earliest description of this fascia was given by Albinius of Leyden in 1734 who mentioned the pretendinous bands and their distal division. Weitbrecht (1742) described the manner in which the palmar fascia spreads out from the flexor retinaculum and stretches between the thenar and hypothenar regions. Bourgery (1834) traced the origin of the palmar aponeurosis from the palmaris longus and from the transverse flexor retinaculum (Figure 2.1). He described the 'bandelette transverse sous-cutanée' (natatory ligament)

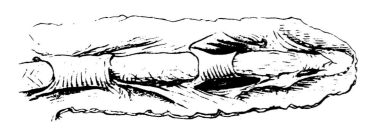

Figure 2.2 Cleland's (1878) original illustration of the cutaneous ligaments of the phalanges. (Reproduced with permission from Milford, 1968.)

and the numerous filamentous prolongations to the skin.

Dupuytren himself did not write about the anatomy of the palmar aponeurosis, his studies being mostly devoted to the clinical findings.

Maslieurat-Lagémard (1839) is probably the earliest author to deal specifically with the anatomy of the palmar aponeurosis. His work emanates from the hospital where Dupuytren was chief surgeon (Hôtel-Dieu) and was published soon after Dupuytren's death. The palmar aponeurosis is regarded as a sheet of varying thickness. The distal fibers extending into the fingers form arcades running from one finger to another.

Cleland (1878) introduced the idea of protection of the skin against sliding. He described a cutaneous ligamentous system in the fingers (Figure 2.2) as a strong fibrous septum arising from the lateral ridges of the proximal phalanx in the distal half of its extent. Joining this band are a few fibers from the base of the middle phalanx, which are inserted into the skin.

Grapow (1887) made a detailed study of the structure of the palmar aponeurosis. He noted the close connections between the skin and the fascia and described the transverse ligament of the thumb web.

He explained the functions of the palmar aponeurosis thus:

1) Maintenance of the curvature of the skeleton;
2) A hydraulic function for the pumping of blood and lymph;
3) Fixation of the skin in order to provide secure grip.

Legueu and Juvara (1892) gave a description of the palmar fasciae, which is considered classical. They divided the fasciae into five parts:

1) The vertical (or longitudinal) superficial palmar aponeurosis with the 'pretendinous languettes' (pretendinous bands)
    The pretendinous languettes present three types of termination:
    a) The fibers going to the skin of the palm and the fingers;
    b) The fibers going to the deep aponeurosis (anterior interosseous fascia);
    c) The perforating fibers.
2) The 'deep transverse fibers of the palmar aponeurosis', later called by Skoog 'superficial transverse palmar ligament.'
3) The interdigital ligament.
4) The deep transverse metacarpal ligament.
5) The fibrous sheaths of the tendons, muscles and neurovascular bundles.

In particular they gave a detailed description of the palmar intertendinous sheaths:

Above the level of the metacarpal heads fibers detach themselves from the principal vertical fascicles, and go backwards in the corresponding intertendinous space [Figure 2.3]. If the palmar aponeurosis is detached from the carpal annular ligament and turned downwards, these fibers can be seen on its

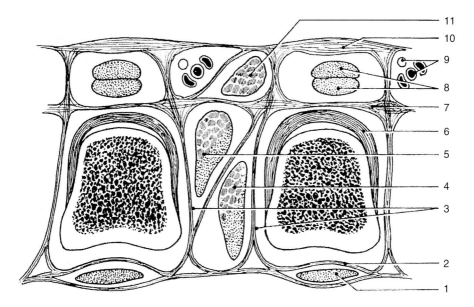

Figure 2.3 Transverse section of two metacarpals at the level of the heads (from Legueu and Juvara, 1892). (1) Extensor tendon; (2) dorsal aponeurosis; (3) perforating fibers; (4) dorsal interosseous muscle; (5) palmar interosseous muscle; (6) proximal part of volar plate; (7) deep palmar aponeurosis; (8) flexor tendons; (9) neurovascular bundles; (10) pretendinous band; (11) lumbrical muscle.

deep surface, passing between the tendons. These make partitions on either side of the tendon...

The arrangement of these sheets in relation to the deep aponeurosis is as follows: on each of the faces of the sheets arciform fibers arise, which pass under the tendons or under the muscles, and join the similar fibers coming from the neighboring partitions. These fibers passing under the muscle or tendon adhere to the deep aponeurosis, and join with it...

Independent of the fibers which each partition sends medially and laterally to the tendon and the neighboring muscle, there are other fibers, which give the third method of termination of the vertical fibers of the pretendinous languettes. These are the fibers which we call the perforating fibers, because instead of ending in the deep aponeurosis,

they traverse it, and perforate it at the level of the deep transverse ligament, in order to surround the metacarpophalangeal articulations with a complete circle.

After perforating the transverse ligament, these fibers travel over the lateral surface of the capsule of the joint, pass backwards and are found as a transverse band passing behind the tendon of the extensors [Figure 2.3]. This is joined by a similar expansion from the perforating fibers of the other peritendinous partitions of the same tendon.

It is, in fact, more complicated than the above description. Detaching itself from the principal peri-articular fascicle of perforating fibers, an oblique fascicle passes between the two interosseous muscles of the space, and joins the periarticular cylinder of the neighboring joint. Hence, the interosseous space, particularly in its articular portion, is divided into two openings, through which the two corresponding interosseous muscles of the same space escape into the fingers.

Grayson (1941) confirmed Cleland's description of the so-called cutaneous ligaments of the human digits lying behind the neurovascular bundles and described a further sheet, which lies in front of the neurovascular bundles and passes from the front of the fibrous flexor tendon sheaths to the skin (Figure 2.4).

Iselin (Marc) in 1955 was one of the first to describe the displacement of the digital nerves, depending on whether the cords had developed from the superficial aponeurosis or from the deep partitions. He distinguished three main variations:

- Type 1: Normal, in which the nerve stays in its normal course under the fascia along the lateral side of the finger.
- Type 2: The nerve is pushed towards the midline of the finger by a cord that has developed from the superficial aponeurosis. The nerve crosses the cord superficially about the level of the web space and, at the level of the middle phalanx, returns to its normal place;
- Type 3: The nerve stays under the cord that is going to insert on the side of the proximal phalanx, when it is crossed the first time by the cord at the level of the web space, and it will be recrossed more distally.

Gosset (1967) described the palmar aponeurosis in a standard fashion. He studied in detail the termination of the pretendinous bands:

Below the inferior border of the superficial transverse ligament, how do the pretendinous bands behave? In the classical descriptions they are drawn as if they are prolonged as far as the anterior surface of the proximal phalanx. In our opinion, this appears to be

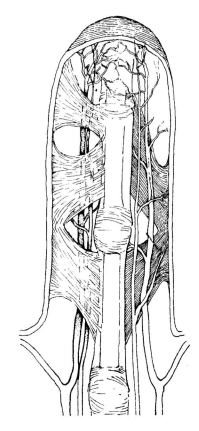

Figure 2.4. Reproduction of the original illustration of Grayson showing the cutaneous ligaments of the digits from the volar aspect.
In the lighter shade, on the left, Grayson's ligament passing volar to the neurovascular bundle. On the right side of the digit, in darker shade, Cleland's ligament passing dorsal to the neurovascular bundle. (Grayson, 1941; reproduced with permission from Milford, 1968.)

incorrect. Arriving at the level of the neck of the metacarpal, the pretendinous bands divide like a 'V' into two bands, which narrow and twist to become sagittal and plunge deep in order to attach to the lateral surface of the metacarpophalangeal joint.

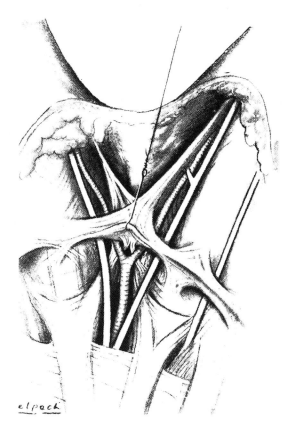

Figure 2.5 In the web space, the origin of the lateral fascia sheets of the finger and crossing between the digital nerves and the aponeurosis, the chiasma of the natatory ligament. (Gosset, 1967; reproduced with permission from Hueston and Tubiana, 1974.)

These fibers spiral around the neurovascular bundle and were later called the 'spiral bands' by McFarlane (1974) (Figure 2.5).

Gosset also defined the upper and lower limits of the Legueu and Juvara partitions:

The proximal limit is falciform, and commences well below the inferior border of the annular ligament on a horizontal plane, which is approximately equidistant from the distal flexion crease of the wrist, and the palmar digital crease. In effect these partitions cannot come above the superficial palmar arch or the tendinous origins of the lumbricals. If the narrow origin of the median palmar aponeurosis is divided, and turned down, as distal as possible, and its attachment at the side to the fascia of the thenar and the hypothenar regions freed, one may see that nothing restrains it on its deep surface. Here, the superficial palmar arch and the widening of the median nerve are found.

As one continues to turn this aponeurosis downwards, this maneuver is stopped by the tension in the origins of the partitions. The flexor tendons and neurovascular bundles are revealed. Release of the aponeurosis from this point onwards necessitates the progressive section of the partitions as far as their distal terminations.

This distal border of the partitions is oblique from proximal to distal, and from volar to dorsal. Its end may be confused with the bands of bifurcation of the pretendinous bundles on the lateral surface of the capsules of the metacarpophalangeal joints.

It is clear that many invaluable dissections of palmar fascia have been made by these previous workers but, as Stack (1971) has rightly noted:

Dissection is, however, an essentially destructive method of examination, and in the main consists of the removal of connective tissue in order to explore other tissues. Thus the study of the palmar fascia by dissection consists essentially of the destruction of the actual tissues under examination. Furthermore, it has always been clear that it is possible by the selective dissection of some fibers to preserve others, and by so doing to demonstrate sheets and bands which may not be entirely valid.

Contemporary research

Contemporary workers have benefited from the magnification of an operating microscope, from special techniques of dissection, and from examination of serial sections of fetal hands. The serial sectioning of the hand, difficult in adults, is relatively simple in the human fetus. By study of the sections, it is possible to follow the fibers. All the tissue present is preserved by fixation and no tissue has to be removed to study the remainder. Investigations by Thomine, Stack and de Frenne have been carried out in the Anatomy Department of the University of Leyden under the supervision of Professor JMF Landsmeer. These surgeons had the opportunity to study several series of serial sections of fetal hands, both transverse, longitudinal and frontal. The sections are 10 μm thick (10 μm per section = 100 sections per millimetre) from embryos of about 15–18 weeks of life (fetal length: 11.5–14.0 cm).

The technique used for dissection is also important. The removal of skin from the hand is first performed as superficially as possible, before beginning the deeper dissection. This is simple enough on the dorsum where the skin is easily detached. It is much more difficult on the palmar aspect 'where, throughout its width, the deep aspect of the dermis is bound to the superficial aspect of the aponeurotic sheet by a multitude of tiny fibrous strands, which enclose the loculi of subdermal fat. This produces a remarkable fixation of the palmar skin and explains the anatomical interdependence between the skin and the fibrous structures of the hand' (Thomine, 1965).

In particular, Thomine studied the digital fascia and de Frenne (1977) the fascia of the radial side of the hand. These descriptions will be reported later.

Stack (1971) studied the relations of the palmar fascia in the MP region and its continuities in the finger. He developed a theory that the fascial layers can be regarded as continuous sheets, covering each layer of muscles or tendons. The volar interosseous fascia covers the interosseous muscles and separates them from the long flexor tendons. This layer is continuous distally with the volar plates and the deep transverse ligament of the palm (deep transverse metacarpal ligament or interglenoid ligament), and more distally still in the fingers with Cleland's ligament or Thomine's retrovascular band (for Stack these are equal; this is not true for McFarlane).

The flexor tendons and the lumbricals lie on this layer and are covered by the flexor retinaculum, the transverse fibers of the palmar aponeurosis and the fibrous flexor tendon sheaths. The next tendinous layer has been modified to become the palmar aponeurosis, arising from the palmaris longus. Over this is the superficial layer, which in the palm is mainly the subcorial fibrous tissue, thickened in the distal palm as the superficial transverse ligament of the palm or natatory ligament, and more distally as the superficial fascia of the fingers.

McGrouther (1982) described an internal anatomical arrangement between the different fiber systems of the palmar fascia in the region of the transverse palmar creases. Anatomists have often viewed the palmar fascia as a static fibrous sheet. McGrouther performed careful dissection with preservation of the overlying skin, which was reflected and removed piecemeal under high magnification, only after definition of the fascial attachments to the skin. The ligamentous system of the palm was considered individually to be transverse, longitudinal and vertical fibers. Normal relative motion between the different fiber systems was confirmed as a constant finding in normal hands. This arrangement will be described later.

Zancolli and Cozzi (1992) have shown in superb dissections that the longitudinal fibers of the midpalmar aponeurosis 'can be divided into two types:

(1) Superficial or cutaneous, which adhere to the palmar skin, some of them inter-

twining distally with the transverse subcutaneous band of the natatory ligament; and

(2) Deep fibers, which along their course to the depth of the palm, form the paratendinous septa at the level of the distal crease of the palm and at the finger base form the "bifurcating fibers"'.

All these valuable studies will be used in the following description of the palmodigital fasciae.

ANATOMY OF THE PALMODIGITAL FASCIAE

The terminology used in this description is listed in Table 2.1.

The fascial anatomy of the palmar aspect of the hand and digits includes four components unequally involved in Dupuytren's disease: the midpalmar, thenar, hypothenar and digital fasciae.

The midpalmar fascia

The midpalmar or central fascia fans out between the thenar and hypothenar fasciae. It has various layers.

The deep layer, or anterior interosseous fascia

This covers the interosseous muscles. It is not involved in Dupuytren's disease. Flexor tendons lie on this fascia. It is reinforced at its distal extremity by transverse fibers at the level of palmar plates forming the deep transverse intermetacarpal ligament or interglenoid ligament.

The superficial palmar aponeurosis

The midpalmar superficial aponeurosis must be considered when studying Dupuytren's disease. It forms a triangular fascial triangle, with the apex proximally attached (Figure 2.6) to the palmaris longus (PL) tendon. Although it is usually thought that the palmar fascia takes its origin from the arborizing terminal fibers of the PL tendon (Wood Jones, 1942; Le Gros Clark, 1958), Kaplan (1938) believed that the PL and the palmar aponeurosis were two separate anatomic entities. This view was reinforced by Caughill et al. (1988) who demonstrated that the two structures have different staining properties, and that their association is only one of proximity.

PL is an inconstant muscle. For Lister (1977) it is present bilaterally in 70% of subjects, unilaterally in 14% and bilaterally absent in a further 16%. For Powell et al. (1986), the

Table 2.1 Nomenclature.

Terminology used in this chapter	Alternative and equivalent terminology
Palmar fascia	Palmar aponeurosis
Deep layer of midpalmar fascia	Anterior interosseous fascia
Pretendinous bands	Longitudinal fibers to skin (McGrouther)
Bifurcated pretendinous band	Bifurcation fibers (Legueu and Juvara)
Deep transverse metacarpal ligament	Interglenoid ligament
Proximal transverse palmar ligament	Superficial transverse palmar ligament (Skoog)
Natatory ligament	Superficial transverse ligament of the palm (Stack)
Septae of Legueu and Juvara	Vertical paratendinous septae (Zancolli and Cozzi)
Spiral band (McFarlane)	Deep extension of pretendinous band (Gosset)
Cleland's ligament	Digital retrovascular osteocutaneous septum
Retrovascular ligament (Thomine)	Longitudinal retrovascular digital band with osteoarticular fixation
Distal transverse commissural ligament of the thumb web	Grapov ligament

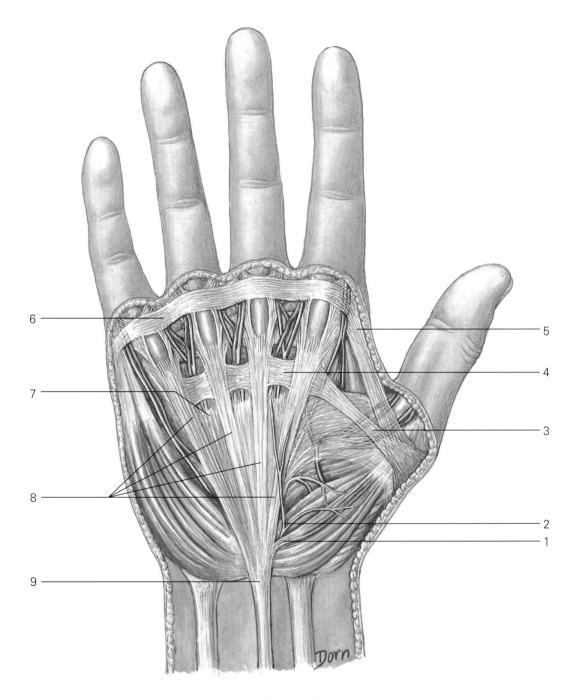

Figure 2.6 The midpalmar fascia. (1) Insertion of the superficial fascicle of the abductor pollicis brevis (APB) on the tendon of palmaris longus; (2) palmar cutaneous branch of the median nerve; (3) proximal commissural ligament of the first web space; (4) proximal transverse palmar ligament or superficial transverse ligament (Skoog); (5) distal commissural ligament of the first web space; (6) natatory ligament; (7) triangular space filled with adipose tissue; (8) pretendinous bands; (9) tendon of palmaris longus.

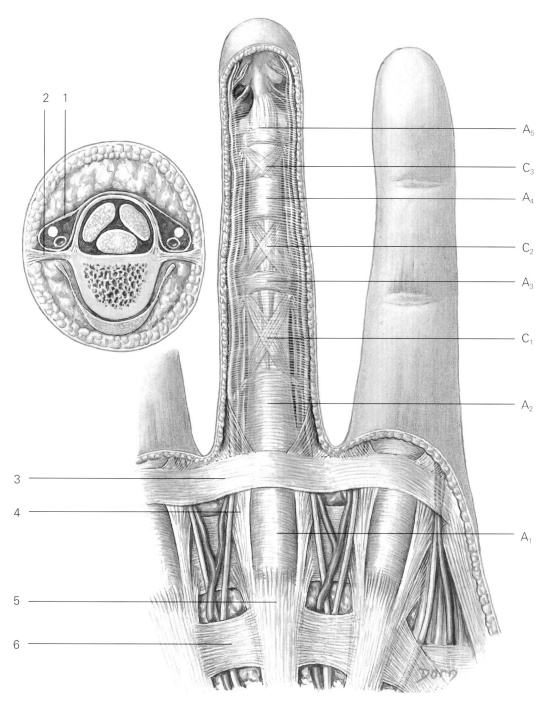

Figure 2.7 (1) Grayson's ligament; (2) Cleland's ligament; (3) natatory ligament; (4) deep extension of the pretendinous band. Some fibers will spiral around the neurovascular bundle; (5) pretendinous band (most of these fibers insert into the deep surface of the dermis); (6) superficial or proximal transverse ligament; A_1–A_5, C_1–C_3 pulleys.

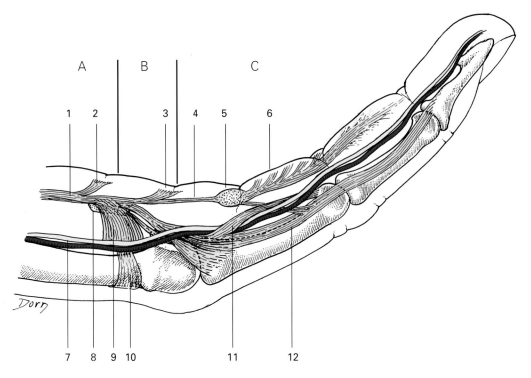

Figure 2.8 Diagrammatic representation of the longitudinal fibers of the midpalmar fascia. (A) preseptal; (B) septal; (C) postseptal: (1) pretendinous band; (2–3) end of the longitudinal fibers inserted on the cutaneous creases of the palm; (4) only some of the longitudinal fibers extend to the natatory ligament; (5) natatory ligament; (6) longitudinal fibers extending to the volar creases of the fingers; most of them originate from the natatory ligament; (7) digital neurovascular bundle; (8) proximal transverse ligament; (9) vertical paratendinous septa; (10) perforating fibers of Legueu and Juvara; (11) spiral band; (12) retrovascular band. (Adapted with permission from Zancolli and Cozzi, 1992.)

incidence of a PL tendon in patients with Dupuytren's disease is significantly greater than in a control group with normal hands.

The midpalmar aponeurosis roofs the compartment of the hand where the flexor tendons and neurovascular bundles diverge. It forms 'a network of fibrous strands that interconnect in a complex multidimentional manner' (Strickland and Leibovic, 1991). Schematically, it comprises longitudinal, transverse and sagittal fibers, which condense in certain zones to form defined fibrous structures.

Karlberg (1935) showed that the superficial palmar aponeurosis is subjected to a considerable number of variations. For Millesi (1986), palmar fascia has the possibility of adapting itself during the patient's lifetime, according to the functional needs.

The longitudinal fibers

These fibers are superficial to the flexor retinaculum to which they adhere and more distally to the finger flexor tendons, thus forming pretendinous bands which run parallel to these. Wood Jones (1942) attributed these to phytogenetically degenerated tendons of an MP joint flexor. Distal fibers of the flexor carpi ulnaris (FCU) tendon may be involved in the formation of the midpalmar fascia (Fahrer, 1980).

The superficial mid-palmar aponeurosis exists even in the absence of the PL (in about 15% of cases); then the fibers blend with the forearm fascia. Dupuytren's disease can still occur under these circumstances. Fahrer has suggested that, in the absence of palmaris longus, the FCU may act as a tensor of the palmar fascia. It must be noted that the number, arrangement and termination of the pretendinous bands varies considerably (Karlberg, 1935).

Distally, the ending insertions of the longitudinal fibers have long been controversial.

On a normal palmar fascia, the pretendinous bands disappear at the level of the distal transverse palmar crease. Most of the longitudinal fibers insert superficially into the deep surface of the dermis, others contribute to form the paratendinous septa of Legueu and Juvara, and only a variable proportion of these longitudinal fibers pass, according to the classical description, deeply to the neurovascular bundle and insert on either side of the MP joints (Figure 2.7).

'The continuity between the palmar aponeurosis and the flexor tendon sheath,' says Landsmeer (which Maslieurat-Lagémard (1839) and Ferrarini (1936) alleged existed), 'has always been a controversial point ... It seems beyond dispute that the palmar aponeurosis extends as a thin fascial layer over the MP segment of the tendon sheath ... but this does not prevent the two structures from being basically different ...'

1) Longitudinal fibers inserted to the palmar skin. These form the retinaculum cutis on the volar aspect of the hand and can be divided (Zancolli and Cozzi, 1992) into three parts, according to vertical paratendinous septa location:

1) Preseptal, inserted proximal to the proximal transverse palmar crease. For McGrouther (1998), the insertion into skin is progressively more proximal on passing from the ulnar to the radial side of the hand, which may be one of many reasons why contracture is more common in the ulnar fingers;

2) Septal, between the two transverse palmar creases;

3) Postseptal (Figure 2.8).

With full extension of the fingers, these insertions of longitudinal fibers into the dermis in the distal part of the palm may be seen as skin depression. Skin pits in Dupuytren's disease result from involvement of these fibers. Some of the superficial longitudinal fibers extend to the creases of the base of the fingers, mingling with the transverse fibers of the natatory ligament (see Figure 2.8). Most of the fibers extending to the volar creases of the fingers originate from the natatory ligament complex.

2) Longitudinal fibers going to the vertical paratendinous septa. These fibers reach the depth of the hand, passing between the transverse fibers of the superficial transverse fibers ligament (proximal transverse ligament) according to Poirier and Charpy (1899). This characteristic has been confirmed by microdissection (Zancolli and Cozzi, 1992).

3) The more distal group of deep longitudinal fibers. These bifurcate on each side of the proximal pulley of the fibrous flexor tendon sheath. Anatomists have given different descriptions and different names to the bifurcating fibers of the pretendinous bands: 'bifurcating fibers' (Legueu and Juvara, 1892), 'languettes divergentes' (Testut, 1893), 'deep extension of pretendinous bands' (Gosset, 1967). They terminate in one of three ways on the deep surface of the web space (Figure 2.9):

1) Blending with the deep palmar fascia over the interossei;

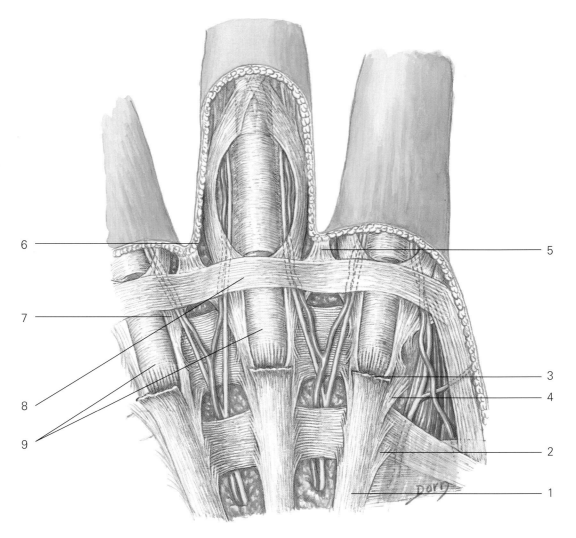

Figure 2.9 Deep longitudinal fibers. (1) Pretendinous band; (2) longitudinal fibers passing between the transverse fibers of the proximal transverse ligament going to the vertical paratendinous septa; (3) superficial longitudinal fibers inserted on the palmar skin; (4) deep longitudinal fibers blending with the deep palmar fascia; (5) web space coalescence; (6) space free of skin adhesion at the lateral aspect of the web; (7) origin of the spiral band; (8) natatory ligament; (9) flexor tendon sheath.

2) Continuing on to the finger on both sides of the digit, contributing to the formation of the retrovascular band;

3) Passing deep to the neurovascular bundles proximally. Some of these fibers attach to the MP joint capsule but the majority continue distally, diving under the neurovascular bundle to join the web space coalescence.

As they spiral around the neurovascular bundle (see Figure 2.8), they rotate 90° from the coronal to the sagittal plane. They are commonly affected in Dupuytren's disease

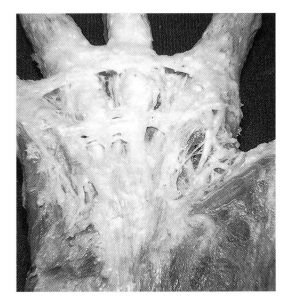

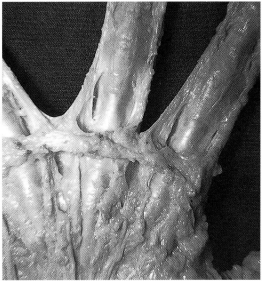

Figure 2.10 Superficial palmar aponeurosis. Note the longitudinal fibers in front of the tendons and the two transverse ligaments; the proximal ligament is called superficial by Skoog (actually these fibers are deep in comparison to the longitudinal fibers) and the distal transverse ligament is called commissural (or natatory).

Figure 2.11 The distal transverse formation and the longitudinal fibrous structures on either side of the fingers, which extend to the distal phalanx.

and are one of the common causes of PIP joint contracture. In these cases with marked spiral cord formation, the neurovascular bundle may be pushed medially, superficially and proximally with increasing PIP contracture.

It is interesting to note that at the base of the finger on the lateral aspect of the web there is a space where the skin does not adhere to the underlying fibrous tissues. This is a useful starting point for the dissection of the digital fibrous structures.

The transverse fibers

There are two sets of transverse fibers in the superficial midpalmar aponeurosis, one proximal and the other distal enclosing the MP joint (Figure 2.10).

The proximal transverse fibers of the palmar aponeurosis, called by Skoog the superficial transverse palmar ligament, are located on the deep surface of the pretendinous bands. The author prefers to call this the 'proximal transverse ligament'. This structure as noted by Skoog is normally not affected by the disease. The distal border of this ligament is situated at approximately the level of the distal palmar skin crease. This means that the dissection of the longitudinal fibers proximal to the distal palmar crease is safe. Distally from this crease, the neurovascular bundles will not be protected by the transverse fibers. The proximal border of the proximal transverse ligament is distal to the superficial palmar arterial arch. This 'ligament' forms a fibrous band approximately 1–5 cm wide. Between the proximal border of the proximal transverse ligament and the diverging borders of the pretendinous bands there are three small triangular spaces in the fascia filled with adipose tissue, deep to which lie the lumbrical muscles with the neurovascular bundles on their surface (see Figure 2.6). On the radial side of the palm, the fibers of the superficial transverse ligament continue to the first web space and form the proximal commissural ligament, which can be affected by Dupuytren's disease.

The distal transverse fibers cross the base of the proximal phalanges superficially and form the fibrous skeleton of the transverse subcutaneous band '*bandelette transverse sous-cutanée*' of Bourgery and Jacob (1832). It was called 'schwimmband' (natatory band) by Braune (1873) and 'superficial transverse ligament of the palm' in the Paris Nomina Anatomica. This appellation leads to confusion with the proximal transverse ligament, called by Skoog 'superficial transverse palmar ligament'. For the distal transverse ligament we shall use the well-accepted term 'natatory ligament'. These fibers course between the web spaces of all digits (Figure 2.11). They are commonly affected in Dupuytren's disease, producing a restriction of separation of the fingers. The proximal border is well defined, extending from the radial border of the index finger to the ulnar border of the little finger. It crosses the proximal pulley (A$_1$) of the flexor tendon sheath, attaching to it. The distal edge extends into the digital fascia forming 'arciform arches' (Bourgery and Jacob's 'gothic arches', 1832) in the interdigital skin folds.

Ferrarini (1936) emphasized that the 'natatorial' ligament and the palmar aponeurosis are basically autonomous structures, a view which Landsmeer (1976) is inclined to support.

The natatory ligament covers the neurovascular bundles of each of the fingers, as well as the flexor tendons. At the base of the little finger, the natatory ligament divides to envelop the abductor digiti minimi muscle and the ulnar neurovascular bundle. At the base of the index finger, the ligament continues into the first web space, where it forms the commissural crest and

becomes the distal commissural ligament, described by Grapow (1887) (see Figure 2.6).

The natatory ligament consists of more than just transverse fibers. Its configuration is three-dimensional (Strickland and Leibovic, 1991). As it crosses each flexor tendon sheath, it sends fibers deep to attach to the sheath overlying the MP joint. In addition, on each side of the finger it sends fibers deep to the web space coalescence. There are additional longitudinal fibers on either side of the finger, extending to the middle and distal phalanx. These fibers lie deep to the digital neurovascular bundles, which are enclosed at the base of the finger by the natatory ligament superficially and the spiral band dorsally. These lateral digital fibers also receive deep fibers originating from the vertical septa. Thus in each web space a chiasma results, which is adherent to the skin of the interdigital fold, except at the lateral part of the web space where the skin is usually free.

The sagittal or vertical fibers

A portion of these originate from longitudinal fibers passing between transverse fibers distally to the superficial palmar arterial arch (Zancolli and Cozzi, 1992). Holland and McGrouther (1997) further identified two different relationships between these fibers and the transverse fibers. These fibers run from the deep surface of the mid-palmar fascia towards the deep palmar fascia, which clothes the metacarpals and the interossei. Their direction is dorsal and at the same time directed proximodistally. They form a series of eight vertical septa, situated on either side of the digital flexor apparatus (Figure 2.12). These septa define the longitudinal compartments, which contain either the flexor tendons or the lumbrical muscles and the digital neurovascular bundles (Legueu and Juvara, 1892). The medial septum for the middle finger is attached upon the entire shaft of the third metacarpal bone (Figure 2.13). To reach the

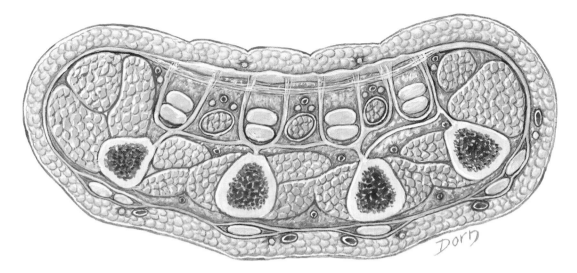

Figure 2.12 Cross-section of the palm of the hand at the distal palmar crease showing the pretendinous bands (just before their bifurcation) to which the transverse fibers of the proximal transverse ligament are seen to run deep, and the eight vertical paratendinous septa limiting the flexor tendon and lumbrical muscle compartments.

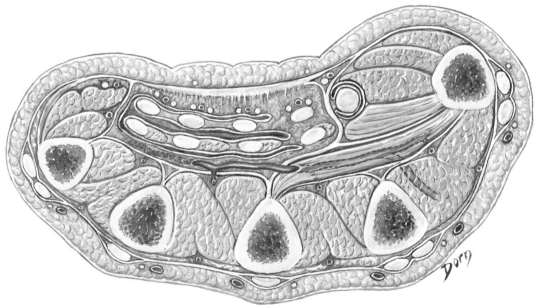

Figure 2.13 Cross-section of the palm of the hand at the level of the deep palmar arch. The superficial midpalmar aponeurosis roofs the central compartment of the hand over the flexor tendons between the thenar and hypothenar compartments. The central compartment is limited by a lateral (thenar) intermuscular septum, a medial (hypothenar) intermuscular septum and a deep fascia. The deep fascia at this level is formed on its radial part by the oblique portion of the thenar fascia and the volar adductor pollicis aponeurosis, which is attached on the third metacarpal longitudinal crest. On its ulnar part, the deep fascia extends over the interosseous muscles (volar interosseous fascia).

volar interosseous fascia, the septa related to the index tendons must pass beyond the distal border of the adductor pollicis and they are correspondingly shorter than those related to the tendons of the middle, ring, and little fingers, which have no adductor pollicis in their path.

Bojsen-Moller and Schmidt (1974) described the septa of the palmar aponeurosis in detail, their relation to the flexor tendon sheaths, their deep anchorages and their proximal extensions. Intercompartmental arthroscopic examination by Rayan (1999) revealed that each of the vertical septa consists of a well-developed fibrous structure that has a sharp and very strong proximal border and lies approximately 1 cm distal to the palmar arterial arch. The length of each septum varies depending upon the digit, from 8–12 mm. The proximal border is proximal to the level of the metacarpal neck, whereas the distal border, which becomes thin and membranous, is at the metacarpal head. When the arthroscope was introduced into the flexor tendon partition, the flexor tendons could be visualized distally to the level of the PIP joint. When it was introduced into each of the neurovascular lumbrical partitions, it stopped at a dead end in each of the three web space areas.

Other, much weaker vertical fibers, described by McGrouther, insert superficially directly into the dermis. They are particularly concentrated for a few millimeters on either side of the palmar skin creases. They run down into the hand from the dermis, between the individual longitudinal fibers and between the individual transverse fibers. They then pass more deeply in the palm to the flexor tendon sheaths and the metacarpal bones.

The digital fascia

The digital fascia has been the object of numerous contemporary studies, notably those of Landsmeer (1949), Thomine (1965) and Milford (1968), reflecting a turn in atten-

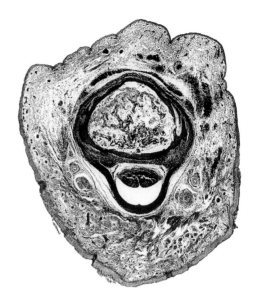

Figure 2.14 Tranverse section of a middle phalanx of a fetal hand. At the level of the posterior angle of the elliptical neurovascular sheath (that is, the plane of the lateral border of the phalanx) there is a more resistant zone of a denser fibrous tissue than anywhere else in the digital fascia (Reproduced with permission from Thomine, 1965).

tion from the palm to the fingers. It is in the fingers that the contractures are most severe, most disabling and most likely to recur.

Individual variation doubtless occurs, which may explain different concepts.

Thomine (1965) bases his description of the digital fascia on an elliptical sheath surrounding the neurovascular bundles. In the fetal hand, the only structure that can be followed continuously from the web space to the base of the distal phalanx is the fibrous sheath of the neurovascular bundles (Figure 2.14). There is a sheet joining these together in front of the fibrous flexor tendon sheath, and also a sheet of fascia on the dorsum, making a complete circular covering of the fingers. The dorsal and palmar sheets of fascia join together along the lateral and medial aspects of the fingers at the line of union of the dorsal and palmar skin, to form a thickened strand that Thomine calls the 'retrovascular digital band'. This digital band has several attachments with the lateral border of the proximal phalanx distal to the interosseous tendon, to the proximal interphalangeal joint and to the middle phalanx.

Communication between volar and dorsal compartments of the finger

This is another controversial subject. It is no longer believed that there is a rigid osteocutaneous transverse septum.

For Thomine, the volar space is separated from the dorsal space by a series of lateral structures located along the side of the phalanges:

The first such structure is a splitting of the most proximal part of the digital fascia behind the neurovascular bundles; one plane passes deeply beneath the terminal layers of interosseous tendon and becomes fixed to the dorsal periosteum of the proximal phalanx, while the more superficial dorsal sheath passes as usual over the extensor apparatus.

Beyond this level, as the interosseous tendon passes dorsally, the dorsal space is only separated from the volar space by a very weak layer of fine connective tissue, amounting to small fibrous spikes joining the lateral border of the bone to the posterior angle of the neurovascular sheath, i.e. to the retrovascular band.

On the volar aspect of these fibers lie the perpendicular branches of the digital artery reaching the fibrous flexor sheaths and tendons. When this first set of fixation has been lifted, the digital fascia and the retrovascular band appears still fixed at the level of the proximal interphalangeal joint by a rather complex arrangement [Figure 2.15].

First the deep aspect of the neurovascular sheath becomes adherent to the fibrous flexor sheath, thus narrowing the volar cleavage space at this level. After incising the digital fascia in the midline where each part is retracted laterally, the points of fixation appear

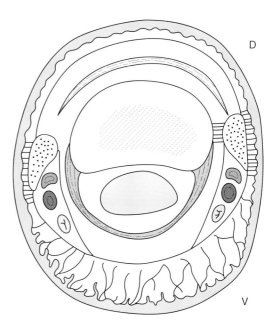

Figure 2.15 The volar space (V) is separated from the dorsal space (D) by a series of lateral structures located along the side of the phalanges.

as two small sets of parallel fibers converging towards the joint line. After dividing these structures it is found that further points of fixation intervene to prevent entry into the dorsal sub-fascial space. At first there are strong adhesions of the deeper aspect of the neurovascular sheath and then of the retrovascular band to the proximal segment of the retinacular ligament extending for several millimeters in the palmar-dorsal direction.

The retrovascular band to the proximal phalanx joins that of the middle phalanx [Figure 2.16] after the zone of adhesion to the retinacular ligament. It appears that at the middle phalanx the retrovascular band is seen as a strong fibrous bundle with a bony attachment at the base of the middle phalanx. This attachment is located deep to the oblique retinacular ligament...

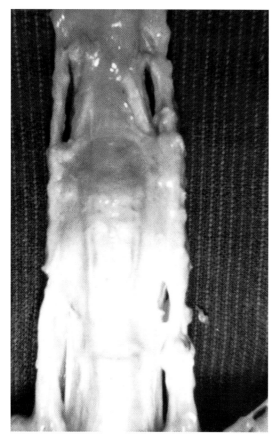

Figure 2.16 The fibers of the retrovascular band have been isolated and only their main attachments preserved on the proximal and middle phalanges.

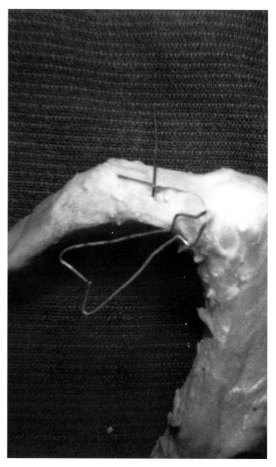

Figure 2.17 Relation of retrovascular band and retinacular ligament. The fibrous bundle of the middle phalanx portion of the retrovascular band fuses at its bony insertion with the oblique retinacular ligament and is separated from the extensor apparatus. (Reproduced with permission from Thomine, 1965.)

Finally at its distal extremity the retrovascular band fuses intimately with the collateral ligaments of the distal IP joint.

Thus the retrovascular band with its fixation superficially to the skin and deeply to the skeleton forms a layer separating dorsal from volar compartments, as first described by Cleland. A slightly different concept from Cleland's is offered. This band is not considered as a roughly transverse osteocutaneous ligament but as a longitudinal structure with points of elective fixation to the skeleton at the base of the prox-

imal phalanx and at the interphalangeal joint level, and having an important continuity with certain volar structures of which the most important is the natatory ligament.

There are numerous openings between the attachments of the digital band, which allow neurovascular branches to pass to the dorsal surface of the fingers and also the oblique

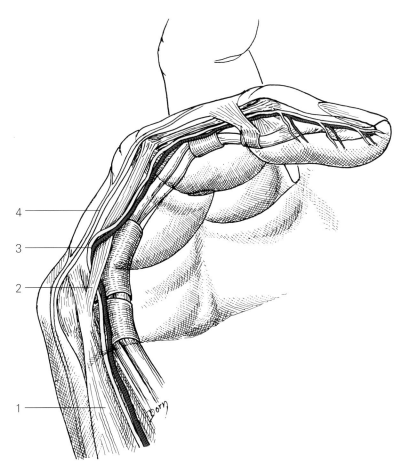

Figure 2.18 The retrovascular band on the ulnar side of the little finger is in continuity with the abductor digiti minimi tendon. (1) Abductor digiti minimi muscle; (2) retrovascular cord; (3) the neurovascular bundle spirals dorsal to the abductor digiti minimi cord; (4) dorsal ulnar sensory nerve.

retinacular ligament, which passes sandwiched between the retrovascular band insertions on the proximal and middle phalanges (Figure 2.17). Grayson's ligament represents the anterior layer of the fibrous sheath surrounding the neurovascular bundles. On the ulnar side of the little finger, the retrovascular cord is usually in continuity with the abductor digiti minimi tendon (Figure 2.18, see also Figure 6.48) and not with the retrovascular band, which can also be contracted.

Relations of the digital fascia to the overlying skin

On the dorsum of the finger, there is only a loose attachment between the skin of the two proximal phalanges and the dorsal fascia. On the contrary, connective tracts divide the palmar subcutaneous fat and fix it to the skin.

At the level of the interphalangeal and digitopalmar flexion creases, the subcutaneous fat gets thinner. The skin is adherent to the digital fascia. There exists an analogous zone of adherence at the level of the line of union of the dorsal and palmar skin of the finger. At the initial part of the proximal phalanx, adherence takes place in the plane of the crest of the web, more distally in the two distal phalanges. This zone of adherence is projected a little behind the collateral palmar bundle and corresponds to the area of the retrovascular digital band (or to the Cleland ligament).

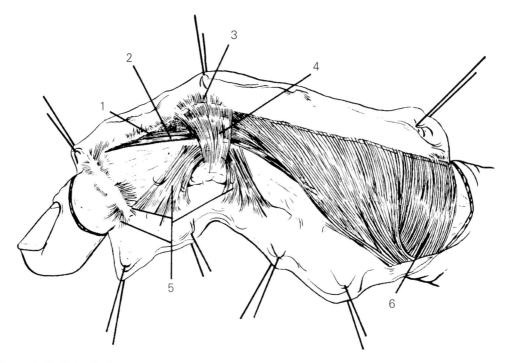

Figure 2.19 Cleland's ligament. (1) Lateral extensor tendon; (2) oblique retinacular ligament; (3) peritendinous fibers; (4) transverse retinacular ligament; (5) Cleland's ligament; (6) sagittal band of the extensor apparatus. (Reproduced with permission from Milford, 1968.)

Milford (1968) has studied retaining ligaments of the digits. The so-called Cleland's cutaneous ligaments (Cleland, 1878) consist of dense fibrous bundles arising from each side of each interphalangeal joint. There are four such structures on each side of each finger. Each bundle is in the shape of a flattened, imperfect cone. The two major sets of bundles or fibers arise on each side of the proximal interphalangeal joint (Figure 2.19). Of these two sets, the more distal set is by far the larger and more prominent. Each set diverges from the joint nearest its origin. This ligament arises from bone, and its fibers diverge as they insert to the skin. The impression can be easily obtained from inaccurate dissection that the ligaments or fibers form a sheet or septum, but such is not the case, since the fibers do not run in one plane. All fibers pass dorsal to the distal nerve and vessels. Functionally, most dorsally originating fibers of these bundles become taut when the proximal interphalangeal joint is flexed. This is because they are stretched over the condyle of the proximal phalanx, thus lending the skin stability. Similarly, the more volar fibers become taut when the proximal interphalangeal joint is extended.

The two lesser and distal bundles of these ligaments take origin from the lateral aspect of the distal interphalangeal joint. They arise from the bone and capsule over a small area of 1–2 mm in the adult finger just proximal and distal to the distal interphalangeal joint.

Grayson's ligament originates on the volar surface of the flexor tendon sheath and projects at right angles to the sheath to insert into the skin (Grayson, 1941). Its fibers are mem-

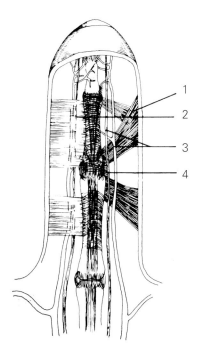

Figure 2.20 Schematic illustration of Cleland's and Grayson's ligaments. Note that the direction of Cleland's ligament is in sharp contrast to the original illustration of Grayson shown in Figure 2.4. (1) Cleland's ligament; (2) Grayson's ligament; (3) artery and nerve; (4) transverse retinacular ligament. (Reproduced with permission from Milford, 1968.)

erally and dorsally to attach to the lateral margin of the extensor mechanism on each side of the proximal interphalangeal joint. The oblique retinacular ligament (Weitbrecht, 1742) or link ligament, is tendinous in character, in contrast to the fascial fibers of the overlying transverse retinacular ligament (Landsmeer, 1949). The oblique retinacular ligaments are not involved in Dupuytren's contracture.

Palmar fascia in the radial side of the hand

The following description includes the thumb, the thenar eminence and the first web space. The study of the anatomy of these fibrous formations was performed by de Frenne in 1977 (Figure 2.21).

The fibrous skeleton of the thenar eminence is thin, and poorly developed in the ulnar and middle areas, while the fascia becomes much thicker at the radial side and superficially to the thumb MP joint where dense crossing fibers exist.

The radial longitudinal fibers of the superficial mid-palmar aponeurosis are in continuation with the PL tendon. This tendon presents, on its radial side, a slip for the insertion of the superficial head of the abductor pollicis brevis (APB). The palmar sensory branch of the median nerve emerges in between the tendinous bifurcation, which constitutes a precious landmark (Fahrer and Tubiana, 1976) (see Figure 2.6).

The most radial longitudinal fibers of the superficial palmar fascia extend towards the thumb. The deeper ones attach on either side of the flexor tendon sheath of the flexor pollicis longus. The more superficial ones attach to the dermis in a similar pattern to the pretendinous bands of the long fingers. Some longitudinal fibers attach to the intermuscular septum between the adductor pollicis and the first dorsal interosseus. Finally, some attach directly to the flexor tendon sheath of the index.

branous in character and pass volar to the distal nerve and artery (Figure 2.20). This ligament helps to keep them from bow-stringing when the finger is flexed. With the more dorsally located Cleland's ligament, it tends to form a tube around the neurovascular bundle. The fibers run parallel to one another and do not diverge as in Cleland's ligament.

The transverse retinacular ligament originates from the volar aspect of the capsule of the proximal interphalangeal joint and flexor tendon sheath at the same level. The fibers pass superficially to the fibers of Cleland's ligament, arising at the same level, and pass lat-

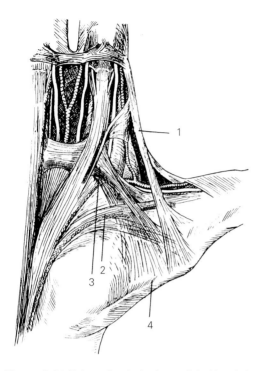

Figure 2.21 Palmar fascia in the radial side of the hand. (1) Distal transverse commissural ligament of the first web (Grapow, 1887); (2) radial longitudinal fibers of the midpalmar aponeurosis to the thumb and index finger; (3) proximal transverse commissural ligament (de Frenne, 1977) (4) fascia of the thenar eminence is thicker at the radial side of the eminence over the thumb MP joint.

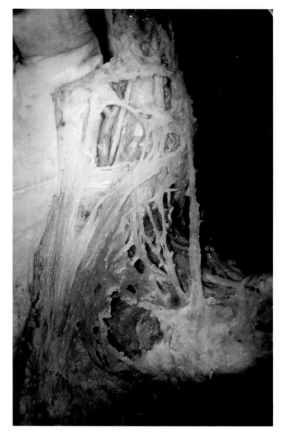

Figure 2.22 Fibrous structure of the first web space.

The pretendinous bands are sometimes poorly developed to both the thumb and index fingers, the longitudinal fibers being inserted into the skin only.

The fascia of the first web space

Two transverse structures cross the thumb web: the distal transverse commissural ligament was described by Grapow in 1887 (Grapow, 1887). It forms a distal transverse band between the thumb and the index finger and is analogous to the natatory ligament of the other web spaces (Figure 2.22). Towards the latter, some fibers join the radial lateral digital sheet of the index finger. In the thumb, the ligament splits on either side of the thumb flexor tendon sheath. Some fibers join the lateral digital sheet of the thumb on both sides.

The proximal commissural ligament (de Frenne, 1977) is the second, more proximal, transverse structure of the first web space. It is similar to the proximal transverse ligament of the midpalmar fascia, and some of its fibers

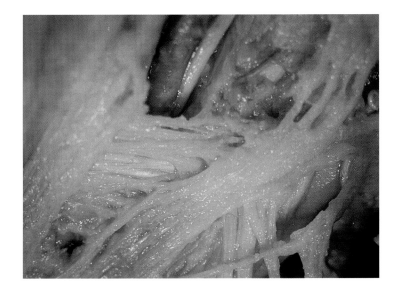

Figure 2.23 Continuity of fibers of the proximal transverse palmar ligament (crossing the index pretendinous band dorsally) with the proximal transverse commissural ligament.

are in continuity with the palmar transverse fibers, crossing the index pretendinous band dorsally (Figure 2.23). Another group of fibers bifurcate on either side of the flexor tendon sheath of the index. It seems that the radial attachments are more developed than the ulnar ones. This shows very well on a cross-section of a fetal hand. Towards the thumb the proximal commissural ligament joins the fibrous crossroad at the palmar radial side of the metacarpophalangeal joint of the thumb. There, just as with the fibers of Grapow's ligament, deep fibers divide on either side of the flexor tendon sheath and other fibers join the lateral sheet of the thumb. In the thumb, the fibrous structures are quite similar to those of the other fingers. There is a prevascular layer and retrovascular fibers attaching respectively to the dermis and to the flexor tendon sheath of the long flexor. These structures extend as far as the distal phalanx. Finally, the index finger fascia is identical to those of the other fingers, with the exception that the lateral digital retrovascular band is reinforced by Grapow's ligament and seems more developed.

Normal relative motion between the different fiber systems

The work of McGrouther has clarified the microscopic anatomy of the palmar aponeurosis: 'Palmar fascia is not fascia, nor it is just palmar! What the hand possesses is a three-dimensional system of fine ligamentous structures, each with a precise origin and insertion and all together constituting a fibrous tissue continuum. This can be regarded as a fibrous skeleton or framework, providing guide channels and retinacular restraint for longitudinally running structures and also as a system that anchors the skin while still allowing it to flex and extend' (McGrouther, 1982).

He described this tridimensional structure, consisting of vertical, longitudinal and transverse fibers (Figure 2.24). The vertical fibers (perpendicular to the skin) are the weakest, and are dispersed throughout the entire palm, but are concentrated for several millimeters on either side of each of the palmar skin creases. The fibers run from the skin, and cross the other two fibers. On transverse

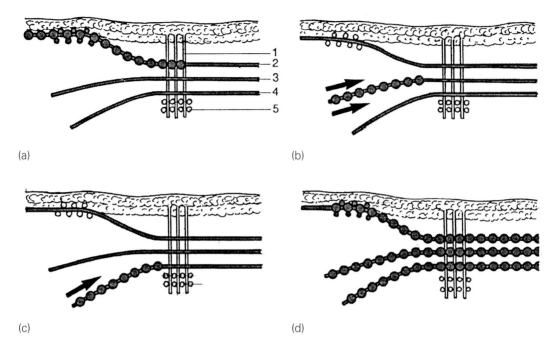

(a)

(b)

(c)

(d)

Figure 2.24 Microscopic tridimensional structure of the palmar fascia (from McGrouther, 1982). (a) Longitudinal section in the distal palmar fascia: (1) vertical fibers; (2) superficial longitudinal fibers inserted into the skin of the distal palm; (3) some longitudinal intermediate fibers turn down into the depth of the hand and pass distally to the fingers; (4) the deepest longitudinal fibers turn down around the sides of the flexor tendon sheath at MP joint level; (5) transverse fibers. (b) The intermediate depth longitudinal fibers are involved with the contracting process; (c) the deepest longitudinal fibers are involved; (d) associated lesions of all longitudinal fibers.

sections of the hand, the vertical fibers appear to run in canals or channels formed by the skin superficially, the transverse fibers deeply, and the longitudinal fibers laterally. The longitudinal fibers insert distally at different sites:

- On the skin, distally, in the region of the PIP joint flexion crease; and
- Deeply on the flexor tendon sheath, in the region of the metacarpal and the proximal phalanx.

The longitudinal fibers provide a system of skin anchorage, which operates irrespective of the position of the underlying joints and acts particularly to resist shearing forces in grip-ping. They have a mobility of 1–2 mm within their channels. It is this mobility that allows structures to slide relative to each other during hand movements. This mobility appears to be lost as part of Dupuytren's disease.

Relationship between the palmodigital aponeurosis and Dupuytren's disease

All the aponeurotic structures in the hand are not clinically affected by Dupuytren's disease. Only specific parts of the palm and digits are involved. Those macroscopically affected tissues are in the superficial layers, and are unevenly affected. The thenar and

Table 2.2 Normal fascia bands and Dupuytren's cords. (Adapted from McFarlane, 1986, and Strickland and Leibovic, 1991.)	
Normal fascia	**Diseased cords**
Pretendinous band	Pretendinous cord
Superficial transverse palmar ligament (proximal)	Not involved, expect in first web
Natatory ligament	Natatory cord
Septae of Legueu and Juvara	Vertical palmar cords
Spiral band	Spiral cord
Grayson's ligament	Part of central, spiral and lateral cords
None	Axial digitopalmar cord
Lateral digital sheath	Lateral digital cord
Cleland's ligament	Not involved (McFarlane)
Retrovascular digital band (Thomine)	Retrovascular cord
Oblique retinacular ligament	Not directly involved

hypothenar eminence aponeurotic tissues are rarely affected.

Almost all the involved tissues lie in the superficially placed layers of the mid-palmar aponeurosis and the digital fascia, that is, in the pretendinous bands and, more specifically, in the distally placed fascia: the natatory ligament and its digital expansions. As commented upon by McFarlane (1990), the deep retinacular tissues, which include the proximal transverse palmar ligament and the fibrous flexor tendon sheaths, are not macroscopically invaded. Skoog (1967) noted that the superficial [proximal] transverse ligament was not affected, possibly because it is not subjected to variations in tension during digital movements. It is noteworthy, however, that the extension of this ligament in the thumb web space (proximal transverse commissural ligament) may be affected and become the site of a contracture. This shows the influence of longitudinal tension on the development of Dupuytren's contracture.

The most troubling aspect of the distribution of lesions in Dupuytren's disease is the frequency of finding lesions in the distal part of the palm, where there is an aponeurotic hiatus (Thomine, 1965). In effect, most of the pretendinous bands insert into the skin here, and the sagittal septa stop at the level of the distal transverse skin crease. Under magnification, it is possible to perceive the longitudinal fibers that insert into the skin and others that run into the fingers. These fibers may constitute an anatomical guide and a mechanical support in the development of the contractile fibrosis. It is important to emphasize that this fibrosis is not proportional to the volume of the affected aponeurotic tissue and that it is not a simple hypertrophy of the normal structure of aponeurotic tissue. It seems that the fibrosis may be able to extend to other parts of the connective tissue of the palm and fingers.

PATHOLOGICAL ANATOMY OF THE DEFORMITIES

Two types of pathological fibrous formation are seen in Dupuytren's disease: nodules and cords. They are histologically different (see their description by Gosset at the beginning of this chapter, pages 13–15). It seems that the nodular formations are independent of the aponeurosis and that the deformities are mainly caused by contractile cords, some of them extending along pre-existing fascia (Table 2.2).

The contractile cords

Following Luck's nomenclature (1959), the normal fibrous tissue will be called 'bands' and the diseased tissue 'cords'.

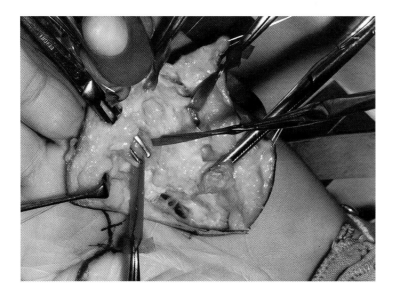

Figure 2.25 Contracture of the natatory ligament.

Deformities are produced by fibrous cords acting on a susceptible mobile osseous segment. Thus the deformities are found most often in the fingers. The pathogenesis of this condition will not be discussed again. The author believes that all diseased Dupuytren's tissue does not derive from normal fascia, but that some of the cords (not all) extend along pre-existing fascia.

In the palm, fibrous diseased tissue only contracts the MP joints. The contracture of the natatory ligament may contract the web spaces, impeding the ability to spread the fingers (Figure 2.25). The invasion by Dupuytren's disease of this ligament, which also has longitudinal extensions into the fingers (Figure 2.26), may also produce a flexion contracture of the PIP joints.

The finger deformities consist essentially of flexion contractures of the three finger joints. These deformities may be the result of the palmar cords or of the digital cords or a combination of the two (Figure 2.27). In the little finger, flexion contractures of the IP joints may be seen without palmar lesions. The distal interphalangeal (DIP) joint may be forced into a hyperextension deformity.

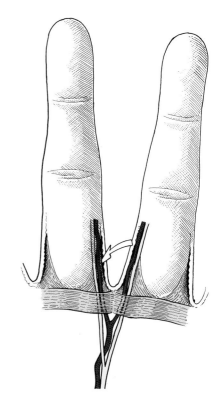

Figure 2.26 Commissural cord. The arrow shows that the skin does not adhere to the underlying fibrous structures at the lateral aspect of the finger web.

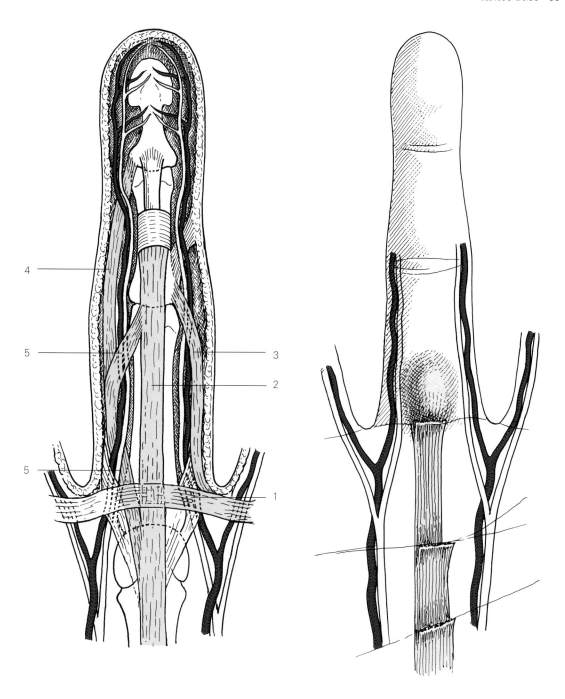

Figure 2.27 Dupuytren's fibrous cords. (1) Natatory ligament; (2) midline or central cord; (3) lateral cord; (4) retrovascular cord; (5) spiral cord.

Figure 2.28 Axial digitopalmar cord (central cord), which ends in a nodule on the proximal phalanx and produces contracture of the MP joint.

Axial digitopalmar cords

These follow the path of the pretendinous band of the palmar aponeurosis and continue into the fingers. The proximal fixation may also be the prolongation of the longitudinal fibers on the sagittal septa and on the deep aponeurotic layers. The distal fixation is placed in the skin or a nodule on the proximal phalanx, adherent to the dermis, distally related to the MP joint, at which the contracture may occur (Figure 2.28). Occasionally this continues to the middle phalanx (Figure 2.29), adherent to the skin on its entire path, and onto the digital fascia and the tendon sheath at the PIP joint, sometimes displacing one or both of the neurovascular bundles superficially toward the axis of the finger.

There are several characteristic features of this axial cord:

• A simple subcutaneous palmar fasciotomy will allow the correction of an MP joint contracture;

• This superficial cord is axial with respect to the neurovascular bundles, which are theoretically safe during a palmar fasciotomy.

When the origin of this cord is deep, the longitudinal cord may cross under the neurovascular bundle or, more commonly, the single collateral nerve (the digital nerve division is more proximal than the homologous artery) (Figure 2.30). The contracture of the cord tends, with respect to the MP joint, to displace the neurovascular bundle more superficially, toward the midline, and proximally (Figure 2.31). The displacement is similar with spiral cords (Figure 2.32). It is thus important to remember that there is a danger, in the presence of these axial digitopalmar cords. Recognition of the deplacement of the digital nerve into the immediate subcutaneous area prior to incision is important. For Short and Watson (1982), the phenomenon is heralded by a circular, soft, pulpy prominence

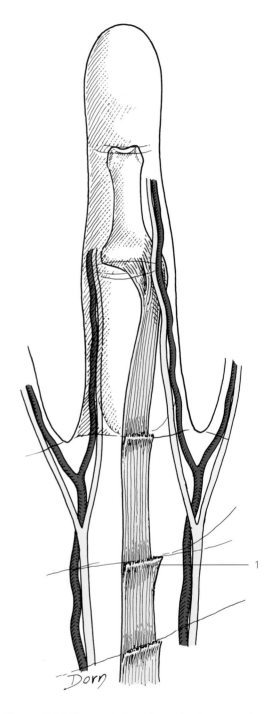

Figure 2.29 The central cord may be longer and continues to the middle phalanx. It may produce contracture of the MP and PIP joints. (1) Fibers inserted into the dermis.

to either side of the pretendinous band at the level of the MP joint. An adequate surgical exposure at the base of the finger is required to visualize the neurovascular bundles before dividing or resecting the cords.

Vertical palmar cords

In severe cases, the vertical septa of Legueu and Juvara may be thickened and contracted.

Digital cords

There are many different types of digital cord, some isolated, but many in combination. These may be symmetrical on the radial and ulnar sides of a finger, but most commonly are asymmetrical, and are more marked on just one side. These cords most commonly cause a contracture of the PIP joint, and occasionally the DIP joint. They alter the usual anatomy of the neurovascular bundles, and produce a difficult dissection. McFarlane (1974) identified four varieties of digital cord: central; lateral; spiral; and retrovascular.

We have already mentioned *central cords* anterior to the proximal phalanx. This cord is one of the usual causes of a PIP contracture.

The *lateral cord* involves the lateral digital sheath. It adheres in its proximal part to the natatory ligament, except on the ulnar side of the little finger, where it is fixed to the tendon of the abductor digiti minimi (Figure 2.33). It lies between the skin and the neurovascular bundle, which it pushes towards the midline of the finger. Distally it is inserted to the skin, and may send a fibrous extension anteriorly to the pedicle, prior to inserting into the tendon sheath at the base of the middle phalanx (see Figure 2.27). The lateral cord causes flexion contracture at the PIP joint. This cord may be extended to the distal phalanx and causes, like the retrovascular cord, a flexion deformity at the DIP joint.

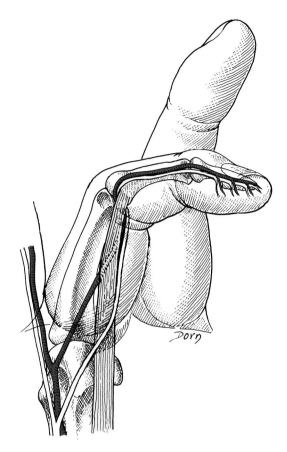

Figure 2.30 Long central cords sometimes combine with spiral cords. With increasing contracture at the MP and PIP joints, they displace the neurovascular bundle or, here, only the collateral nerve, superficially, proximally and toward the midline, where it may be easily injured.

The *spiral cords* pass in a spiral manner around a neurovascular bundle. There are several varieties of spiral cord, according to the proximal origin (see Figure 2.32), which may be in continuity, as it is usually described with the bifurcating fibers of the pretendinous band. Spiral cords that blend with the deep palmar fascia over the interosseous in continuity with the distal end of the vertical

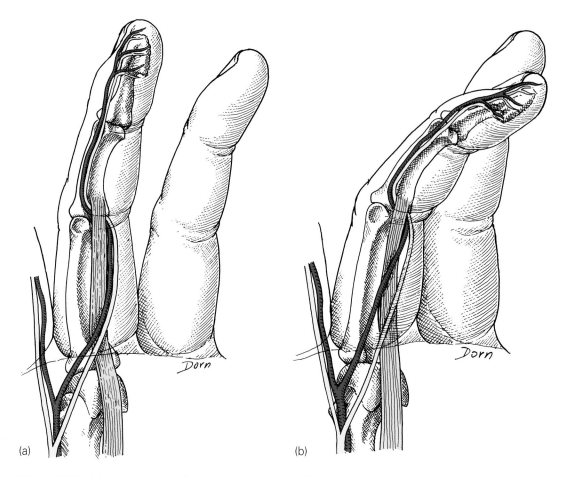

(a)   (b)

Figure 2.31 (a) Long central cords may have a deep origin from the continuation of the deep longitudinal fibers of the pretendinous band; (b) with further contraction of the PIP joint the cord displaces the neurovascular bundle toward the midline.

septa have also been seen. The cord then passes under the neurovascular bundle, becomes axial and then recrosses the bundle before inserting into the fibrous tendon sheath or the bony skeleton. The cord has a tendency to become progressively straight, and in fact it is the bundle that 'spirals' around the cord. With further contraction of the PIP joint, the bundle is displaced towards the midline, proximally and superficially, which increases the risk of damage during surgical dissection at the level of the proximal phalanx. However, in most cases, the neurovascular bundles will be found superficially on either side of the PIP joint. McFarlane (1974) suggested several interpretations for these spiral cords, which involve several normal fascial elements. These are the pretendinous bands, the 'spiral' band, which passes in front of the MP joint, the lateral digital fascia and Graysons's ligament. Other combinations are possible.

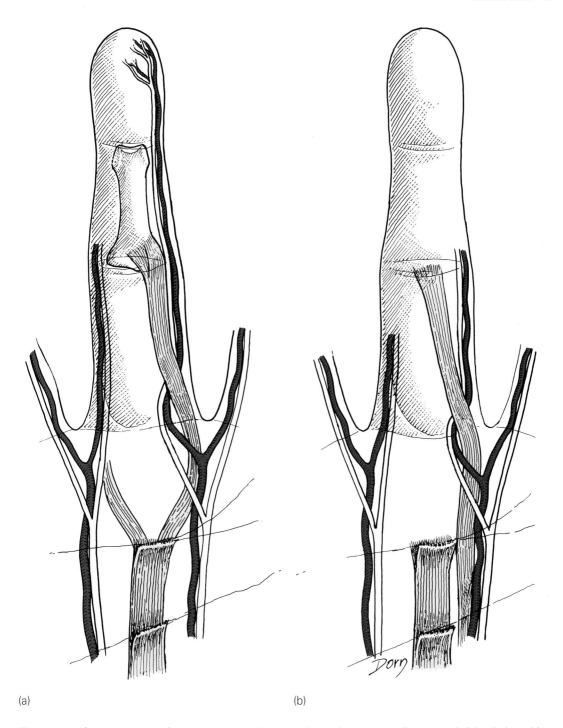

(a)   (b)

Figure 2.32 Spiral cords. (a) Spiral cord in continuity with a palmar pretendinous cord; (b) spiral cord in continuity with the deep longitudinal fibers. As the spiral cord shortens, the PIP joint is contracted in flexion and the neurovascular bundle is drawn toward the midline.

The *retrovascular cords* are longitudinal cords that arise in the retrovascular band, which runs as far as the distal phalanx (see Figure 2.27). McFarlane believes that this cord is separate from the oblique fibers of Cleland's ligament, which is not affected by Dupuytren's disease. A retrovascular cord can cause a contraction of both the PIP and the DIP joints. Retrovascular fibers that are left in situ may be the cause of recurrent contracture.

Little finger deformities

There are several unique features of the retractile cords in the little fingers. Isolated disease in the finger, with no continuity to any palmar disease, is seen most commonly in the little finger (Strickland and Bassett, 1985). All the types of cords previously described may be found, but the most specific and almost constant finding is that of the ulnar-sided cord attached to the tendon of abductor digiti minimi (ADM). At the base of the finger, the ulnar neurovascular bundle is always pushed towards the midline (Figure 2.33). The dorsal ulnar sensory branch may be closely applied to the ADM cord and can be damaged when dissecting this cord (Hurst, 1996) (see Figure 2.18). The cord may remain laterally, or may spiral around the bundle. This cord, which is occasionally very thick, may produce a contraction of the MP joint or produce an abduction deformity of the finger, if the little finger/ring finger web space is not affected by the disease.

The little finger usually produces the most marked contractures, and not infrequently the PIP joint is flexed beyond 90°, combined with a DIP joint contracture in flexion or hyperextension.

The extent of involvement of the little finger, where often all the different cords will be found together, explains why the surgical correction is sometimes incomplete and recurrences are more common.

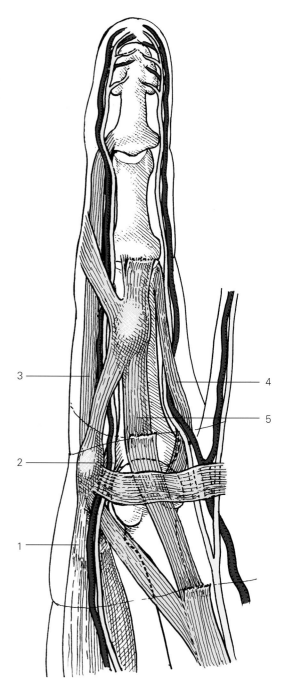

Figure 2.33 Little finger cords. (1) Tendon of abductor digiti minimi; (2) the ulnar collateral bundle is displaced radially at the MP level; (3) retrovascular cord; (4) spiral cord on the radial side; (5) central cord.

(a)

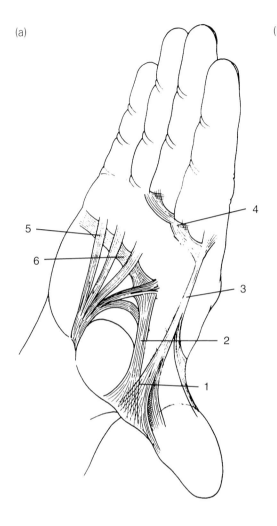

(b)

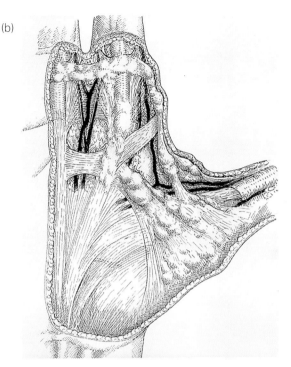

Figure 2.34 Dupuytren's locations in the radial side of the hand. (a) Fibrous contracture at the radial part of the hand: (1) fibrous complex in front of the metacarpophalangeal joint of the thumb; (2) proximal commissural ligament of the first web space; (3) distal commissural ligament of the first web space (Grapow); (4) interdigital or natatory ligament; (5) pretendinous bands; (6) transverse superficial ligament. (b) Localization of Dupuytren's disease in the radial part of the hand.

Hyperextension of the distal interphalangeal joint

This is seen most often in the little finger, usually accompanying a severe contracture of the PIP joint (see Figure 6.51).

This is not, as has been thought, a contracture of Landsmeer's oblique retinacular ligament, which is not actually affected. Thomine suggested that it is the result of traction forces transmitted on the distal part of the extensor apparatus, which is not invaded, from contracted digital fascia.

Hueston (1991) also supported the proposition that DIP hyperextension is not produced by the involvement of Landsmeer's ligament. DIP hyperextension is not seen in the absence of severe PIP fixed flexion, and the DIP joint becomes 'flail' when the PIP is held fully flexed; thus hyperextension is passively inflicted. Joint and retinacular ligaments, along with the extensor apparatus (sometimes creating a boutonnière-type deformity), become secondarily fixed in this shortened position.

Pathologic fibrous formations in the radial side of the hand

Four locations were observed corresponding to the anatomical structures (Figure 2.34):

1) A longitudinal fibrous cord on the radial side of the thenar eminence, extending into the thumb and having the tendency to pull the metacarpophalangeal joint of the thumb into radial deviation and flexion;
2) A longitudinal cord to the first web and flexor sheath of the thumb corresponding to the longitudinal fibers of the palmar aponeurosis, causing a flexion contracture of the thumb;
3) A distal transverse interdigital cord, corresponding to Grapow's ligament, producing an adduction and retroposition contracture (Figures 2.35 and 2.36);
4) A transverse proximal cord in the first web, corresponding to the proximal transverse commissural ligament, resulting in a web space contracture.

Contracture of the digital joints

We have seen that, initially, digital joint contracture occurs as a consequence of the fibrous tissue contracture. During the evolution both the fascia and the skin are involved.

With long-standing deformities, associated lesions develop in the structures surrounding the joints. They are not caused by infiltration of Dupuytren's tissue but are the consequence of chronic joint contracture. Secondary changes are as follows (Crowley and Tonkin, 1999):

- Contracture of the flexor sheath;
- Shortening of the flexor muscles;
- Lesions of the extensor mechanism;
- Contracture of the volar plate;
- Contracture and adhesion of accessory collateral ligaments;
- Contracture of collateral ligaments.

Even intra-articular changes are involved: obliteration of the dorsal joint space and lesions of articular cartilage. Also, scarring is present in recurrences.

The effects of these secondary lesions are different on each digital joint.

In the MP joint, the collateral ligaments are slack in extension and tight in flexion because of the eccentric insertion of the ligaments and the shape of the metacarpal head, which has a condylar protuberance volarly. Also, the MP volar plate attachments are more mobile than at the volar plate of the PIP. As a result of this anatomical configuration, long-standing flexion contractures are easily corrected. This is not true for the interphalangeal joints, which are of the trochlear type. Tension of the collateral ligaments is almost the same throughout the whole range of movement. They rapidly contract in flexion.

At the PIP joint level, because of the joint flexion deformity, the central extensor tendon is elongated and the lateral extensor tendons are displaced volarly. Contracture of the transverse retinacular ligament inserted on the lateral slip will fix this boutonnière-type deformity. This explains why the correction of PIP joint deformity is difficult and also the possibility of relapse (see the section on correction of PIP joint contracture, pages 161–63, and Chapter 7).

At the DIP joint, flexion contractures are caused by the distal insertion of the retrovascular cords. Hyperextension contractures are possible, usually accompanying a severe PIP joint contracture, and thus passively inflected (the DIP joint becomes 'flail' in the normal hand when the PIP is held fully flexed). Dorsal plaques of Dupuytren's tissue, distinct from knuckle pads, at the level of the middle phlanx, are extremely rare (Hueston, 1982). It is important to realize that joint contractures induce all the soft tissues to become shortened. This is particularly true of the vessels and nerves, which can lose a centimeter of length for each 60° of contracture at the MP joint (Brand and Hollister, 1999). Care should

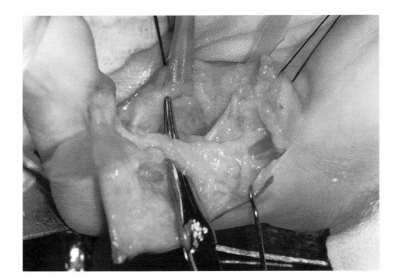

Figure 2.35 Distal commissural cord of the first web.

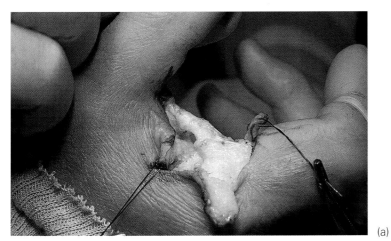

Figure 2.36 Very severe distal commissural cord (a) before and (b) after resection.

(a)

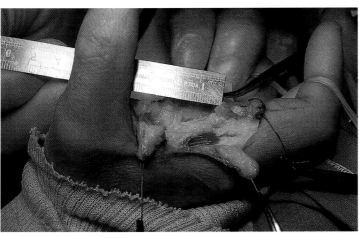

(b)

be taken to protect the nerves and vessels from being overstretched (see 'Fasciectomy', pages 157–59).

References

Albinius BS (1734) *Historia Musculorum Hominis. Leidae batavorum.* Bibliothèque de Chirurgie, Paris.

Bojsen-Moller F, Schmidt L (1974) The palmar aponeurosis and the central spaces of the hand. *J Anat* **117**: 55–68.

Bourgery JM, Jacob NA (1832) *Traité Complet de l'Anatomie de l'Homme Comprenant la Médecine Opératoire.* CA Delauney, Paris.

Brand PW, Hollister AM (1999) *Clinical Mechanics of the Hand*, 3rd edn, 253–54. Mosby, St Louis.

Braune WA, Trübiger A (1873) *Die Venen der menschlichen Hand.* Leipzig. (Cited by Grapow, 1887.)

Cannanus G (1543) *Musculorum Humani Corporis – Picturata Dissecto.* Ferrara.

Caughill KA, McFarlane RM, McGrouther DA *et al.* (1988) Developmental anatomy of the palmar aponeurosis and its relationship to the palmaris longus tendon. *J Hand Surg* **13A**: 485–93.

Cleland J (1878) On the cutaneous ligaments of the phalanges. *J Anat Physiol* **12**: 526.

Crowley B, Tonkin MA (1999) The proximal interphalangeal joint in Dupuytren's disease. *Hand Clin* **15**: 137–47.

De Frenne HA (1977) Les structures aponévrotiques au niveau de la première commissure. *Ann Chir* **31**: 1017–19.

Dupuytren G (1831) De la rétraction des doigts par suite d'une affection de l'aponeurose palmaire. *Journal Universel et Hebdomadaire de Médecine et de Chirurgie Pratiques et des Institutions Médicales, Paris.* **25**: 349–65. (Reprinted in *Medical Classics 1939–1940*, Vol. 4. Royal Society of Medicine, London.)

Fahrer M (1980) The proximal end of the palmar aponeurosis. *Hand* **12**: 33.

Fahrer M, Tubiana R (1976) Palmaris longus, anteductor of the thumb. An experimental study. *Hand* **8**: 287.

Ferrarini M (1936) Morphogenesi della aponevrosi palmare. *Arch Ital Anat Embryol* **37**: 203–68.

Gosset J (1967) Maladie de Dupuytren et anatomie des aponévroses palmodigitales. *Ann Chir* **21**: 554–65.

Gosset J (1972) Anatomie des aponévroses palmo-digitales. In: Tubiana R, Hueston J, eds, *Maladie de Dupuytren*, 23–38. L'Expansion Scientifique, Paris.

Gosset J (1985) Dupuytren's disease and the anatomy of the palmodigital aponeuroses. In: Hueston JT, Tubiana R, eds, *Dupuytren's Disease*, 2nd edn, 13–26. Churchill Livingstone, London.

Goyrand G (1833) Nouvelles recherches sur la rétraction permanente des doigts. *Mémoires Acad Med* **3**: 489.

Goyrand G (1834) Nouvelles recherches sur la rétraction permanente des doigts. *Mémoire Acad R Med* **3**: 489–96.

Grapow M (1887) Die Anatomie und Physiologische Bedeutung der Palmaraponeurose. *Arch Anat Physiol* **143**: 2–3.

Grayson J (1940) The cutaneous ligaments of the digits. *J Anat* **75**: 164.

Holland AJ, McGrouther DA (1997) Dupuytren's disease and the relationship between the transverse and longitudinal fibers of the palmar fascia. A dissection study. *Clin Anat* **10**: 97–103.

Hueston JT (1982) Dorsal Dupuytren's disease. *J Hand Surg* **7**: 384–87.

Hueston JT (1991) Comment on 'Anatomy and pathogenesis of the digital cords and nodules'. *Hand Clin* **7**: 659–60.

Hueston JT, Tubiana R (1974) *Dupuytren's Disease.* Churchill Livingstone, Edinburgh.

Hurst LC (1996) Dupuytren's fasciectomy: zig-zag-plasty technique. In: Blair WF, ed., *Techniques in Hand Surgery*, 518–29. Williams and Wilkins, Baltimore.

Iselin M (1955) *Chirurgie de la Main*, Vol. 2. Livre de Chirurgien, Masson, Paris.

Kaplan EB (1938) The palmar fascia in connection with Dupuytren's contracture. *Surgery* **4**: 415–22.

Karlberg W (1935) Zur Anatomie der palmaraponeurose. *Anatomischer Anzeiger* **81**: 149–59.

Landsmeer JMF (1949) The anatomy of the dorsal aponeurosis of the human finger and its functional significance. *Anat Rec* **104**: 31–44.

Landsmeer JMF (1956) Les aponévroses dorsales de la main. *Compte Rendu de l'Association des Anatomistes* **43**: 443.

Landsmeer JMF (1976) *Atlas of Anatomy of the Hand.* Churchill Livingstone, Edinburgh.

Legueu F, Juvara E (1892) Des aponévroses de la paume de la main. *Bull Soc Anat Paris* **6**: 383.

Le Gros Clark W (1958) *The Tissues of the Body*, 4th edn. Oxford University Press, London.

Lister G (1977) *The Hand: Diagnosis and Indications.* Churchill Livingstone, Edinburgh.

Luck JV (1959) Dupuytren's contracture – a new concept of the pathogenesis correlated with surgical management. *J Bone Joint Surg* **41A**: 635–64.

MacCallum P, Hueston JT (1962) The pathology of Dupuytren's contracture. *Aust N Z J Surg* **31**: 241–53.

Maslieurat-Lagémard GE (1839) De l'anatomie descriptive et chirurgicale des aponévroses et des membranes synoviales de la main, de leur application à la thérapeutique et à la médecine opératoire. *Gazette Med Paris* **7**: 273–80.

McFarlane RM (1974) Pattern of the diseased fascia in the fingers in Dupuytren's contracture. *Plast Reconstruct Surg* **54**: 31.

McFarlane RM (1985) The anatomy of Dupuytren's disease. In: Hueston JT, Tubiana R, eds, *Dupuytren's Disease*, 2nd edn. Churchill Livingstone, Edinburgh.

McFarlane RM, McGrouther DA, Flint MH (1990) *Dupuytren's Disease. Biology and Treatment.* Churchill Livingstone, Edinburgh.

McGrouther DA (1982) The microanatomy of Dupuytren's contracture. *Hand* **13**: 215–36.

McGrouther DA (1998) Dupuytren's contracture. In: Green DP, Hotchkiss RN, Pederson WC, eds, *Green's Operative Hand Surgery*, Vol. 1, 4th edn, 563–91. Churchill Livingstone, New York.

Meyerding HW, Black JR, Broders AC (1941) The etiology and pathology of Dupuytren's contracture. *Surg Gynecol Obstet* **72**: 582–90.

Milford L (1968) *Retaining Ligaments of the Digits of the Hand.* WB Saunders, Philadelphia.

Millesi H (1986) Evolution clinique et morphologique de la maladie de Dupuytren. In: Tubiana R, Hueston JT, eds, *Maladie de Dupuytren*, 3rd edn, 115–21. L'Expansion Scientifique, Paris.

Nezelof C, Tubiana R (1958) La Maladie de Dupuytren: étude histologique. *Sem Hop Paris* **34**: 1102–109.

Poirier P, Charpy A (1899) *Traité d'anatomie humaine*, Vol. 2. Masson, Paris.

Powell BW, McLean NR, Jeffs JV (1986) The incidence of a palmaris longus tendon in patients with Dupuytren's disease. *J Hand Surg* **11B**: 382–84.

Rayan GM (1999) Palmar fascia complex. Anatomy and pathology in Dupuytren's disease. *Hand Clin* **15**: 73–86.

Short WH, Watson HK (1982) Prediction of the spiral nerve in Dupuytren's contracture. *J Hand Surg* **7A**: 84–86.

Skoog T (1967) The superficial transverse fibers of the palmar aponeuroses and their significance in Dupuytren's contracture. *Surg Clin North Am* **47**: 443.

Stack HG (1971) The palmar fascia and the development of deformities and displacements in Dupuytren's contracture. *Ann R Coll Surg Engl* **48**: 230.

Stack HG (1973) *The Palmar Fascia.* Churchill Livingstone, Edinburgh.

Strickland JW, Bassett RL (1985) The isolated digital cord in Dupuytren's contracture. Anatomy and clinical significance. *J Hand Surg* **10A**: 118–24.

Strickland JW, Leibovic SJ (1991) Anatomy and pathogenesis of the digital cords and nodules. *Hand Clin* **7**: 645–57.

Testut L (1893) *Traité d'anatomie humaine.* Octave Doin, Paris.

Thomine J-M (1965) Conjonctif d'enveloppe des doigts et squelette fibreux des commissures interdigitales. *Ann Chirurg Plast* **3**: 194–203.

Weitbrecht J (1742) Syndesmologia sive Historia Ligamentorum Corporis Humani. Translated by EB Kaplan (1969). In: *Syndesmology.* WB Saunders, Philadelphia.

Wood Jones F (1942) *The Principles of Anatomy as Seen in the Hand*, 2nd edn. Williams and Wilkins, Baltimore.

Zancolli EA, Cozzi EP (1992) The retinaculum cutis of the hand. In: Zancolli EA, Cozzi EP, eds, *Atlas of Surgical Anatomy of the Hand.* Churchill Livingstone, New York.

3

Epidemiology

Caroline Leclercq

RACE AND COUNTRY

Legend has it that the MacCrimmons, who ran the Scottish College of Bagpiping from the 15th–18th Centuries, had a high incidence of Dupuytren's contracture, which prevented them from playing the pipes in later life. The disease became known as 'the curse of the MacCrimmons' (Elliot, 1988). Comparisons of different series actually seem to show a genuine high prevalence of Dupuytren's disease in north-east Scotland (Lennox et al., 1993; Ling, 1963). Aside from this, the disease has been traced back to Icelandic Middle Ages literature (Whaley and Elliot, 1993), but is not described in Roman or Greek ancient literature. In France the disease was described by Baron Dupuytren in 1831.

The global prevalence of Dupuytren's disease in today's Caucasian population is estimated to be 3–6% (Early, 1962; Murrell and Hueston, 1990; Yost et al., 1955) with the highest prevalence being in Scandinavia (Hueston, 1960, 1962, 1987; Lund, 1941; Mikkelsen, 1990; Yost et al., 1955). This has led to the theory of a Northern origin of Dupuytren's disease, disseminated by the Vikings during their invasions (Early, 1962). The three directions of their expeditions were to Canada through Iceland, down the Western European coast, including the British Isles, and east into Poland and so far as the Ukraine and the Volga basin (Hueston, 1987). For instance, the disease is rather common in Spain (Quintana Guitian, 1988; Saez Aldana et al., 1996), whereas it is almost unknown in Greece (Hueston, 1987).

An interesting study performed by Brouet (1986) in southern France (Toulon) where the population is a mixture of local Mediterranean people, and descendants of Northern European seamen who have migrated, has shown that the prevalence of Dupuytren's disease in persons with blue eyes (i.e. of Northern origin) is several times that in persons with brown eyes (i.e. of local origin).

In Australia the high level of immigration from Scotland and Ireland accounts for the high figures, as 30% of people aged 60 years and over are involved (Hueston, 1960, 1962).

The disease is much less frequent in non-Caucasian populations as attested by the scarcity of case reports in those populations.

In the black races all reports included single cases (Furnas, 1979; Haeseker, 1981; Mennen and Gräbe, 1979; Plasse, 1979; Rosenfeld et al., 1983; Simons et al., 1996; Zaworski and Mann, 1979) or series with fewer than 10 patients (Brenner et al., 1994; Mennen, 1986; Mitra and Goldstein, 1994; Muguti and Appelt, 1993; Sladicka et al., 1996; Yost et al., 1955) until a recent 14-year retrospective review performed in Chicago (Illinois, USA) by Gonzalez et al. (1998) identifying 17 black patients who had undergone a Dupuytren's release.

In his international epidemiological study by questionnaire based on 812 patients, McFarlane (1985) reported nine black Americans (1%) and five black Africans (0.5%).

In African-American patients, there is always a question as to whether they might have some Caucasian ancestry. However, reports by Mennen (1986) and Furnas (1979) on Africans seem to indicate a small, but definite incidence of Dupuytren's disease in pure blacks. Furnas's case was a tribesman from Tanzania, and the only Caucasian settlement in the area (a Lutheran Mission) did not exist at the time of the patient's birth, the chances that he had carried any Caucasian genes being 'virtually nil'.

Although some of the cases reported in black patients seem to involve a strong diathesis (Simons et al., 1996), results of the largest series (Gonzalez et al., 1998; Mitra and Goldstein, 1994) suggest that the presentation and outcome of surgical release in black patients is very similar to that found in North Europeans.

In Asia, Dupuytren's disease is extremely uncommon, with the notable exception of Japan. In China, for instance, the first case to be reported was published by Ma in 1964 (cited by Chow et al., 1984) and the next three cases in 1984 by Chow et al. from Hong Kong. Maes (1979), during a mission in Vietnam, performed a fasciectomy on a 30-year-old Vietnamese. Later, Liu and Chen (1991) reported a series of 41 Taiwan Chinese with Dupuytren's disease.

The Japanese distribution is much higher: according to Egawa et al. (1990) 16–28% of males and 3–10% of females are involved. This higher prevalence could be due, according to Hueston (Hueston, 1988; Hueston and Seyfer, 1991), to an invasion of Northern Japan by Uro-Baltic populations through the Bering Pass. Study of a Japanese old peoples' home tends to show that the disease has a low rate of evolution, with spontaneous resorption of nodules in a few cases (Egawa et al., 1990).

This lesser severity of Dupuytren's disease in Asian populations was also noted in Liu's series. Within recent years, more cases have been reported from the Asian continent. In India, Srivastava et al. (1989) have gathered 10 cases, and in Thailand Brenner et al. (1994) have observed 19 cases.

FAMILY HISTORY

Goyrand (1833) was the first author to mention that Dupuytren's disease at times showed a familial appearance.

Since Couch's description in 1938 there have been many reports of Dupuytren's disease in identical twins, and in 1948, Skoog reviewed the relevant literature and presented his own studies relating to the hereditary nature of the condition.

Average figures show a family incidence of 10–30% (Brouet, 1986; James, 1985; McFarlane, 1985). These figures rise significantly, however, when specific enquiries are made into the patient's relatives, as demonstrated by Skoog (1948) with a 44% family incidence, and more so by Ling (1963) who examined 832 relatives of 50 Dupuytren patients. When asked, 16% of the 50 patients gave a positive family history, and after examination of the 832 relatives this rate had risen to 68%. Inspection of the pedigrees led him to the conclusion that a single gene is probably involved in the production of Dupuytren's disease. It is suggested that expression of this gene is almost complete in males over 75 years, but less than complete in females. Later, Burch (1966) suggested that transmission of this gene was recessive autosomal, but larger studies performed by Thieme (quoted by James, 1985) on first-degree relatives of 131 Dupuytren's disease patients in Edinburgh favor a dominant autosomal transmission with incomplete penetrance.

Anecdotally, Demers and Blais (1960) report on eight members of the same family affected over four generations.

GENDER

There is an obvious higher prevalence of Dupuytren's disease in men. However, the female to male ratio varies much with series, from 1:10 (Brouet, 1986) to more than 1:2 (Hueston, 1987). These differences are probably related to several factors. First, Dupuytren's disease occurs later in life in women than in men, with a peak incidence at around 60–70 years in women and around 50 years in men (Early, personal communication, 1962; Ling, 1963; Brouet, 1986). Secondly, progression of the disease is usually slower in women, and many of them probably never reach the level where medical advice is sought. In Brouet's series of 1000 patients the female to male ratio is 1:10 for the operated group versus 1:3 for the non-operated group (one-third of whom were referred for another problem). Therefore the proportion of women is probably more accurate in epidemiological series than in surgical statistics (Mikkelsen, 1976). If one sums up the largest epidemiological series (Ling, 1963; Early, 1962; Brouet, 1986; Mikkelsen, 1976) the average female to male ratio is close to 2:10.

Isolated involvement of the little finger seems more frequent in women than in men (Brouet, 1986), with a higher rate of recurrence after surgery.

A study by Wallace (1965) of 46 women who underwent surgery for Dupuytren's disease showed that the results were globally poorer than in men, and especially so when a palmar fasciectomy was performed (versus a digital fasciectomy or an amputation) and when the patient was between 39 and 59 years old. Moreover, Zemel (1991) found that reflex sympathetic dystrophy was twice as frequent in women (24.5%) than in men (12.5%) following operation. However, two different retrospective studies, by Tonkin et al. (1984) and by Zemel et al. (1987) showed a rate of recurrence after operation that was significantly lower in women than in men.

AGE

Dupuytren's disease usually starts in adult life, with a peak incidence in the forties and fifties, as shown by James and Tubiana (1952) and by Ling (1963) from the combination of his series with that by Early. Figure 3.1, reproduced from Ling's article, relates numbers of cases to ages of onset of Dupuytren's disease in men and women, showing a later age of onset in women. In fact, the real average age of onset is probably younger than reported because of the insidiousness of early symptoms. Palmar nodules are frequently overlooked by the patients and when asked about the time of onset of the disease their answer is often very imprecise.

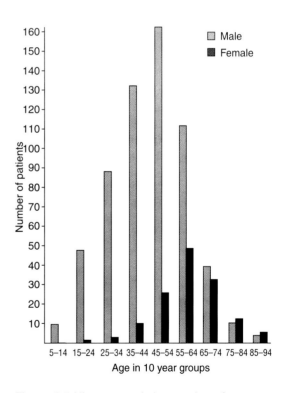

Figure 3.1 Histogram relating number of cases to ages of onset of Dupuytren's disease. (Reproduced with permission from Ling, 1963.)

Although the condition is very rare in young people, it has been reported by various authors as far back as Dupuytren himself (1832) who described the case of a 6-year-old boy and by Kanavel et al. (1929). There are over 100 cases reported where the disease began during the teenage years, although some of the early cases are questionable and are more likely, according to the clinical description, to be other conditions such as camptodactyly or congenital ulnar drift of the fingers (Bunch, 1913; Hutchinson, 1897). Urban et al. (1996) have collected from the literature (Pickren et al., 1951; Goetzee and Williams, 1954–55; Aviles et al., 1971; Rao and Luthra, 1988), and from their own series, 22 cases where the disease had begun before the age of 13, and was either certain (histological confirmation) or very likely.

There is significance in the age of onset on the course of the disease: an early onset (before the age of 30) is more likely to follow a severe course, leading to early and severe contractures, than a late onset (after the age of 60). These early-onset cases are also more prone to recurrence after surgery (Leclercq and Tubiana, 1986; Brouet, 1986; McFarlane, 1985).

This epidemiological survey shows that there are many variations in the occurrence and evolution of Dupuytren's disease. These variations are linked to several factors, which influence greatly the course of the disease in each individual, and have led Hueston to the concept of a Dupuytren's 'diathesis', which groups all the detrimental prognostic factors (see Chapter 5, pages 117–18). When several of these factors are present in the same patient, the course of the disease is likely to be severe, with multiple involvement, early and severe contractures, and a high rate of recurrence after surgery.

References

Aviles E, Arlen L, Miller T (1971) Plantar fibromatosis. *Surgery* **69**: 117–20.

Brenner P, Mailänder P, Berger A (1994) Epidemiology of Dupuytren's disease. In: Berger A, Delbrück A, Brenner P, Hinzmann R, eds, *Dupuytren's Disease*, 244–54. Springer Verlag, Berlin.

Brouet JP (1986) Etude de 1000 dossiers de maladie de Dupuytren. In: Tubiana R, Hueston JT, eds, *La Maladie de Dupuytren*, 98–105. L'Expansion Scientifique Française, Paris.

Bunch JL (1913) Hereditary Dupuytren's contracture. *Br J Dermatol* **25**: 279–83.

Burch PRJ (1966) Dupuytren's contracture: an autoimmune disease? *J Bone Joint Surg* **48B**: 312–19.

Chow SP, Luk KDK, Kung TM (1984) Dupuytren's contracture in Chinese. *J R Coll Surg Edin* **29**: 49–51.

Couch H (1938) Identical Dupuytren's contracture in identical twins. *Can Med Assoc J* **39**: 225.

Demers R, Blais JA (1960) Le caractère familial et héréditaire de la contracture de Dupuytren. *Union Med Can* **89**: 1238–49.

Dupuytren G (1831) De la rétraction des doigts par suite d'une affection de l'aponévrose palmaire. *Journal Universel et Hebdomadaire de Médecine et de Chirurgie Pratique et des Institutions Médicales Paris* **25**: 349–65. (Reprinted in *Medical Classics 1939–1940*, Vol. 4. Royal Society of Medicine, London, 1940.)

Dupuytren G (1832) Rétraction permanente des doigts. In: Dupuytren G, *Leçons orales de clinique chirurgicale faites à l'Hôtel-Dieu de Paris*, 2–24. Germer Baillière, Paris.

Early PF (1962) Population studies in Dupuytren's contracture. *J Bone Joint Surg* **44B**: 602–13.

Egawa T, Senrui H, Horiki A, Egawa M (1990) Epidemiology of the oriental patient. In: McFarlane RM, McGrouther DA, Flint MH, eds, *Dupuytren's Disease*, 239–45. Churchill Livingstone, Edinburgh.

Elliot D (1988) The early history of contracture of the palmar fascia. Part 1. *J Hand Surg* **13B**: 246–53.

Furnas DW (1979) Dupuytren's contractures in a black patient in east Africa. *Plast Reconstr Surg* **64**: 250–51 (letter).

Goetzee AE, Williams HO (1954–55) A case of Dupuytren's contracture involving the hand and foot in a child. *Br J Surg* **42**: 417–20.

Gonzalez MH, Sobeski J, Grindel S et al. (1998) Dupuytren's disease in African-Americans. *J Hand Surg* **23B**: 306–307.

Goyrand G (1833) Nouvelles recherches sur la rétraction permanente des doigts. *Mem Acad R Med* **3**: 489.

Haeseker B (1981) Dupuytren's disease and the sickle-cell trait in a female black patient. *Br J Plast Surg* **34**: 438–40.

Hueston JT (1960) The incidence of Dupuytren's contracture. *Med J Aust* **2**: 999–1002.

Hueston JT (1962) Further studies on the incidence of Dupuytren's contracture. *Med J Aust* **1**: 586–88.

Hueston JT (1987) Dupuytren's contracture: medicolegal aspects. *Med J Aust* **147** (special supplement): 1–11.

Hueston JT (1988) Dupuytren's contracture. *Curr Orthop* **2**: 173–78.

Hueston JT, Seyfer AE (1991) Some medicolegal aspects of Dupuytren's contracture. *Hand Clin* **7**: 617–32.

Hutchinson J (1897) On the juvenile form of the Dupuytren's contraction. *Arch Surg* **8**: 20–21.

James JIP (1985) The genetic pattern of Dupuytren's disease and idiopathic epilepsy. In: Hueston JT, Tubiana R, eds, *Dupuytren's Disease*, 2nd edn, 94–99. Churchill Livingstone, Edinburgh.

James JIP, Tubiana R (1952) La maladie de Dupuytren. *Rev Chir Orthop* **38**: 352–406.

Kanavel AB, Koch SL, Mason ML (1929) Dupuytren's contraction. *Surg Gynecol Obstet* **48**: 145–90.

Leclercq C, Tubiana R (1986) Résultats à long terme des aponévrectomies pour maladie de Dupuytren. *Chirurgie* **112**: 195.

Lennox IA, Murali SR, Porter R (1993) A study of the repeatability of the diagnosis of Dupuytren's contracture and its prevalence in the Grampian region. *J Hand Surg* **18B**: 258–61.

Ling RSM (1963) The genetic factor in Dupuytren's disease. *J Bone Joint Surg* **45B**: 709–18.

Liu Y, Chen WY (1991) Dupuytren's disease among the Chinese in Taiwan. *J Hand Surg* **16A**: 779–86.

Lund M (1941) Dupuytren's contracture and epilepsy. *Acta Psychiatr Scand* **16**: 465–82.

Maes J (1979) Dupuytren's contracture in an oriental patient. *Plast Reconstr Surg* **64**: 251 (letter).

McFarlane RM (1985) Some observations on the epidemiology of Dupuytren's disease. In: Hueston JT, Tubiana R, eds, *Dupuytren's Disease*, 2nd edn, 122–28. Churchill Livingstone, London.

Mennen U (1986) Dupuytren's contracture in the Negro. *J Hand Surg* **11B**: 61–64.

Mennen U, Gräbe RP (1979) Dupuytren's contracture in a Negro. A case report. *J Hand Surg* **4**: 451–53.

Mikkelsen OA (1976) Dupuytren's disease – a study of the pattern of distribution and stage of contracture in the hand. *Hand* **8**: 265–71.

Mikkelsen OA (1990) Epidemiology of a Norwegian population. In: McFarlane RM, McGrouther DA, Flint MH, eds, *Dupuytren's Disease*, 191–200. Churchill Livingstone, Edinburgh.

Mitra A, Goldstein RY (1994) Dupuytren's contrac-

ture in the black population: a review. *Ann Plast Surg* **32**: 619–22.

Muguti GI, Appelt B (1993) Dupuytren's contracture in black Zimbabweans. *Centr Afr J Med* **39**: 129–32.

Murrell GAC, Hueston JT (1990) Aetiology of Dupuytren's contracture. *Aust N Z J Surg* **60**: 247–52.

Pickren JW, Smith AG, Stevenson TW, Stout AP (1951) Fibromatosis of the plantar fascia. *Cancer* **4**: 846–56.

Plasse JS (1979) Dupuytren's contractures in a black patient. *Plast Reconstr Surg* **64**: 250 (letter).

Quintana Guitian A (1988) Epidemiological features of Dupuytren's disease. *Ann Chir Main* **7**: 256–62 (in French).

Rao GS, Luthra PK (1988) Dupuytren's disease of the foot in children: a report of three cases. *Br J Plast Surg* **41**: 313–15.

Rosenfeld N, Mavor E, Wise L (1983) Dupuytren's contracture in a black female child. *Hand* **15**: 82–84.

Saez Aldana F, Gonzales del Pino J, Delgado A, Lovic A (1996) Epidemologia de la enfermedad de Dupuytren: analisis de 314 casos. *Rev Ortop Traum* **40**: 15–21.

Simons AW, Srivastava S, Nancarrow JD (1996) Dupuytren's disease affecting the wrist. *J Hand Surg* **21B**: 367–68.

Skoog T (1948) Dupuytren's contraction with special reference to aetiology and improved surgical treatment. Its occurrence in epileptics – Note on knuckle pads. *Acta Chir Scand* **96** (suppl 139): 1.

Sladicka SJ, Benfanti P, Raab M, Becton J (1996) Dupuytren's contracture in the black population: a case report and review of the literature. *J Hand Surg* **21A**: 898–99.

Srivastava S, Nancarrow JD, Cort DF (1989) Dupuytren's disease in patients from the Indian sub-continent. Report of ten cases. *J Hand Surg* **14B**: 32–34.

Tonkin MA, Burke FD, Varian JP (1984) Dupuytren's contracture: a comparative study of fasciectomy in one hundred patients. *J Hand Surg* **9B**: 156–62.

Urban M, Feldberg L, Janssen A, Elliot D (1996) Dupuytren's disease in children. *J Hand Surg* **21B**: 112–16.

Wallace AF (1965) Dupuytren's contracture in women. *Br J Plast Surg* **13**: 385–86.

Whaley DC, Elliot D (1993) Dupuytren's disease: a legacy to the North? *J Hand Surg* **18B**: 363–67.

Yost J, Winters T, Fett HC (1955) Dupuytren's contracture. A statistical study. *Am J Surg* **90**: 568–71.

Zaworski RE, Mann RJ (1979) Dupuytren's contractures in a black patient. *Plast Reconstr Surg* **63**: 122–24.

Zemel NP (1991) Dupuytren's contracture in women. *Hand Clin* **7**: 707–11.

Zemel NP, Balcomb TV, Skark HH et al. (1987) Dupuytren's disease in women: evaluation of long-term results after operation. *J Hand Surg* **12A**: 1012–16.

4

Histopathology and cell biology

Lawrence C Hurst and Marie A Badalamente

HISTORY OF THE SCIENCE OF DUPUYTREN'S DISEASE

The landmarks in the science of Dupuytren's disease are many and varied. Surprisingly, it was not until the 1970s that the definitive report was published by Gabbiani and Majno on the specialized fibroblast, termed a myofibroblast, which they believed was important to the pathogenesis of the disorder. They postulated that the contraction of the palmar fascia and overlying skin and fingers was directly related to the contractile abilities of myofibroblasts. Many investigators have since substantiated this finding including Tomasek et al. in 1986, identifying the presence of nonmuscle myosin, actin, and fibronectin. Tomasek et al., in 1987, produced another landmark study, which defined the cellular basis of contracture of the palmar fascia in Dupuytren's disease. Their work suggested that the transmission of intracellular force from myofibroblasts to each other and the surrounding tissue was due to close association with intracellular bundles of actin microfilaments resulting in specialized transmembranous associations. Bundles of the filamentous extracellular material were found to extend from the surface of the myofibroblast, connecting it with the surrounding matrix and, also, with adjacent myofibroblasts. This group went on further to identify that the chemical nature of the filamentous material was fibronectin and coined the term 'anchoring strands'.

Brickley-Parsons et al., in the early 1980s, provided us with great insight as to the nature of the collagen in Dupuytren's disease. Her group identified that Type III collagen was important to the pathogenesis of Dupuytren's disease in that it is proportionately increased in relation to Type I collagen within the affected palmar fascia (Brickley-Parsons et al., 1981). They also proposed that the active cellular process of contraction draws the distal extremities of the affected tissue closer together at the same time that the original tissue is being replaced. The result is a shorter, smaller piece of tissue fabric with collagen fibers and fibrils of normal length. Interest in how myofibroblasts are regulated led many investigators into studies on growth factors. Several growth factors, including platelet-derived growth factor (PDGF), transforming growth factor beta (TGF-β), and basic fibroblast growth factor (bFGF), have been implicated in the pathways involved, which allow myofibroblasts to proliferate in great numbers. TGF-β, especially, has received great attention, not only for its ability to induce proliferation of myofibroblasts but, also, to increase production of collagen. It has been proposed that myofibroblasts are quite sensitive to these growth factors owing to increased expression of growth factor receptors. Thus, the cells may proliferate and produce abundant amounts of collagen without normal regulatory controls. As our understanding of this mechanism increases, it may be possible to interfere with either the production of the growth factors themselves or a blockade of cellular receptors as clinical interventions in the treatment of Dupuytren's disease.

At present, a non-operative medical injection therapy for Dupuytren's disease, using Clostridial collagenase injection, is currently in clinical trials for safety and efficacy. The injection of collagenase induces a wide area of lysis in the collagen cord allowing rupture and thus extension of the injected finger. Early results of this clinical trial indicate an approximately 94% success rate in both MP and PIP joints. The injection therapy has proven extremely safe in that the adverse effects it induces are minimal and very local. The injection therapy also does not seem to be of concern with regard to potential immune adverse effects. Patient satisfaction is high using this injection therapy as, obviously, patients are able to avoid sometimes major hand surgery with resultant postoperative rehabilitation, which can also be trying and painful. It remains to be seen whether the results of collagenase injection therapy for Dupuytren's disease will stand the test of time, since long-term follow-up is ongoing and potential recurrence is under study.

HISTOPATHOLOGY OF DUPUYTREN'S DISEASE

The histopathology of Dupuytren's disease was correctly described in 1941 by Meyerding et al. They suggested that the disorder not only affected the palmar fascia but also involved fibromatosis, which extended to the subcutaneous tissues and to the dermis. Meyerding observed that 'the characteristic change is a

proliferation of fibroblasts in nodules of the contracture'. He also correctly observed that the cell density could be variable in tissue in Dupuytren's disease. Thus, Meyerding was the first to suggest that the histopathological changes in Dupuytren's disease with regard to the cellularity of the nodules related to the activity of the disease. Meyerding also suggested a grade scale from 1 to 4 to indicate the activity of the cellular process. He also gave a very accurate account of the histopathological changes of adjacent subcutaneous tissue and overlying skin, which was more accurate than all previous reports. He noted that in long-standing cases of Dupuytren's disease, 'evidence of subcutaneous adipose tissue is not revealed and sweat glands are rare or completely absent...' He attributed this to an increase in the size and number of connective tissue bands, which are normally separated by adipose tissue. He also noted that there were increased numbers of capillaries in the connective tissue and that the capillaries were associated with and infiltrated by lymphocytes.

It was not until 1959 that Luck developed a histopathological classification of Dupuytren's disease into three stages (Luck, 1959). This classification is still in use today. Luck's three stages are known as the proliferative, involutional and residual disease stages. In the proliferative disease stage, Luck noted that the tissue is essentially composed of fibrous nodules that are a focus of proliferating fibroblasts in which he stated: '... in this focal fibroplasia, the fibroblasts do not align themselves with lines of stress and have, in fact, no purposeful arrangement.' The second disease stage, termed involutional disease stage, is characterized by fibroblasts aligning themselves with the major lines of stress that go through the nodules. In the residual disease tissue, essentially composed of fibrous cord tissue material, Luck suggested that the fibrous cords were in response to reactive functional hypertrophy to the repeated tension stresses on the hand of fascia from which the nodule took its origin. With complete involution, Luck wrote,

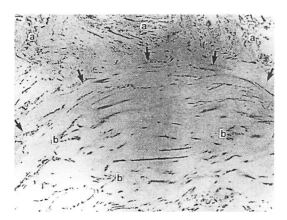

Figure 4.1 A Dupuytren's nodule during the proliferative stage of the disease. The section was reacted with antibodies against factor VIII in order to demonstrate the endothelial cells of the capillaries (factor VIII antibodies peroxidase stain; × 10 original). (a) Normal vessels in surrounding subcutaneous tissue; (b) arborescent network of vessels in Dupuytren's disease. Arrows: nodular boundary of Dupuytren's nodule. (Reproduced with permission from McFarlane et al., 1990.)

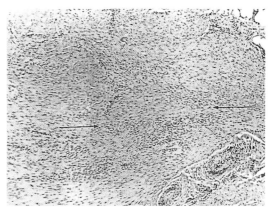

Figure 4.2 Reactive tissue during the involutional stage of Dupuytren's disease. The nodular configuration of the proliferative lesion is lost. (Hematoxylin and eosin; × 25 original). Arrows: alignment of fibroblasts along lines of stress with loss of the nodular configuration of initial lesion. (Reproduced with permission from McFarlane et al., 1990.)

'... the nodule disappears leaving only a focus of dense adhesions and the reactive proximal fibrous cord, which is almost acellular and tendon like' (Figures 4.1–4.3).

It was not until 1972 that Gabbiani and Majno reported on a specialized or adapted type of fibroblast, which they termed a myofibroblast, which, they believed, was important to the pathogenesis of Dupuytren's disease and the contraction of the palmar fascia and the overlying skin and fingers (Gabbiani and Majno, 1972). In their study, electron microscopy was used to describe the ultrastructural features of this new cell type. They reported that myofibroblasts had distinctive ultrastructural characteristics. First, there was a system of intercellular myofibrils with associated dense areas very similar to the so-called dense bodies of smooth muscle cells. Secondly, they noted that the nuclei of myofibroblasts had indentations and folds which they thought might be because of the contractile ability of the myofibroblasts. Lastly, these authors described some

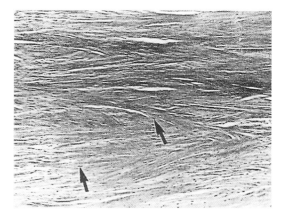

Figure 4.3 Dense fibrous cord of residual stage. (Hematoxylin and eosin; × 25 original). Arrows: spindle-shaped nuclei of fibrocytes in between dense collagenous fibres. (Reproduced with permission from McFarlane et al., 1990.)

surface features of the myofibroblasts, which they noted were composed of basement membrane and hemidesmosomal structures. The important point of Gabbiani and Majno's work was that myofibroblasts had all the component intracellular features, such as the bundles of intercellular fibrils, and the cell surface characteristics for transmission of contractile forces. In 1975, a study was published on the significance of histopathological findings in Dupuytren's contracture (Tyrkko and Viljanto, 1975). In this study, clinical and histopathological data were compared in a series of 59 patients with Dupuytren's disease in order to clarify whether histopathological findings were in accordance with the clinical development of the disease. They concluded that the most valuable prognostic signs seem to be the appearance of several active nodules, indicating a rapid development of the disease with a high frequency of postoperative recurrence in these patients. They noted that lack of active nodules did not exclude the possibility of recurrence but made it less likely. They also noted other occasional findings that are typical of Dupuytren's disease, such as the number of mitoses, microhemorrhages and perivascular lymphocytic infiltrations, but these seemed to be of minor prognostic value.

In 1978, Chiu and McFarlane also reported on a correlative clinical–pathological study. These authors examined tissue from 38 patients with Dupuytren's disease using light and electron microscopy. The clinical and pathological data were correlated so that three stages of disease were recognized, that is, early, active and advanced. The cell of the early disease was the perivascular fibroblast and the myofibroblast was the cell of the active disease. Since the myofibroblasts have cell–cell and cell–stroma attachments, the authors concluded that collagen not only becomes oriented as it is formed but also is subjected to a contractile force. Gelberman et al. (1980) also reported on the electron microscopic, biochemical and clinical aspects in a correlative study. In their work, specimens of fascia were obtained from 24 patients with Dupuytren's disease. The clinical course and response to operative treatment were then correlated with the tissue findings. Ultrastructural analysis revealed myofibroblasts in the nodules of seven of the 24 patients. Fibroblasts containing prominent microtubules were found in 10 patients. The authors noted that the fascia contained type III collagen, increased amounts of collagen per unit dry weight and an increase in reducible cross-links of collagen. While nodules were noted to contain a greater increase in reducible cross-links than the cords, there was little variation of the biochemical findings from patient to patient. These authors concluded that clinical recurrence was not related to the age of the patient at onset, duration or severity of disease. They suggested, however, that recurrence was related to the electron microscopic findings of myofibroblasts in the nodules and fibroblasts containing prominent microtubules in the fascia of these patients. Also, in 1980, other workers (Salamon and Hamori, 1980a,b) published research on the possible role of myofibroblasts in the pathogenesis of Dupuytren's disease. These authors also confirmed that the myofibroblasts have abnormal foldings of the nucleus; microfilaments resembling the myofilaments of smooth muscle cells; rough endoplasmic reticulum; free ribosomes; a well-developed Golgi apparatus; numerous mitochondria and occasional lipid droplets; as well as cilia-like formations; hemidesmosomes and desmosomes; and formation of basement membrane. They suggested that, according to data in the literature, the myofibroblast may contain actin and have contractile properties.

In the early 1980s the relationship of the skin to nodules and cords in Dupuytren's disease was investigated (Vandeberg et al., 1982). These authors noted that the interface of skin and nodule or cord had four distinct anatomic zones in the skin/nodule specimens and three zones in the skin/cord specimens. Skin/nodule specimens had a horizontally layered dense band just underneath the dermis, which was a feature not found in the skin/cord specimens. They performed ultra-

---

Table 4.1 Histologic features of Dupuytren's disease lesions by disease stage. (Adapted with permission from McFarlane et al., 1990.)

Features of early lesions (proliferative disease stage)
1) Focal increase in vascularity with growth of capillaries and proliferation of endothelial cells.
2) Proliferation of perivascular cells, many of which are desmin-positive and probably akin to perivascular smooth muscle cells.
3) Formation of angiocentric, nodular lesion by centrifugal spread of proliferating cells.
4) Extravasation of red cells focally from the newly formed capillaries.
5) Production of reticulum but not elastic fibers.

Features of intermediate lesions (involutional disease stage)
1) Proliferating cells are undergoing metamorphosis from cells with round nuclei and scanty cytoplasm to spindle-shaped cells with indented, elongated nuclei and moderate amount of cytoplasm. These are the morphological features of myofibroblasts.
2) Lesions become less cellular with increasing stromal collagen.
3) Alignment of cells along lines of stress.
4) Fibrous infiltration of adjacent skin and subcutaneous tissue.
5) Focal deposition of hemosiderin pigment as a result of degeneration of extravasated red cells.
6) Lymphocytic infiltration.

Features of late lesions (residual disease stage)
1) Relatively acellular cords of densely packed and aligned collagen fibers.
2) Cells appear as typical fibrocytes with hyperchromatic, wavy and spindle-shaped nuclei between dense collagen bundles.
3) Few cells are positive for desmin-type intermediate filaments.

---

structural studies, which showed that the active contractile myofibroblasts in the lower two zones in the skin/nodule had clusters of active and degenerating cells side by side. They noted that there were no myofibroblasts in either the skin/cord samples or in any skin sample. They concluded that skin overlying both nodule and cord appears to be drawn passively by underlying contractile forces and they suggested that a local defect in palmar skin may prevent normal inhibition of myofibroblast contraction and more aggressive resection of fascia and dermis may be indicated in skin/nodule areas. The skin cell known as a dermal dendrocyte has also been implicated in the pathogenesis of Dupuytren's disease (Sugden et al., 1993). The dermal dendrocyte is a factor XIIIa-positive cell. Many factor XIIIa-positive cells were shown by Sugden's group in affected as well as surrounding Dupuytren's tissue.

In 1984, Kischer and Speer were the first to report on microvascular changes in Dupuytren's disease. These authors hypothesized that lower oxygen tension was considered to be a stimulus to excessive collagen production in scar tissue. Since the characteristics are similar to Dupuytren's disease, it appeared to be a good model with which to confirm the presence of occluded microvessels. Therefore, these authors examined six cases of Dupuytren's disease by light, electron and polarization microscopy. Most of the microvessels from the precontracture band area throughout the periphery of the body of the nodules were occluded by bulging endothelial cells into the lumen of the vessel. The microvessels were surrounded by extensive reduplicated layers of basement membrane. On the basis of many of these studies, Shum published a summary of histopathological changes in Dupuytren's disease based upon disease stage as shown in Table 4.1.

CELL BIOLOGY OF DUPUYTREN'S DISEASE

In the mid-1980s, two reports stand out as superior descriptions of the myofibroblast, its cytoskeleton and extracellular matrix. In 1986, Tomasek et al. published a paper entitled 'The cytoskeleton and extracellular matrix of the

Dupuytren's disease 'myofibroblast': an immunofluorescence study of a non-muscle cell type'. These authors examined the diseased palmar fascia using indirect immunofluorescence. Primary antibodies that were used as probes in this study were directed against:

1) Smooth muscle myosin;
2) Non-muscle myosin – components of the cytoplasmic contractile apparatus in smooth muscle and non-muscle cells;
3) Laminin; and
4) Fibronectin – extracellular glycoproteins mediating cell matrix attachment in smooth muscle and non-muscle fibroblastic cells, respectively.

The Dupuytren's nodular cells stained for non-muscle myosin and fibronectin but not for smooth muscle myosin or laminin. This indicated that, at the level of differentiation, these cells are a *non-muscle* type. Staining for fibronectin between cells was dramatically increased over that seen between fibroblasts in control normal palmar fascia. In a landmark study in 1987, Tomasek et al. defined the cellular basis of contracture of the palmar fascia in patients with Dupuytren's disease. As had been well established in several previous studies, the myofibroblast was capable of generation of intracellular force. However, the transmission of this force to the surrounding tissue of the extracellular matrix remained unexplained. Since their prior studies demonstrated that the cytoskeleton of myofibroblast contained non-muscle myosin, not smooth muscle myosin, it suggested that non-muscle contractile systems were important. In addition, their prior studies identified the extracellular glycoprotein, fibronectin, not the basal lamina-specific glycoprotein, laminin, at the surface of myofibroblasts, suggesting that the transmission of intracellular force to the surrounding tissue may also occur by a non-muscle mechanism. To determine the mechanism by which the intracellular force might be transmitted to the surrounding tissues, these authors exam-

ined the ultrastructure of the connection of the cytoskeleton of the myofibroblast to the surrounding extracellular matrix. Using ultrastructural means, an extracellular filamentous material was identified at the surface of the myofibroblast. These extracellular fibrils were found to be in close association with intracellular bundles of actin microfilaments, resulting in specialized transmembranous associations at the surface of the myofibroblast. Bundles of the filamentous extracellular material were found to extend from the surface of the myofibroblast connecting it with the surrounding matrix and also with adjacent myofibroblasts. This group further went on to identify the biochemical nature of the filamentous material as fibronectin and coined the term 'anchoring strands'. Thus, on the basis of this pioneering work, it was apparent that myofibroblasts could indeed generate contractile force, not only between the cells themselves, but also between the cells and the extracellular matrix in inducing contracture of the palmar fascia. Shum and McFarlane (1988) and Shum (1990) also suggested a theory on the histogenesis of Dupuytren's disease myofibroblasts. These authors examined 37 specimens from the hands of 30 patients using light microscopy after histochemical staining for the presence of desmin-intermediate filaments. Their results indicated that desmin-positive cells were present in the proliferative Dupuytren's nodules and that the number of desmin-positive cells decreased significantly in the fibrous phase of the disease. Also, on the basis of the pattern of distribution of the desmin-positive cells around vessels, these authors postulated that desmin-positive cells in Dupuytren's nodules were migrating perivascular smooth muscle cells from the vessel wall. The exact fate of these cells was uncertain according to the authors' conclusion but they hypothesized that these displaced perivascular smooth muscle cells were capable of transforming into collagen-producing, desmin-negative myofibroblasts that formed the cellular basis of Dupuytren's lesions. Tomasek and

Haaksma (1991) went on to further define the close transmembrane association between fibronectin filaments and actin microfilaments of the myofibroblast. In this study, the authors used immunoelectron microscopy to demonstrate that the extracellular filaments that participate in this close transmembrane association contained fibronectin. The authors coined the term 'fibronexus', describing it as a dominant adhesive structure at the surface of the myofibroblasts in Dupuytren's disease. Thus, the fibronexus, by mediating cell–cell and cell–matrix attachments, may serve to transmit contractile forces generated by actin microfilaments in these cells throughout the diseased tissue. Tomasek and Rayan (1995) went on to further correlate the expression of alpha smooth muscle actin with contraction in myofibroblasts. The authors studied 11 nodules from patients with Dupuytren's disease to determine whether alpha smooth muscle actin expression in myofibroblasts was related to the generation of contractile force. Tissue was placed into explant culture and cell strains were obtained. The mean percentage of cultured Dupuytren's myofibroblast expressing alpha smooth muscle actin, as determined by immunofluorescence, was 14 ± 8 and ranged from 1–26%. The ability of myofibroblasts to generate contractile force was determined by using a collagen lattice contraction assay. The authors observed a significant positive correlation between the expression of alpha smooth muscle actin and degeneration of contractile force in the cell strains. In addition, six cell strains from palmar fascia of individuals undergoing carpal tunnel release as controls, were examined. In the six strains of palmar fibroblasts the mean percentage of cells expressing alpha smooth muscle actin was 5 ± 3 and ranged from 1–9%. The authors found that six Dupuytren's cell strains in which more than 15% of the cells expressed alpha smooth muscle actin were significantly more contractile than that of palmar fibroblasts. The authors suggested that Dupuytren's myofibroblasts can acquire smooth muscle charac-

teristics and that the acquisition of a smooth-muscle-like phenotype correlates with increased contractility of the myofibroblasts. The results of this study were in agreement with a prior work indicating that the myofibrils within myofibroblasts contained a pH-dependent adenosine-triphosphase (ATPase) capable of inducing cellular contraction (Badalamente and Hurst, 1983).

Magro et al. (1995a) were among the first to describe the expression of an integrin, as well as fibronectin, as important to the contractile process occurring in Dupuytren's disease. These authors examined the expression of alpha 5 beta 1 integrin and its extracellular ligand fibronectin in 23 cases of Dupuytren's disease using immunohistochemistry and light microscopic methods. These authors staged the disease, on histological appearance, into proliferative, involutional and residual stages. Alpha 5 beta 1 integrin was detected in the highly cellular areas of both the proliferative and involutional stages where fibronectin was simultaneously expressed in the extracellular matrix. Alpha 5 beta 1 integrin and fibronectin disappeared from the hypocellular areas of the involutional phase undergoing fibrotic transformation and also from fibrotic connective tissue of the residual phase. These findings indicated that the expression pattern of alpha 5 beta 1 integrin correlates with the presence of the extracellular matrix of the corresponding ligand fibronectin during the different phases of Dupuytren's disease. The authors suggested that, for alpha 5 beta 1 integrin, linking fibronectin to stromal cells of both the proliferative and involutional disease stages may be involved in the contractile processes of Dupuytren's disease.

Several authors have published reports regarding the influence of both endogenous and exogenous chemical regulation of myofibroblast contraction in Dupuytren's disease. Badalamente and Hurst and colleagues performed both an in vitro study and an examination of Dupuytren's disease tissue with special emphasis on the vasoactive prostaglandins,

$PGE_2\alpha$ and $PGF_2\alpha$ (Hurst et al., 1986; Badalamente et al., 1988). $PGF_2\alpha$ in vitro was shown to have significant contractile influence on cultured myofibroblasts, whereas $PGE_2\alpha$ had significant relaxation properties in vitro. Using ultrastructural immunocytochemical techniques with antibodies specific for these prostaglandins, these authors confirmed their association with myofibroblasts of Dupuytren's disease. Further, radioimmunoassay was used to quantify prostaglandin levels. Radio-immunoassay of prostaglandins in plasma of patients with Dupuytren's disease revealed mean increases of 23% of $PGE_2\alpha$ and 16% of $PGF_2\alpha$ when compared with controls. In nodules, radioimmunoassay showed a mean increase of 40% in $PGE_2\alpha$ and 55% in $PGF_2\alpha$ in patients with Dupuytren's disease when compared with control fascia. The specific prostaglandins shown in this study are well known to influence smooth muscle, especially vascular contractility. These authors concluded that prostaglandins may exert similar contractile responses on myofibroblasts in Dupuytren's disease to contribute to collagen deformation and ultimately to the joint contracture. The significant increase in $PGF_2\alpha$ in Dupuytren's nodules would appear to indicate that this substance may be locally available. Its availability may derive from the microcirculation, since nodules are known to be highly vascular. Presumably, prostaglandin E_2 may be available from the same source within nodules.

Rayan et al. (1996) went on to define further the pharmacologic regulation of Dupuytren's myofibroblast contraction in vitro. These authors evaluated pharmacologic agents for their availability to promote or inhibit contraction of myofibroblasts in vitro using a collagen lattice contraction assay. In the first part of their study, lysophosphatidic acid (LPA), serotonin, angiotensin II and $PGF_2\alpha$ were tested for their ability to promote myofibroblast contraction. LPA was found to significantly promote cell contraction when compared with controls. This response to LPA was dose dependent, with half maximal response at a concentration of 0.07 µmol. Angiotensin II, serotonin and $PGF_2\alpha$ at 1 mmol concentration also induced a significant amount of contraction as compared with controls. However, the amount of contraction was at least six times less than that observed for LPA. In the second part of the study, prostaglandin E_1 and E_2 or the calcium-channel blockers nifedipine and verapamil were tested for their ability to inhibit LPA-promoted contraction. It was found that both types of inhibitors partially blocked LPA-promoted contraction of myofibroblasts. The effect of the various pharmacologic agents on normal palmar fibroblasts was not evaluated in this study. Thus, this study showed that LPA was a potent agonist of myofibroblast contraction and this contraction can be inhibited by specific pharmacologic agents. These authors went on to suggest that this study provided a rational basis for investigating the further clinical use of the calcium-channel blockers nifedipine or verapamil and PGE_1 and PGE_2 to control Dupuytren's disease and possibly other fibrotic conditions.

GROWTH FACTORS

In recent years, there has been great interest in a variety of growth factors that may enhance proliferation of myofibroblasts or affect collagen synthesis and thus be important in the pathobiology of Dupuytren's disease. In the early 1990s, Badalamente et al. (1992) investigated whether platelet-derived growth factor (PDGF) was identifiable in association with myofibroblasts in Dupuytren's disease. In this study, samples of palmar fascia were obtained at surgical release from 28 patients who had had partial fasciectomy. Control fascia was obtained from 18 patients who had undergone hand surgery for other reasons such as carpal tunnel release. This study used light microscopic methods to histologically stage each patient's sample. Next, both light and electron microscopic immunocytochemistry for PDGF was utilized. The results of this study showed that PDGF was associated with myofibroblasts in the hypercellular, proliferative and involutional stages of Dupuytren's disease. The results suggested that PDGF is bound to a cell membrane surface receptor on myofibroblasts. It is known that PDGF may induce a wide variety of cellular responses. These reactions include an increase in the rate of protein synthesis, including type III collagen synthesis. Platelet-derived growth factor can promote reorganization of cytoskeletal actin filaments, which is characteristic of myofibroblasts. This growth factor also stimulates increased synthesis in release of arachidonic acid. By a complex cascade, arachidonic acid may be converted to prostaglandin. It was shown in previous studies (Hurst et al., 1986; Badalamente et al., 1988) that levels of both PGE_2 and $PGF\alpha$ are increased in affected palmar fascia of Dupuytren's disease. Platelet-derived growth factor is a polypeptide carried in the alpha granules of human platelets, and Dupuytren's nodules are known to be highly vascular. Finally, it was noted that PDGF is known as a competence factor and is known to act in synergistic association with other growth factors to cause cell proliferation by progression into the S phase of DNA synthesis from a state of G_0/G_1 growth arrest. Other investigators have also demonstrated that the beta chain PDF gene is expressed in Dupuytren's disease tissue but not in normal fascia (Terek et al., 1995).

In 1994, Alioto et al. performed an in vitro cell study of both normal palmar fascia fibroblasts and Dupuytren's myofibroblasts and examined a variety of growth factors. The cells were exposed separately to basic fibroblast growth factor (bFGF), transforming growth factor beta (TGF-β) and PDGF. Thereafter, the effects of these growth factors on the proliferation rate and collagen production were assayed. This study found that bFGF and PDGF were mitogenic for both the cells of the normal palmar fascia and Dupuytren's myofibroblasts. It was found that TGFβ was a very potent stimula-

tor of collagen production for both cell types. This study also concluded that the Dupuytren's cells were more metabolically active and more sensitive to the growth factors tested. In another report, Dupuytren's lesions and samples of normal palmar fascia were examined for the presence of the angiogenic protein bFGF. This study reported that all the cells of the lesion contained this growth factor, that is endothelial cells, fibroblasts and myofibroblasts (Gonzalez et al., 1992). In situ hybridization using an antisense probe for human bFGF and its receptor mRNA showed a major difference between normal palmar fascia and Dupuytren's disease tissues; that is, the levels of the factor were significantly higher than in the normal palmar fascia. Thus, the cells in Dupuytren's tissue, since they express both bFGF and its receptor, may function in a potential autocrine-paracrine role in the pathogenesis of the disorder. This study was purported to be the first description of a nontumoral proliferative disease that was directly associated with an increased level of bFGF mRNA. Baird's group confirmed the results of this study, as well as identifying other growth factors that may be important to the pathogenesis of Dupuytren's disease (Baird et al., 1993). In Baird's study, tissue samples from 12 patients with Dupuytren's disease and 12 controls were investigated using reverse transcription/polymerase chain reaction (RT-PCR). These authors reported that the tissues from patients with Dupuytren's disease expressed a higher percentage of cytokine peptide regulatory factors than those of controls. This study went on to further identify the cytokine factors as interleukin-1α, interleukin-1β, TGF-β and bFGF. This study also identified that PDGFs of both the alpha and beta type were also expressed in Dupuytren's disease tissue in comparison with the controls but that the differences were not significant.

TGF-β, especially, has received the attention of several investigators with regard to its importance in the pathogenesis of Dupuytren's disease. In a study published by Badalamente et al. (1996), two isoforms of $TGF-\beta_1$ and $TGF-\beta_2$

were investigated with regard to their intra- and/or extracellular sites of localization within the specific disease stages of Dupuytren's disease. In addition, the effect of TGF-β on myofibroblast proliferation was studied using explant cultures from Dupuytren's nodules in the proliferative or involutional disease stages. This study found that, regardless of the disease stage, TGF-β_1 showed a non-specific but intense intracellular marking pattern associated with fibroblasts, myofibroblasts and capillary endothelial cells in all the Dupuytren's disease samples studied. In the control samples, TGF-β_1 also showed a non-specific but intense intracellular marking pattern associated with fibroblasts and capillary endothelial cells. TGF-β_2 showed an intense intracellular localization within the myofibroblasts of the proliferative stage and the involutional disease stage. Capillary endothelial cells in all Dupuytren's and control samples were also intensely marked for TGF-β_2. Fibroblasts from the samples of the patients in the residual disease stage and in all control palmar fascia samples did not show TGF-β_2 immunocytochemical localization. This study also investigated the in vitro effects of exogenous TGF-β_1 and TGF-β_2 addition to explant cultures at various plating densities. The rationale for using low and high plating densities in this study was to simulate the proliferative disease stage (low-density) and the involutional disease stage (high-density). Results of cell culture indicated that, compared with control samples of myofibroblasts, the addition of TGF-β_1, TGF-β_2 and TGF-β_1 plus β_2 had significant effects on myofibroblast proliferation, especially at higher plating densities. However, TGF-β_2 had the most significant proliferative effect. This suggested that TGF-β_2 may be important in cell proliferation within the involutional disease stage where the cell density is known to be high. Kloen et al. (1995) have also identified that there are three types of TGF-β receptors in Dupuytren's disease tissue. His group showed in vitro that TGF-β_1 stimulated DNA synthesis and cellular proliferation significantly. TGF-β_1 in synergistic association with epidermal growth factor also stimulated DNA synthesis in cell proliferation in this investigation.

A possible model for the pathogenesis of Dupuytren's disease based on prior works of several authors and relating to the contribution of growth factors was put forward by Alioto et al. (1994). (Figure 4.4). The model proposed that the palmar fascia is exposed to repeated microhemorrhages due to ischemic vascular disease, liver pathology, trauma or other undetermined cause. Based on a genetic predisposition, normal palmar fascia fibroblasts may respond abnormally to the release of platelets and inflammatory cells. Cells in the normal palmar fascia are then exposed to certain growth factors such as PDGF and TGF-β, both of which are known to be released in high quantities from this cell type. PDGF may stimulate fibroblast proliferation, and exposure to TGFβ may initiate the production of collagen synthesis and other non-collagenous proteins. In addition, proteolytic enzymes, including collagenase and heparinase, may be released from inflammatory cells, endothelial cells and the extracellular matrix. This, in turn, may result in the release of bound bFGF from the extracellular matrix and bFGF may stimulate additional fibroblast proliferation, as well as angiogenesis. In the normal physiologic response, for example to injury, when the amount of bFGF reaches its critical threshold, a negative feedback loop may occur on endothelial cells. Fibroblast proliferation is halted while healing is completed through additional collagen synthesis. In the case of patients who develop Dupuytren's disease, however, the genetically altered fibroblasts are more sensitive to both bFGF and TGF-β owing to increased expression of their growth factor receptors. Thus, the fibroblasts may proliferate and produce abundant amounts of collagen without the normal regulatory controls. Endothelial cells may also remain activated and become unresponsive to normal feedback mechanisms and may continue signaling fibroblast proliferation. As this cell proliferation continues unabated, the thickened fascia

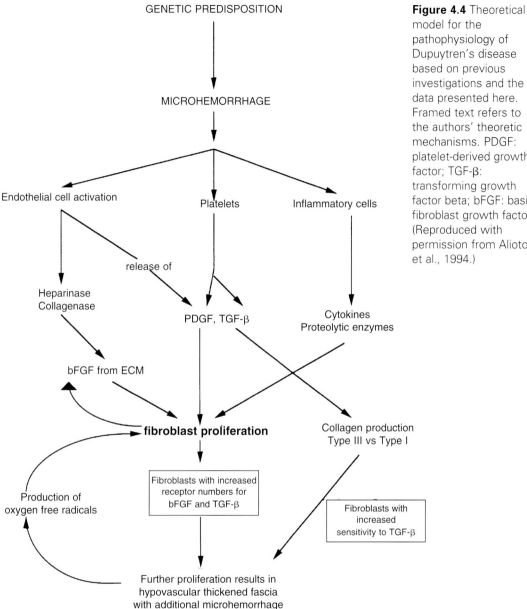

Figure 4.4 Theoretical model for the pathophysiology of Dupuytren's disease based on previous investigations and the data presented here. Framed text refers to the authors' theoretic mechanisms. PDGF: platelet-derived growth factor; TGF-β: transforming growth factor beta; bFGF: basic fibroblast growth factor. (Reproduced with permission from Alioto et al., 1994.)

eventually becomes less vascular and more prone to hypoxia and microhemorrhages. Additionally, the production of oxygen free radicals (Murrell, 1991) may further stimulate proliferation of abnormal fibroblasts. The cycle continues with the final result being a contracture of the palmar fascia with increased collagen synthesis and production into the well known cord of Dupuytren's disease.

COLLAGEN

As is well known, the excess deposition and proliferation of fibrous collagen is the major biochemical defect characteristic of Dupuytren's disease in inducing contracture of the fingers.

Collagen is a protein that has a triple helix of three peptide chains (alpha chains), the amino acid sequence of which is the repeating tripeptide gly-X-Y where X is often proline and Y is often hydroxyproline. The position of the amino acid glycine at every third residue is a prerequisite for the helical formation because glycine is the only amino acid small enough to fit into the interior of the helix. The larger amino acids, proline and hydroxyproline, are located on the exterior of the helix. The triple helix is stabilized by hydrogen bonds involving hydroxyl groups of hydroxyproline.

The different types of collagen have been assigned roman numerals and they differ in their amino acid sequence, in the length of their alpha chains, and in the presence or absence of globular domains in the molecule. Collagens Type I, II and III are the major fibrous collagens. Type I collagen is, by far, the most abundant type of collagen. It consists of two alpha 1 chains that are identical and an alpha 2 chain. Type I collagen is the most abundant structural type in skin, tendon and bone.

Type II collagen is contained in articular cartilage and nucleus pulposis. This collagen is composed of three identical alpha chains and these chains have relatively high contents of hydroxylysine and carbohydrate. The carbohydrate consists of a galactose residue or a glucose galactose disaccharide attached to the hydroxyl group of hydroxylysine.

Type III collagen usually exists with Type I with the exception of bone where Type III is absent. Type III collagen is present in increased amounts in tissues such as the intestines, larger blood vessels and the uterine wall. Type III collagen is composed of three identical chains and it differs from Type I and II collagen in having a pro-collagen extension peptide with disulfide bonds when it is deposited in the extracellular matrix spaces. Type III collagen usually gives rise to very thin fibrils in relation to Types I and II collagen.

Other collagen types include the non-fibrous collagen, such as Type IV collagen, which is associated with the basal lamina of such cells as epithelial and endothelial cells. The Type IV collagen molecule has a longer triple helix than do Types I–III and the terminal globular regions are retained. The filamentous collagens such as Type VI and IX usually form aggregates of microfibrils rather than a tightly packed striated fiber. Type IX collagen is usually distributed with Type II in the extracellular spaces of articular cartilage. Type VI collagen has been identified in several tissue types, such as cornea skin and tendon. The Type VI molecule is small. Many other collagen types have been identified and 13 collagen types have been reported on.

The biosynthesis of collagen follows the same mechanism of mRNA and ribosomes as other proteins. A noteworthy feature of the gene's coding for the alpha chains of Type I collagen is their very large size. Each gene is about 10 times the size of the functional small mRNA. The gene encoding for the alpha 2 (I chains) of Type I collagen has 40 kilobases and contains 52 exons or coding regions that are separated from each other by large introns (intervening sequences that range in size from 80–2000 kilobases). The RNAs are spliced after transcription to generate the specific mRNAs for each chain. These mRNA chains are translocated to the cytoplasm where translation occurs in the rough endoplasmic reticulum on membrane-bound ribosomes.

The alpha chains are synthesized in the form of large precursors called pro alpha chains, with extra procollagen extension peptides at both the N- and C-terminals. These chains then undergo an extensive array of post-translational modifications before they are formed into the fully mature collagen fibril in the extracellular matrix compartment. Certain enzymes are extremely important to this, such as prolyl and lylsylhydroxylase as they hydroxylate appropriate residues to hydroxyproline and hydroxylysine respectively. Ascorbic acid is also an extremely important co-factor for these enzymes. Glycosylation of specific hydroxylysine residues then occurs and interchain disulfide bond formation occurs at the C-terminal. Three pro alpha chains intertwine around one another to form the procollagen molecule within the cell. This is extruded into the extracellular matrix space where the N- and C-terminal peptidases cleave off the procollagen extension peptide. The collagen molecules thus generated can form and assemble by aligning themselves into a microfibril. It has been reported that changes in the synthesis of Type I and III collagens can be caused by both transcriptional and post-transcriptional mechanisms (Crombrugghe et al., 1990). It has been speculated that a number of protein factors, such as TGF-β, interact with sequences upstream of this transcription start in the alpha 1 (I), alpha 2 (I), and alpha 1 (III) collagen genes. It may be that similar or other factors bind to other regulatory sequences such as those in the first intron of the alpha 1(I), and alpha 1 (III) collagen genes.

Cross-linking

It is well established that the individual collagen molecules have little tensile strength. Therefore, covalent cross-links are quite essential for the formation of the mature collagen fibril. The start of the cross-linking process begins with the enzyme lysloxidase that oxidatively deaminates selective lysine residues on the collagen molecule, with the formation of an aldehyde. The aldehydes then react with free amino groups. The aldehyde generated reacts with neighboring amino groups on the triple helical portion of neighboring collagen molecule to form an N=C bond (Schiff base). The Schiff bases then undergo spontaneous chemical reactions to form temporary cross-links that are called reducible cross-links. The reducible cross-links will form chemically stable mature cross-links. Stable cross-links are composed of a ring

of five carbons and one nitrogen, called a pyridinium ring.

Collagen in Dupuytren's disease

The major collagen of the normal palmar fascia is Type I, although small amounts of Type III collagen have also been detected. In the late 1970s and early 1980s it became apparent that there was a change in collagen type associated with affected palmar fascia in Dupuytren's disease. Numerous investigators have all confirmed that there is an increase in the ratio of Type III to Type I collagen (Bailey et al., 1977; Menzel et al., 1979; Bazin et al., 1980; Gelberman et al., 1980). It has been reported that there was an increase of 1–2% Type III collagen in the apparently uninvolved palmar fascia of Dupuytren's patients, while there was a 10–20% increase of Type III collagen in the nodules and a 30–40% increase in Type III collagen in the fibrous bands of the cord. These changes have been noted to be similar to those that occur in hypertrophic scars and granulation tissue to skin wounds.

It was Brickley-Parsons and her group in 1981 who gave some clear insight as to the importance of Type III collagen to the pathogenesis of Dupuytren's disease. She suggested that there was a very rapid synthesis of the so-called immature collagen Type III but with no evidence of collagen fibril contraction. She also demonstrated that the Type III collagen produced is of normal length and suggested that the collagen tissue fabric is shortened in a progressive manner by contractile forces of cells acting on each other, as well as collagen fibrils as they are synthesized. Brickley-Parsons also reported that major biochemical changes in the palmar fascia included increased hexosamine content in the presence of galactosamine in the most severely involved tissue. She further stated that post-translational modifications included a very elevated hydroxylysine content, an increase in the total number of reducible cross-links and the appearance of hydroxylysino-hydroxynor-lucine, which is essentially absent from normal palmar fascia. She identified this as a major reducible cross-link. Quite interestingly, she noted that apparently uninvolved fascia from Dupuytren's patients showed the same biochemical changes, although to a lesser extent. With these biochemical changes in mind, Brickley-Parsons proposed that the active cellular process draws the distal extremities of the affected tissue closer together, at the same time as the original tissue is being replaced. The result of these two processes is simply a shorter, smaller piece of tissue fabric containing collagen molecules, fibrils and fibers of normal length and organization but with pre- and post-translational modifications similar to those observed in collagens during the active stages of connective tissue repair. Another report also suggested that the enzyme transglutaminase was important to the cross-linking of Type III collagen propeptide in Dupuytren's disease (Dolynchuck and Pettigrew, 1991). This result has not been substantiated by other investigators.

Berndt's group published a report of a study that attempted to define further the extracellular matrix into various collagen types in Dupuytren's disease (Berndt et al., 1994). Up to this point, as reported in the literature, investigations had shown a fibronectin matrix but had failed to demonstrate a laminin. The study by Berndt et al. examined the composition of the extracellular matrix in Dupuytren's samples for fibronectin, laminin and collagen Type IV and tenascin, which is an adhesion glycoprotein. Using immunohistochemistry, staining for fibronectin was positive within the whole palmar fascia and was particularly intense in the proliferative areas. Laminin, collagen Type IV and tenascin labeling was restricted to the alpha-smooth-muscle-actin-positive proliferative nodules. Thus, Berndt suggested that his results substantiated the theory that the extracellular matrix formation by myofibroblasts contained fibronectin, laminin, collagen Type IV and tenascin as important constituents. In 1995, Magro et al. (1995b) showed that another collagen type, Type VI, exists as thin, extracellular matrix fibers in association with proliferating cells of the first two disease stages. Using a combined study approach of identifying myofibroblasts by cellular phenotype, and identifying constituents of the extracellular matrix, Magro et al. (1995a) demonstrated that the distribution of collagen Types IV and VI, laminin and fibronectin followed the distribution of myofibroblasts, while they were not expressed in areas devoid of these cells, such as the residual cord stage (Magro et al., 1997).

A non-operative therapy targeting collagen

Badalamente and Hurst (1996) have employed a non-operative injection treatment of collagen cords using Clostridial collagenase in the treatment of Dupuytren's disease. The purpose of their study was to test the clinical safety and efficacy of this enzyme as an injection treatment for Dupuytren's disease in a Phase II open-label trial. Their methods included entering 28 Dupuytren's patients into the study, 26 males and two females, mean age 67.3 ± 10 years. Using a dose-escalation protocol, the first six study patients received 300, 600, 1200, 2400, 4800 and 9600 units of collagenase, respectively, which was injected into the cord causing contractures of the metacarpophalangeal (MP) joint. The remaining 22 patients had collagenase injections (27 MP joints and two PIP joints) at a dose level of 10 000 units, followed by a 10–12-hour period of hand immobilization. Patients were instructed to manipulate the finger gently. The surgeon was also allowed to assist the patient with this manipulation at the first follow-up visit the day after the injection. Patients were seen the next morning, fitted with a night-time extension splint to be worn for 4 months, and instructed in at-home extension exercises. One patient was lost to follow-up. The results indicate that in the first six patients, treated under the dose-escalation protocol, there was involvement of two ring and four little fingers with a mean degree of initial MP joint contracture of $49.2 \pm 11°$. Collagenase injections had no effect in reducing the degree of MP joint contracture. In the remaining 22 patients, the mean degree of initial MP joint contracture was $42.4 \pm 13.4°$. Twenty-seven cords, causing MP joint contracture, were injected with 10 000 units collagenase (four long, 16 ring, 10 little fingers and one thumb web cord). The mean degree of initial PIP joint contracture in two patients was $45°$ in one ring and one little finger. Twenty-six of the 27 MP joint contractures corrected to normal $(0°)$ with full range of motion within 1–7 days of the injection. The patient injected in the thumb web cord achieved only a 10-degree correction of an initial thumb web contracture of $45°$. In patients with PIP joint contractures, one joint corrected to normal $(0°)$ and the other PIP joint corrected to within five degrees of normal $(0°)$, both within days of the injection. Minor adverse reactions included tenderness to pressure at the injection site with minimal palmar, and sometimes dorsal, edema, which resolved within 1–2 weeks after the injection. Mean follow-up in this patient series was at 4 months, ranging from 7 days to 1 year. The conclusions of this ongoing study indicate that Clostridial collagenase injection of Dupuytren's cords involving MP and PIP joints appears to have merit as a non-operative treatment to correct these contractures. Disease recurrence in long-term follow-up is currently being assessed. Injection of increased numbers of PIP joint contractures is also planned. It must be borne in mind that this study was designed as an open-label investigation in consultation with the US Food and Drug Administration, prior to initiating a placebo-controlled random double-blind study. Pending further study, collagenase injection for Dupuytren's disease may be a safe and effective alternative to surgical fasciectomy and a cost-effective, non-invasive treatment for this disorder (Starkweather et al., 1996).

GENETICS

The work of Ling in the 1960s (Ling, 1963) and the follow-up work by James in the 1980s (James, 1985) both support the concept that Dupuytren's disease is an inherited disorder. Their studies show that the Dupuytren's disease inheritance follows an autosomal dominant pattern but that penetrance is variable (McKusick, 1983). Why the gene for Dupuytren's disease has an incomplete (partial) penetrance is unknown. Sometimes incomplete penetrance is caused by 'skipped generations' or by observations made before the disease expressed itself. Why the inheritance of Dupuytren's disease fails to express itself is not known but may be related to the delayed onset age that is so typical of Dupuytren's disease (Bridge, 1994). Furthermore, Dupuytren's disease gene is associated with collagen formation but it is not sex-linked (Walsh and Spencer, 1990). Given this inheritance pattern, if a man (Dd) with Dupuytren's disease marries a woman with no disease (dd), then each child would have a 75% chance of becoming a carrier of the Dupuytren's gene (Figure 4.5). Owing to the variable penetrance, however, the child's chance of having a symptomatic Dupuytren's contracture would be considerably less (James, 1985; Ling, 1963). An accurate measurement of this variability in penetrance is impossible but only 10% of patients with Dupuytren's disease have a positive family history of the disorder. On the other hand, Ling found that 68% of the families from his 50 index cases had signs of Dupuytren's disease when age-corrected data were used. The use of age-corrected data is important because Dupuytren's disease clearly occurs more often in the elderly and rarely in children (Urban et al., 1996). Thieme's work also supports the theory that Dupuytren's disease is inherited by an autosomal dominant pattern (James, 1985). Ling and Mikkelsen's works also support the concept that the frequency of the clinical expression of Dupuytren's disease is age-related. Children

Female gametes

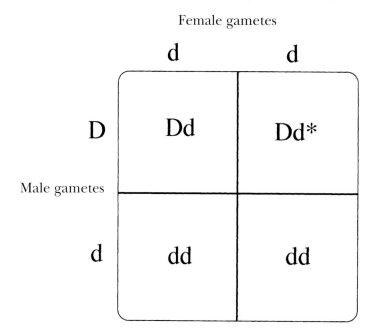

Figure 4.5 Dupuytren's disease follows an autosomal dominant Mendelian inheritance pattern with incomplete penetrance. In this example, the affected male (Dd) mating with the unaffected female (dd) would be expected to produce offspring with a 50% chance of Dupuytren's disease (Dd). However, the incidence of Dupuytren's disease in the offspring will be less than 50% because Dd* has a high likelihood of not expressing the disease.

occasionally develop Dupuytren's contracture but such cases are rare (Ling, 1963; Urban et al., 1996; Mikkelsen, 1972).

Given an autosomal dominant pattern of inheritance, it is probable that patients who present with an aggressive form of the disease, i.e. a diathesis, are homozygous for this gene, which affects collagen metabolism (McFarlane et al., 1990). The interplay of the genes and this disease is emphasized by the recent study of Halliday and co-workers, the results of which suggested that the alternate splicing of a single gene transcript in a cell can lead to different fibronectin (FN) isoforms in Dupuytren's disease (Halliday et al., 1994).

Twin studies in Dupuytren's disease have usually shown the presence of Dupuytren's disease in both twins (McGrouther, 1990). McDowell has recently verified this in 85-year-old identical female twins. These two ladies had exactly the same Dupuytren's deformities. Their disease occurred at the same age and progressed approximately at the same rate

(McDowell, personal communication, 1997). Despite these reports, Lyall's report of two pairs of identical twins in which only one twin had Dupuytren's disease demonstrates the variable penetrance of this disorder and suggests that environmental triggers are important components to the expression of the disease (Lyall, 1993).

Although there is no evidence that Dupuytren's disease is a sex-linked disease there are considerable data showing that it is both more common and more severe in men. Sex ratios vary from 10:1 to 2:1 (male:female) (Mikkelsen, 1972, 1976; Quintana, 1988). In elderly patient populations, however, the ratio approaches 1:1 (McFarlane, 1983). Furthermore, one family pedigree study has shown Dupuytren's disease to be predominantly manifested in the female side of the family tree (Matthews, 1979). Zemel has reported an increased incidence of flare reactions in women after fasciectomies but others have disputed this (Zemel, 1991).

Initial chromosomal karotyping performed on myofibroblasts cultured from excised Dupuytren's tissue showed a trisomy abnormality on chromosome eight (Sergovich et al., 1973). Additional studies have shown marked chromosomal instability in Dupuytren's disease with trisomies on chromosomes 7 and 8, as well as random structural aberrations. These changes were found in the diseased tissue, in the clinically uninvolved transverse fascia, and in the flexor retinaculum from carpal tunnel cases. The significance of these abnormalities is debatable but perhaps chromosomal changes play an important role in this pathological fibromatosis (Wurster-Hill et al., 1988; Madden, 1976; Bonnici et al., 1992).

Despite the genetic basis of Dupuytren's disease, early studies did not find a specific human leukocyte antigen (HLA) associated with this disease (Spencer and Walsh, 1984; Tait and Mackay, 1982). This is in contrast to many autoimmune diseases such as some rheumatic disorders, which show HLA-antigen markers. A study in 1994 by Neumuller et al. has shown a higher frequency of autoantibodies against elastin (ELAB) and autoantibodies against collagen (ACA) in Dupuytren's patients who demonstrate the HLA-DR3 antigen. They conclude that immune cells in conjunction with mast cells play an important role in the pathogenesis of Dupuytren's disease (Neumuller et al., 1994).

The relationship of race and Dupuytren's disease has also been studied extensively. The incidence is clearly the highest in the Caucasian races of northern Europe (McFarlane, 1983). Early's study and the more recent work of Elliot give great support to the theory that Dupuytren's disease is a disorder of Viking origin, which the Vikings brought to northern Scotland centuries ago (Early, 1962; Elliot, 1988; Lennox et al., 1993). It follows that Dupuytren's disease has been brought to Australia, Canada, the USA and New Zealand by the emigrations of these Celtic races (Hueston, 1985).

Nevertheless, Dupuytren's disease is not solely a Caucasian disease. It has been reported in blacks from Africa and the Americas (Muguti and Appelt, 1993; Mitra and Goldstein, 1994; Sladicka et al., 1996). These studies have frequently noted a history of trauma in these black patients. The disease has also been noted in patients from the Indian subcontinent (Srivastava et al., 1989), from Japan, China, Taiwan, Thailand and the Arab countries (Hueston, 1985). In the Japanese, the disease rarely causes severe contractures requiring surgery.

References

Alioto RJ, Rosier RN, Burton RI et al. (1994) Comparative effects of growth factors on fibroblasts of Dupuytren's tissue and normal plantar fascia. *J Hand Surg* **19A**: 442–52.

Badalamente MA, Hurst LC (1983) The pathogenesis of Dupuytren's contracture: contractile mechanisms of the myofibroblasts. *J Hand Surg* **8A**: 235–43.

Badalamente MA, Hurst LC (1996) Enzyme injection as a non-operative treatment for Dupuytren's disease. *J Drug Delivery* **3**: 35–40.

Badalamente MA, Hurst LC, Sampson SP (1988) Prostaglandins influence myofibroblast contractility in Dupuytren's disease. *J Hand Surg* **13A**: 867–71.

Badalamente MA, Hurst LC, Sampson SP (1992) Platelet derived growth factor in Dupuytren's disease. *J Hand Surg* **17A**: 317–23.

Badalamente MA, Sampson SP, Hurst LC (1996) The role of transforming growth factor beta in Dupuytren's disease. *J Hand Surg* **21A**: 210–15.

Bailey AJ, Sims TJ, Gabbiani G et al. (1977) Collagen of Dupuytren's disease. *Clin Sci Mol Med* **53**: 499–502.

Baird KS, Crossan JF, Ralston SH (1993) Abnormal growth factor and cytokine expression in Dupuytren's contracture. *J Clin Pathol* **46**: 425–28.

Bazin S, LeLous M, Duance VC (1980) Biochemistry and histology of the connective tissue of Dupuytren's disease lesions. *Eur J Clin Invest* **10**: 9–16.

Berndt A, Kosmehl H, Katenkamp D et al. (1994) Appearance of the myofibroblastic phenotype in Dupuytren's disease is associated with a fibronectin, laminin, collagen type IV and tenascin extracellular matrix. *Pathobiology* **62**: 55–58.

Bonnici A, Birjandi F, Spencer J et al. (1992) Chromosomal abnormalities in Dupuytren's contracture and carpal tunnel syndrome. *J Hand Surg* **17B**: 349–55.

Brickley-Parsons D, Glimcher MJ, Smith RJ et al. (1981) Biochemical changes in the collagen of the palmar fascia in patients with Dupuytren's disease. *J Bone Joint Surg* **63A**: 787–97.

Bridge P (1994) *The Calculation of Genetic Risks*. Johns Hopkins Press, Baltimore.

Chiu HF, McFarlane RM (1978) Pathogenesis of Dupuytren's contracture: a correlative clinical–pathological study. *J Hand Surg* **3**: 1–10.

Crombrugghe BD, Karsenty G, Maity S (1990) Transcriptional mechanisms controlling Types I and III collagen genes. *Ann N Y Acad Sci* **580**: 88–96.

Dolynchuk KN, Pettigrew NM (1991) Transglutaminase levels in Dupuytren's disease. *J Hand Surg* **16A**: 787–90.

Early P (1962) Population studies in Dupuytren's contracture. *J Bone Joint Surg* **44A**: 602–13.

Elliot D (1988) The early history of contracture of the palmar fascia, part 1. *J Hand Surg* **13B**: 246–53.

Gabbiani G, Majno G (1972) Dupuytren's contracture: fibroblast contraction? An ultrastructural study. *Am J Pathol* **66**: 131–46.

Gelberman RH, Amiel D, Rudolph RM et al. (1980) Dupuytren's contracture. An electron microscopic, biochemical, and clinical correlative study. *J Bone Joint Surg* **62A**: 425–32.

Gonzalez AM, Buscaglia M, Fox R et al. (1992) Basic fibroblast growth factor in Dupuytren's contracture. *Am J Pathol* **141**: 661–71.

Halliday N, Rayan G, Zardi L et al. (1994) Distribution of ED-A and ED-B containing fibronectin isoforms in Dupuytren's disease. *J Hand Surg* **19A**: 428–34.

Hueston J (1985) Overview of etiology and pathology. In: Hueston JT, Tubiana R, eds, *Dupuytren's Disease*, 2nd edn, 75–81. Churchill Livingstone, Edinburgh.

Hurst LC, Badalamente MA, Makowski J (1986) The pathobiology of Dupuytren's contracture: effects of prostaglandins on myofibroblasts. *J Hand Surg* **11A**: 18–23.

James JIP (1985) The genetic pattern of Dupuytren's contracture. In: Hueston JT, Tubiana R, eds, *Dupuytren's Disease*, 94. Churchill Livingstone, Edinburgh.

Kischer CW, Speer DP (1984) Microvascular changes in Dupuytren's contracture. *J Hand Surg* **9A**: 58–62.

Kloen P, Jenning CL, Gebhardt MC et al. (1995) TGF beta: possible roles in Dupuytren's contracture. *J Hand Surg* **20A**: 101–108.

Lennox I, Murali S, Porter R (1993) A study of the repeatability of the diagnosis of Dupuytren's contracture and its prevalence in the Grampian region. *J Hand Surg* **18B**: 258–61.

Ling R (1963) The genetic factor in Dupuytren's disease. *J Bone Joint Surg* **45B**: 709–18.

Luck JV (1959) Dupuytren's contracture – a new concept of the pathogenesis correlated with surgical management. *J Bone Joint Surg* **41A**: 635–64.

Lyall H (1993) Dupuytren's disease in identical twins. *J Hand Surg* **18B**: 368–70.

Madden J (1976) Chromosomal abnormalities in Dupuytren's disease. *Lancet* **1**: 207 (letter).

Magro G, Colombatti A, Lanzafame S (1995a) Immunohistochemical expression of Type VI collagen in superficial fibromatoses. *Pathol Res Pract* **191**: 1023–28.

Magro G, Lanzafame S, Micoli G (1995b) Co-ordinate expression of alpha 5 beta 1 integrin and fibronectin in Dupuytren's disease. *Acta Histochem* **97**: 229–33.

Magro G, Fraggetta F, Colombatti A et al. (1997) Myofibroblasts and extracellular matric glycoproteins in palmar fibromatosis. *Gen Diagn Pathol* **142**: 185–90.

Matthews P (1979) Familial Dupuytren's contracture with predominantly female expression. *Br J Plast Surg* **32**: 120–23.

McFarlane R (1983) The current status of Dupuytren's disease. *J Hand Surg* **8A**: 703–708.

McFarlane R, McGrouther D, Flint M (1990) *Dupuytren's Disease. Biology and Treatment*, Vol. 5. Churchill Livingstone, Edinburgh.

McGrouther D (1990) Is Dupuytren's disease an inherited disorder? In: McFarlane R, McGrouther D, Flint M, eds, *Dupuytren's Disease*, 280–81. Churchill Livingstone, Edinburgh.

McKusick V (1983) *Mendelian Inheritance in Man*. Johns Hopkins University Press, Baltimore.

Menzel EJ, Piza H, Zielinski C et al. (1979) Collagen types and anticollagen antibodies in Dupuytren's disease. *Hand* **11**: 243–48.

Meyerding H, Black J, Broders A (1941) The etiology and pathology of Dupuytren's contracture. *Surg Gynecol Obstetr* **72**: 582–90.

Mikkelsen O (1972) The prevalence of Dupuytren's disease in Norway. *Acta Chir Scand* **138**: 695–700.

Mikkelsen O (1976) Dupuytren's disease – a study of the pattern of distribution and stage of contracture in the hand. *Hand* **8**: 265–71.

Mitra A, Goldstein R (1994) Dupuytren's contracture in the black population; a review. *Ann Plast Surg* **32**: 619–22.

Muguti G, Appelt B (1993) Dupuytren's contracture in black Zimbabweans. *Central Afr J Med* **39**: 129–32.

Murrell GA (1991) The role of the fibroblast in Dupuytren's contracture. *Hand Clin* **7**: 669–80.

Neumuller J, Menzel J, Millesi H (1994) Prevalence of HLA-DR3 and autoantibodies to connective tissue components in Dupuytren's contracture. *Clin Immunol Immunopathol* **71**: 142–48.

Quintana GA (1988) Various epidemiologic aspects of Dupuytren's disease. *Ann Chir Main* **7**: 256–62.

Rayan GM, Parizi M, Tomasek JJ (1996) Pharmacologic regulation of Dupuytren's fibroblast contraction in vitro. *J Hand Surg* **21B**: 1065–70.

Salamon A, Hamori J (1980a) The role of myofibroblasts in the pathogenesis of Dupuytren's contracture. *Hand Chir* **12**: 113–17.

Salamon A, Hamori J (1980b) Possible role of myofibroblasts in the pathology of Dupuytren's disease. *Acta Morphol Acad Sci Hung* **28**: 71–82.

Sergovich F, Botz J, McFarlane R (1973) Nonrandom cytogenetic abnormalities in Dupuytren's disease. *N Engl J Med* **308**: 162–63.

Shum DT (1990) Histopathology. In: McFarlane RM, McGrouther DA, Flint MH, eds, *Dupuytren's Disease*, 25–30. Churchill Livingstone, New York.

Shum DT, McFarlane R (1988) Histogenesis of Dupuytren's disease: an immunohistochemical study of 30 cases. *J Hand Surg* **13A**: 61–67.

Sladicka M, Benfanti P, Raab MB (1996) Dupuytren's contracture in the black population: a case report and review of the literature. *J Hand Surg* **21A**: 898–99.

Spencer J, Walsh K (1984) Histocompatibility antigen patterns in Dupuytren's contracture. *J Hand Surg* **9B**: 276–78.

Srivastava S, Nancarrow JD, Cort DF (1989) Dupuytren's disease in patients from the Indian sub-continent. Report of ten cases. *J Hand Surg* **14B**: 32–34.

Starkweather K, Lattuga S, Hurst LC et al. (1996) Collagenase in the treatment of Dupuytren's disease: an in vitro study. *J Hand Surg* **21A**: 490–95.

Sugden P, Andrew JG, Andrew SM (1993) Dermal dendrocytes in Dupuytren's disease: a link between skin and pathogenesis? *J Hand Surg* **18B**: 662–66.

Tait B, Mackay L (1982) HLA phenotypes in Dupuytren's contracture. *Tissue Antigens* **19**: 240–41.

Terek RM, Jiranek WA, Goldberg MJ (1995) The expression of platelet derived growth-factor gene in Dupuytren's contracture. *J Bone Joint Surg* **77A**: 1–9.

Tomasek JJ, Haaksma CJ (1991) Fibronectin filaments and actin microfilaments are organized into a fibronexus in Dupuytren's diseased tissue. *Anat Rec* **230**: 175–82.

Tomasek JJ, Rayan GM (1995) Correlation of alpha-smooth muscle actin expression and contraction in Dupuytren's disease fibroblasts. *J Hand Surg* **20A**: 450–55.

Tomasek JJ, Schultz RJ, Episalla CW et al. (1986) The cytoskeleton and extracellular matrix of the Dupuytren's disease 'myofibroblast': an immunofluorescence study of a non-muscle cell type. *J Hand Surg* **11A**: 365–71.

Tomasek JJ, Schultz RJ, Haaksma CJ (1987) Extracellular matrix–cytoskeleton connections at the surface of the specialized contractile fibroblast (myofibroblast) in Dupuytren's disease. *J Bone Joint Surg* **69A**: 1400–407.

Tyrkko J, Viljanto J (1975) Significance of histopathological findings in Dupuytren's contracture. *Ann Chir Gynaecol Fenniae* **64**: 288–91.

Urban M, Feldberg L, Janssen A et al. (1996) Dupuytren's disease in children. *J Hand Surg* **21B**: 112–16.

Vandeberg JS, Rudolph R, Gelberman R, Woodward MR (1982) Ultrastructural relationship of skin to nodule and cord in Dupuytren's contracture. *Plast Reconstr Surg* **69**: 835–44.

Walsh K, Spencer J (1990) Immunology and genetics. In: McFarlane R, McGrouther D, Flint M, eds, *Dupuytren's Disease*, 99–103. Churchill Livingstone, Edinburgh.

Wurster-Hill D, Brown F, Park J et al. (1988) Cytogenetic studies in Dupuytren's contracture. *Am J Hum Genet* **43**: 285–92.

Zemel N (1991) Dupuytren's contracture in women. *Hand Clin* **7**: 707–12.

5

Clinical aspects

CLINICAL PRESENTATION

Caroline Leclercq

The diagnosis of Dupuytren's disease relies almost exclusively on clinical findings. There is no related blood test anomaly, and radiological investigations are not specific. Only histological examination will secondarily confirm the diagnosis. However, this diagnosis is simple in most cases, since the clinical presentation of Dupuytren's disease is usually straightforward. It is generally agreed to be based on the finding of a thickening of the palmar aspect of the hand or fingers as a nodule or cord (Lennox et al., 1993; Mawhinney et al., 1999).

Palmar lesions

Palmar lesions are the most frequent and early symptoms of the disease. They present either as nodules, skin pits, distorsion of palmar creases and cords, isolated or in association.

Nodules

Nodules are more frequent on the ulnar half of the palm. They lie on top of the longitudinal bands of the palmar fascia, along the axis

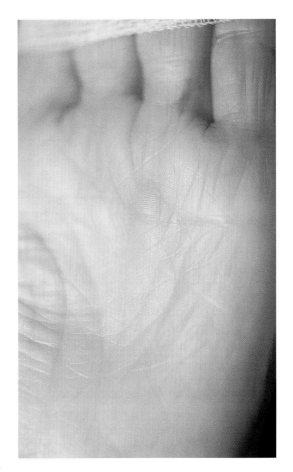

Figure 5.1 Typical aspect of a palmar nodule.

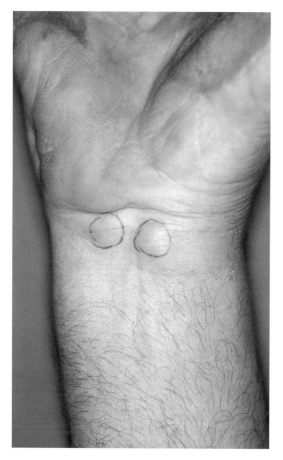

Figure 5.2 Unusual location of nodules at the wrist.

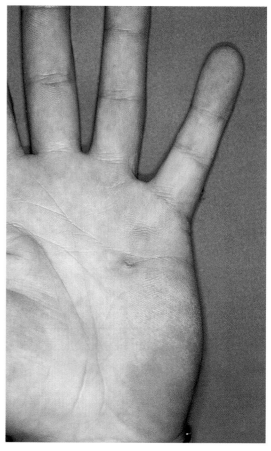

Figure 5.3 Skin pit located near the distal palmar crease.

of the digital rays. They are typically located in the vicinity of the proximal and distal palmar creases (Figure 5.1). They may also be found off the finger axis, overlying the natatory ligament. Localization on the radial side of the palm is less frequent. Nodules may then either sit in the distal palmar crease, as for the ulnar nodules, or superficially in the first web, either distally or proximally located in the web.

A few cases of nodules around the wrist crease have been reported, usually surrounding the insertions of flexor carpi ulnaris or palmaris longus (Boyes and Jones, 1968; Hueston, 1965; Simons et al., 1996). The author has observed this localization on two occasions (Figure 5.2) and in both cases the diathesis was strong with multiple involvement, as reported in the literature.

Nodules are firm, solid and usually painless, even under pressure. Proximally there is often a layer of adipose cellular tissue between the skin and the nodule but distally the nodule may be intimately adherent to the skin.

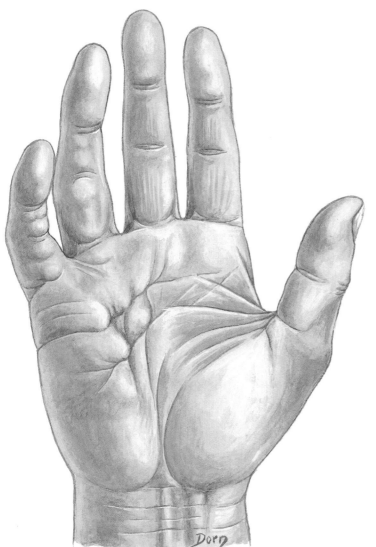

Figure 5.4 Distortion of the proximal and distal palmar creases.

Skin pits

Skin pits are mostly located around the distal palmar crease (Figure 5.3). They usually appear in the earliest phases of the disease but can remain at later stages in conjunction with nodules and cords. They are initially more visible in certain specific positions (maximal extension of metacarpophalangeal (MP) joints with maximal flexion of proximal interphalangeal (PIP)

joints) and then become permanent (Millesi, 1985). McGrouther (1986), who has dissected 48 of them, states that they are probably caused by adhesions between longitudinal and vertical fibers of the fascia. Obstruction to the orifice of a palmar skin pit has been seen to lead to acute abscess formation requiring drainage (Wylock and Vansteenland, 1989).

When isolated, nodules and skin pits do not lead to any functional impairment, although

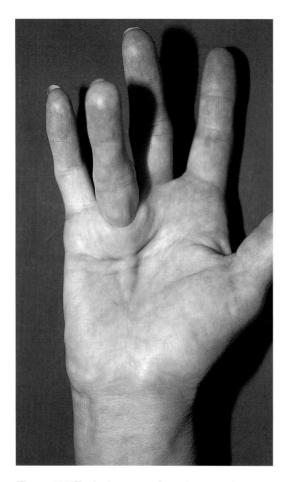

Figure 5.5 Typical aspect of a palmar cord.

patients may complain of unusual palmar tension when passively hyperextending their fingers.

Distortion of skin creases

Distortion of skin creases has been emphasized by McGrouther (1982, 1986). It can occur in isolation as a deepening of the crease, noticeable in full extension of the hand, or as a broadening of the crease, as described by Johnson (1980) in his own hand (the 'Hugh Johnson sign') (Figure 5.4). Skin

pits and nodules concur to aggravate it, by proximal or distal attraction of the crease.

Cords

Cords (sometimes referred to as 'bands', although this term should be restricted to the normal fascial structures) usually occur at a later stage, developing from a pre-existing nodule; however they can also occur de novo. Proximal palmar cords are usually easy to delineate by attentive palpation. This is not so easy when dealing with distal cords, which are often more deeply located.

Proximal cords are longitudinal along the axis of the ray, with little skin involvement until the palmar creases. There, a nodule can be embodied in the cord (Figure 5.5).

These cords, when running distally, may follow different paths according to the depth of involvement of the longitudinal fibers. They can terminate in the dermis at the point of insertion of the longitudinal fibers, forming a skin pit. They can also continue along the axis of the finger to form a digital central cord as described by McFarlane (1974) or continue obliquely towards the finger. McGrouther (1982), through microscopic dissection, has shown that these three patterns indicate involvement limited to the superficial longitudinal fibers. A cord running obliquely towards the finger may pass underneath the neurovascular bundle. As it retracts and straightens over time, it forces the neurovascular bundle into a more superficial and midline position, putting it at risk during the skin incision (see Figure 6.9, page 133). Short and Watson (1982) have emphasized the clinical recognition of this situation – there is a circular, soft, and pulpy prominence to either side of the pretendinous cord at the level of the MP joint (the 'Short–Watson sign').

The cord can also run towards the lateral sides of the finger through the latero-digital fascia, leading to a retraction of the PIP joint, indicating involvement of the deeper longitu-

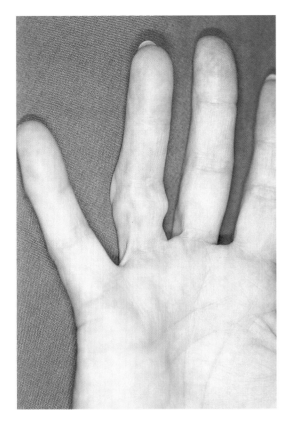

Figure 5.6 Digital nodule over the proximal phalanx.

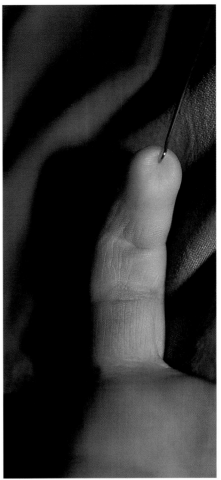

Figure 5.7 Unusual distal digital cord.

dinal fibers, or else run laterally on each side of the MP joint, where they can no longer be palpated, leading to MP joint contracture (involvement of the deepest fibers).

Digital lesions

Digital involvement can consist of nodules, cords and joint contractures.

Nodules

Nodules are usually central, on the volar aspect of the proximal phalanx, large, with

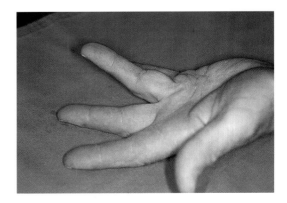

Figure 5.8 MP joint contracture.

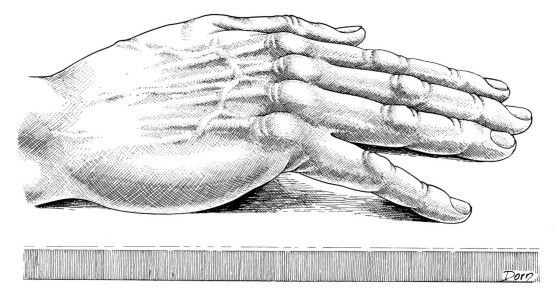

Figure 5.9 The 'table-top' test: flexion contracture of the fifth MP joint leads to a loss of contact of the palmar skin with the table.

massive skin involvement (Figure 5.6). They often produce a proximal attraction of the PIP flexion crease and may lead to some degree of PIP flexion contracture, even if no actual cord is palpated.

Digital cords

Digital cords are often subtle and ill defined. Careful palpation may identify a central cord running longitudinally along the axis of the finger, disappearing at the PIP level, or an anterolateral cord running from the proximal MP area to the distal PIP area ('pre-vascular' cord), but often one only palpates a broad thickening of the volar and lateral aspects of the proximal phalanx. Cords are rarely found distal to the middle phalanx, but patients may occasionally present a lateral cord running across the distal interphalangeal (DIP) joint (Figure 5.7). A cord at finger level leads shortly to finger contracture.

Joint contracture

Joint contracture primarily affects the MP joint in most cases. Limited to a restriction of MP joint hyperextension in the early phase of the disease, it turns progressively into a permanent and uncorrectable lack of extension, unmodified by the position of adjacent joints (Figure 5.8). Occurrence of this contracture can be monitored by the patient through the table-top test described by Hueston: when the hand lies flat on a table, palm downward, any limitation of extension of an MP joint will lead to loss of contact of the overlying palmar skin pad with the table (Figure 5.9).

Progression of the contracture is usually slow, over the course of years. Occasionally, however, the joint may retract rapidly, within months. There is often an accompanying inflammatory reaction with temporary pain and swelling along a pre-existing nodule or cord, or formation of a new cord.

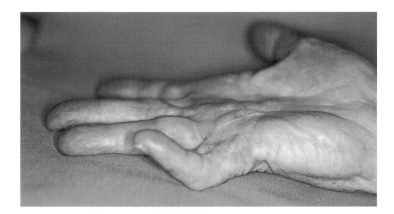

Figure 5.10 Isolated PIP joint contracture with compensatory MP joint hyperextension.

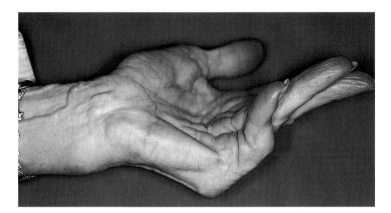

Figure 5.11 DIP joint hyperextension.

MP joint contracture, as stated earlier, is related to contraction of a palmar cord, and can occur without any digital involvement. When isolated, it progresses very rarely beyond 60° of flexion. It is then usually well tolerated, and causes only minimal functional impairment. Involvement of the natatory ligaments will eventually produce a concomitant limitation of abduction of the two adjacent fingers. This limitation often goes unnoticed because of the MP flexion deformity, and must be sought during clinical examination.

Involvement of the PIP joint usually occurs later in the course of the disease. It is a progressive limitation of extension of the joint, uncorrectable either actively or passively. This contracture can progress until full flexion, stopping only when the base of the middle phalanx comes into contact with the neck of the proximal phalanx. This will lead to skin crease maceration and even nail incrustation in severe cases.

PIP joint flexion produces disability more readily than MP joint flexion and when both are present the disability is greatest.

When isolated, PIP joint contracture is usually compensated for by hyperextension of the MP joint, so that the flexed fingertip does not protrude into the palm (Figure 5.10). Functional impairment is noted in fitting gloves, putting the hand in a tight pocket, or handling certain tools. Another complaint is the dorsum of the flexed joint being repeatedly traumatized, owing to the compensatory hyperextension of the MP joint.

When combined with MP joint contracture the flexed phalanges protrude into the palm, becoming caught in clothing, often hurting the skin while washing, especially the face, impinging on hand-shaking, and tending to push away large objects such as bottles while the patient attempts to grasp them with the other fingers. These hooked digits may even constitute a danger to the patient's life in the inability to release objects rapidly (Hueston, 1963).

The DIP joint may assume two different types of deformity. The most frequent is a hyperextension deformity at the DIP level consecutive to the PIP joint flexion contracture. Passive flexion of the joint is initially unimpaired, but with the passage of time a hyperextension contracture may develop (Figure 5.11), leading to a boutonnière-type deformity. The joint may less frequently be attracted in flexion by a volar cord. These distal cords are usually lateral, on either side of the flexor tendon, and may be isolated, without PIP joint contracture (see Figure 5.7).

Functional impairment is more important with the flexion type of deformity as it interferes more with grasping, and as the fingers are more readily caught in clothes and handles.

Whatever deformity occurs, the joints are usually not affected by any other symptom. They remain pain free, without any swelling or other inflammatory sign. Occasionally, some patients complain of tension or mild pain on attempted full extension. Moreover, there is never any limitation of active or passive flexion of the MP and PIP joints. Except for cases of DIP hyperextension contracture, active flexion of the fingers always remains complete in Dupuytren's disease. One should otherwise question the responsibility of Dupuytren's disease for the deformity and search for another cause (previous trauma, etc.).

Other symptoms may be present, as reported by Galambo (quoted by Viljanto, 1973) in his series of 766 patients. He reported pain in 19.8%, tingling in 17.9%, sweating in 6.5%, freezing in 5.2%, edema in 4.2%, changing color in 2.6%, and difference in skin temperature in 1.5%. However, most of these symptoms are usually related to another simultaneous pathology (such as carpal tunnel syndrome, Raynaud's phenomenon, etc.) rather than to Dupuytren's disease.

X-rays do not show any skeletal abnormalities, except for the flexed position of phalanges in cases of contractures. Sometimes a bony spur, amounting to an exostosis, may be found on the lateral aspect of a proximal or middle phalanx (Andrew, 1987). It stands at the distal end of a cord, at the level of its bony insertion.

Differential diagnosis

In its typical form, the diagnosis of Dupuytren's disease is easy. In doubtful cases a positive family history, bilaterality or ectopic lesions are helpful. But in a few cases the diagnosis may remain difficult.

A study of the repeatability of the diagnosis of Dupuytren's disease carried out by Lennox et al. (1993) showed that interobservers agreement was perfect when there was a flexion contracture, but for skin-tethering agreement existed in only 80%, and for nodules in only 76%. Ling (1963) also mentioned the difficulty of being certain whether Dupuytren's disease was present or not, while searching for it in relatives of Dupuytren's patients.

In some cases, one may be hesitant with other conditions.

Occurrence of an isolated nodule, whether palmar or digital, may mimic a tumor of the hand, such as lipoma, inclusion dermoid, sebaceous cyst, or a foreign body. Differentiation from a callosity may also be difficult, but changes in the superficial keratinic skin layers, and knowledge of the

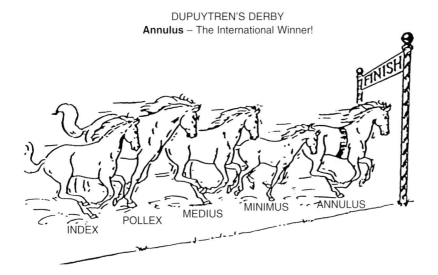

DUPUYTREN'S DERBY
Annulus – The International Winner!

INDEX POLLEX MEDIUS MINIMUS ANNULUS

Figure 5.12
Schematic representation by Bruner of the distribution of the disease in each finger. (Reproduced with permission from Bruner, 1970.)

patient's occupation (heavy manual labor with handling of tools) will usually be helpful. Finally, a Dupuytren's nodule may mimic any other fibrous tumor (desmoid fibroma, nodular fasciitis, fibrosarcoma). In doubtful cases, especially if the growth expands rapidly, a positive diagnosis should be made histologically.

Congenital flexion deformity of the fingers ('camptodactyly'), generally localized on the little and ring fingers, occurs much earlier in life and shows no evidence of fascial retraction.

Flexion contracture of the PIP joint due to a retraction of the flexor tendons may be misleading, but a history of trauma and/or previous surgery will help to establish the correct diagnosis.

Distribution

Topography

Fingers are not equally involved in Dupuytren's disease. Thumb and index involvements are rare, whereas the ring and little finger are most frequently involved, as illustrated in an 'equestrian' drawing by Bruner in 1970 (Figure 5.12).

A review of the largest series of the literature (5273 hands) shows that the fourth ray is slightly more frequently involved than the fifth (Table 5.1). Then frequency decreases from the third to the second and first rays; all authors agree that involvement of the index finger is very rare. For the first ray, however,

Table 5.1 Involvement of individual rays in large series of Dupuytren's disease.						
	No.	I (%)	II (%)	III (%)	IV (%)	V (%)
James and Tubiana, 1952	3251	3	5	22	65	52
McFarlane, 1985	812	25	13	33	65	71
Brouet, 1986	1014	7	3	15	38	36
De la Caffinière, 1986	196	1	5	27	90	31
Total	**5273**	**7**	**5.8**	**22.5**	**60.7**	**51**

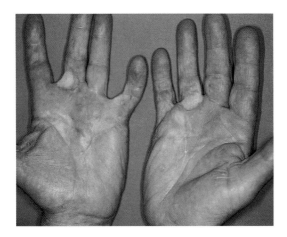

Figure 5.13 Severe case of Dupuytren's disease with involvement of both hands.

The most common combination of affected fingers are ring and little finger, then middle and ring, and then middle, ring and little fingers. In severe cases, all fingers may be affected, with massive involvement at the palmar and digital level (Figure 5.13).

Two localizations, namely radial and little finger, have special clinical features and require a specific description.

Radial involvement

Involvement of the radial aspect of the hand, i.e. thumb, first web space and index finger, is considered rare; however, it has been demonstrated to be rather frequent when it is looked for systematically (Tubiana et al., 1982; Tubiana, 1999). Four different types of cord may occur in the thumb and first web:

1. A longitudinal thenar cord, prolonged on the lateral aspect of the thumb, which may lead to MP and possibly IP joint retraction of the thumb;
2. A longitudinal commissural cord, prolonged on the lateral aspect of the index finger, which may retract the index MP and possibly PIP joints;
3,4. Two transverse commissural cords, one proximal and one distal, which may lead to web contracture and thumb adduction (Figure 5.14).

A central cord may also be found on the volar aspect of the thumb, as in the fingers, leading to IP joint contracture (Figure 5.15) (Cleland and Morrison, 1986).

All of the above may combine in the same hand. They are usually limited to a slowly progressing cord in a patient presenting with the usual involvement of the ulnar side of the palm, leading to little or no disability; but they can also present as an aggressive involvement occurring in young individuals early in the course of the disease, leading to a disabling contracture of the web and the thumb.

there is disagreement regarding the rate of involvement as it varies from 1 to 25% in different series. If one excludes the first web, involvement of the thumb itself is probably infrequent but if the first web is included, and systematically assessed, figures rise significantly. This was demonstrated by Tubiana et al. who found a 63% involvement of the first ray in 94 patients where it was systematically examined (Tubiana et al., 1982; Tubiana, 1999).

Although the disease is initially limited to a single ray, it usually progresses to other rays but not necessarily adjacent to the ray of onset. The number of rays involved will depend greatly on the stage at which the patient is examined. In McFarlane's (1985) multicenter study the distribution was roughly even between involvement of a single ray, of two rays and of more than two rays, at one-third each. But in Tubiana et al.'s (1982) series, which includes many severe and recurrent cases, involvement was limited to one or two rays in 8%, to three rays in 20%, extended to four rays in 32%, and to all five rays in 40%.

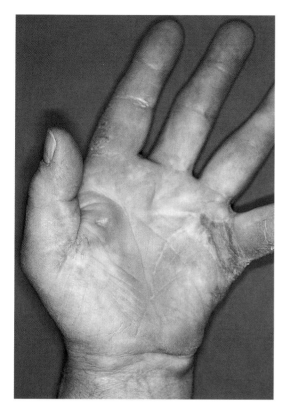

Figure 5.14 Thumb involvement with commissural cord and adduction of the thumb.

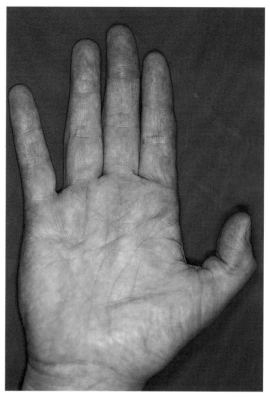

Figure 5.15 Thumb involvement with central digital cord and IP joint contracture.

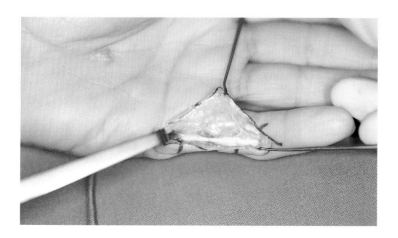

Figure 5.16 Intraoperative view of a hypothenar cord inserting proximally on the hypothenar muscles.

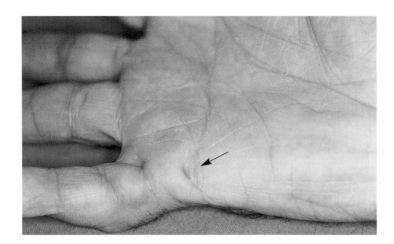

Figure 5.17 Nodule and skin pit (arrow) over the distal insertion of the hypothenar muscles.

Little finger involvement

This may occur in isolation, without the palm or any other fingers being involved. It often follows a more severe course, with significant joint retractions and a high incidence of recurrence after surgery. In Brouet's series of 1000 patients, all cases of Dupuytren's disease limited to a single digit involvement occurred on the little finger. As shown in his series, it is more frequent in women (Brouet, 1986).

The digital cord is often located laterally, originating from the hypothenar muscles and fascia at the MP joint level (Figure 5.16). There, a large nodule overlying the abductor digiti minimi tendon often puckers the adherent skin (Figure 5.17). Then the cord reaches the lateral side of the PIP joint, flexing the joint, and sometimes abducting the little finger.

The finger usually assumes a hyperextended position at MP level, compensating for the PIP flexion contracture. Involvement of the DIP is more frequent than in other fingers with a higher incidence of hyperextension deformities (see Figure 5.11) (James and Tubiana, 1952).

Bilaterality

Dupuytren's disease is usually bilateral, with figures varying from 42 to 98% in the literature. These differences are probably due to the difficulty of ascertaining the diagnosis in very early nodular forms, and to the evolutive pattern of the disease. Millesi (1985) followed a population of 113 patients operated on for unilateral Dupuytren's disease. This invaded the contralateral hand in 9% after 1 year, in 39% at 5 years, and in 48% after 6 years. When unilateral, the disease involves the right hand a little more frequently than the left (McFarlane, 1985; de la Caffinière, 1986). But there is no relationship to handedness (Zachariae, 1971; Boyes, 1954; Fisk, 1985). Data derived from patients who have undergone surgery will always show the right hand to be operated on more commonly, for the obvious reason that the deformity is more functionally impairing in the right-handed majority.

McFarlane (1985), in his study of 812 patients, found that the 36% unilateral involvement differed in many respects from the bilateral ones, i.e. there was a lower inci-

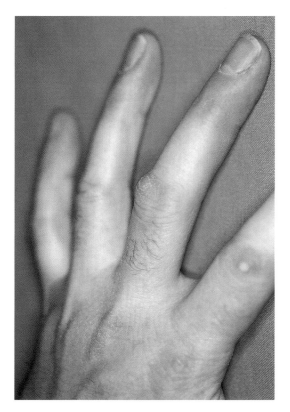

Figure 5.18 Multiple knuckle pads over the dorsum of the PIP joints.

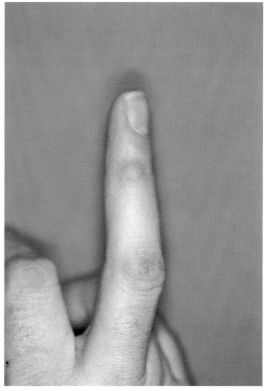

Figure 5.19 Unusual location of a knuckle pad over the DIP joint.

dence of a family history and fewer ectopic lesions or associated diseases. However, the age at onset and at first operation were similar to those with bilateral involvement, indicating that the disease was very likely to progress to the other hand.

Ectopic lesions

It has long been known that other fibrotic lesions could occur with Dupuytren's disease, and Dupuytren himself was aware that knuckle pads and plantar lesions could occur as well as palmar lesions. Anderson, in 1891, used the term 'diathesis' to indicate the predisposition of certain patients for multiple site involvement

of the contracture. Touraine and Ruel, in 1945, coined the term 'hereditary polyfibromatosis' in which they grouped Dupuytren's disease, spontaneous keloids and induratio penis plastica as the main lesions, and no fewer than 11 other cutaneous locations as secondary lesions. Hueston was the first to use the term 'ectopic lesions' for knuckle pads and plantar lesions.

Knuckle pads

Knuckle pads are fibrous processes localized on the extensor side of the PIP joint. They are fairly firm, somewhat irregular on palpation, adherent to the skin and to the underlying extensor tendons (Figure 5.18). However, they usually cause little or no impairment of flexion. They may be a little tender when appearing, or later when knocked, but are otherwise fairly painless. Their appearance may be preceded by a depression over the dorsum of the PIP joint, suggesting, according to Hueston (1984), 'a role of the dermis in the subcutaneous space.' They are not exclusively found on the dorsum of the PIP joint, occurring sometimes over the DIP or MP joints, or over the thumb IP joint (Figure 5.19) (Hueston, 1982, 1984).

The first note of knuckle pads in connection with Dupuytren's disease was probably made by Garrod in 1893 and they were subsequently referred to as Garrod's nodes (as well as helodermia, keratosis supracapitularis, etc.). They are quite frequent in Dupuytren's disease, but are not always located on the involved finger(s). Prevalence ranges from 7% (Iselin et al., 1988) to 44% (Skoog, 1948), with most series averaging 15% (Early, 1962). As for Dupuytren's disease, and other ectopic lesions, they are more frequent in men than in women. They are more frequent in younger patients (average 48 years) than in older ones, which led some authors to wonder whether they may undergo spontaneous regression (Hueston, 1963; Hoet et al., 1983).

Hueston (1963) has shown them to be present in 75% of patients with a recurrence of Dupuytren's disease (average age 45 years) and in only 20% of patients remaining clear of the disease after surgery (average age 58 years), this indicating a greater potential severity of the disease when knuckle pads are present.

Knuckle pads may also occur in patients free of the disease, as shown by Mikkelsen (1977, 1990) who examined 1871 adults of a Norwegian town and found knuckle pads in 9% of men and 8.6% of women. However, they were four times more frequent in patients with Dupuytren's disease than in the general population. McIndoe (1958) stated that 'the clinician who observes a patient to have knuckle pads may be quite sure that that

patient either has a Dupuytren's disease contracture or that one will develop in the future,' but Hueston (1963) replies more prudently that 'their presence indicates a definite predisposition to the production of similar tissue in the palm and possibly elsewhere.'

When isolated they can be mistaken for Bouchard's nodes (PIP equivalent of Heberden's nodes), joint synovitis, villonodular synovitis, or occupational keratoses. Hueston and Wilson (1973) have reported similarities with occupational nodes (shearing, carpet-laying) but the latter regress during vacation from work.

A different type of dorsal node has been reported both by Hueston (1982: one case) and by Iselin et al. (1988: two cases), located over the middle phalanx between PIP and DIP joints. These lesions, as opposed to knuckle pads, lead to an extension contracture, with loss of active and passive flexion of the DIP joint. This contracture is relieved after removal of the node, further supporting, for Hueston, the 'extrinsic' theory of the pathogenesis of Dupuytren's disease.

Plantar lesions

Changes similar to Dupuytren's disease of the palm may be seen in the sole of the foot. Although Ledderhose's name is often connected with it, he was not the first to report this condition (Ledderhose, 1897): Madelung (1875) was probably the first. These lesions are not infrequent. In 1951, Pickren et al. searched the literature and found 104 cases, to which they added 18 personal cases.

Plantar lesions occur as painless lumps in the non-weight-bearing part of the sole, usually near the highest point of the arch. They usually produce no symptoms other than because of their size, and patients may be unaware of them. Pain is infrequent, usually limited to mild discomfort after standing or walking for long periods (Allen et al., 1955). They have occasionally been reported to be so painful that walking becomes almost impossible (Lettin, 1964). The skin is generally mobile over the lump, which is fixed to the plantar fascia. A few cases of adhesion of the nodule to the overlying skin have been described (Gordon, 1964; Pickren et al., 1951). A lump commonly appears in the fourth to fifth decades (Pentland and Anderson, 1985), reaches a certain size, and then, unlike palmar lesions, does not progress further (Hueston, 1963, 1974) and does not lead to any toe contracture. Toe contractures have been reported twice, by Classen and Hurst (1992), and by Donato and Morrison (1996). The latter researchers state that the reason for the absence of toe contracture may lie in the anatomy of the plantar fascia, which divides into very thin and 'insignificant' digital slips.

Other locations have been reported in the foot: namely in the great toe (Hueston, 1963); beneath the first metatarsal head (Gordon, 1964); and the bases of the other toes (Reynolds and Bostram, 1975; Donato and Morrison, 1996).

Plantar lesions may be isolated, without any palmar involvement. Allen et al. (1955) reviewed the files of the Mayo Clinic and found 24 isolated cases among 69 plantar fibromatoses; similarly Aviles et al. (1971) found in the files of the NY Memorial Hospital 20 isolated cases among 22 plantar fibromatoses. Haedicke and Sturim (1989) reported four personal cases of isolated plantar fibromatosis, although the patients were followed for 13–21 months only. In Allen's report (1955), from the 45 cases with plantar and Dupuytren's disease, nearly half of the cases had an isolated plantar lesion initially, with occurrence of the palmar disease after an interval of up to 10 years. It is therefore difficult to determine the percentage of plantar fibromatoses that remain isolated.

The prevalence of plantar fibromatosis in Dupuytren's disease varies greatly in the literature, from 5% (James and Tubiana, 1952) to 20% (Hueston, 1963). The figures depend on the population studied, whether it is a series of operated patients, a survey of a Dupuytren's disease population, or a general survey of a population. Results also vary according to whether the feet are examined or whether the patient is only asked about it in general terms.

In the past, dramatic confusions have been made with a malignant process, mainly when the plantar lesion was isolated and unilateral. The histologic features (non-encapsulated, highly cellular lesion with numerous mitotic figures) associated with early recurrence have sometimes led to the erroneous diagnosis of sarcoma (Allen et al., 1955; Aviles et al., 1971; Haedicke and Sturim, 1989) and several foot amputations have even been reported.

Peyronie's disease

Peyronie's disease (also known as induratio penis plastica) is an inflammatory disease affecting the tunica albuginea of the corpora cavernosa of the penis. It is characterized by the development of a circumscribed plaque, commonly situated on the dorsum of the penis, usually in its middle third. The plaque may range from a few millimeters to a broad sheet. Uncommonly it may lie ventrally or laterally, or encircle the corporea (Vorstman et al., 1986). There may occasionally be more than one plaque. On palpation the plaque is best felt when the penis is flaccid; it is hard and usually painless. On erection, the plaque may lead to pain and bending of the penis. The degree of bending varies according to the site of the plaque, being worse with more distal lesions (Hueston, 1963).

Peyronie's disease affects mostly middle-aged men, but occurrence as early as 14 years has been reported (Vorstman et al., 1986). It predominates in Caucasians. Its incidence is probably far greater than reported, as many patients are not aware of it or do not report it. The acute process tends to have a self-limiting course, with lesions becoming stationary after 2–5 years then sometimes regressing.

According to James and Tubiana (1952), its association with Dupuytren's disease was first mentioned by Kirby in 1849. It is much less frequent than with knuckle pads or plantar lesions, with a reported prevalence of 1–3% (Viljanto, 1973; McFarlane, 1985; Hueston, 1963; Brouet, 1986). Skoog (1948) reported seven cases of Peyronie's disease in 207 epileptics. Ciniewicz (1956, quoted by Hueston, 1963) reported eight cases of Dupuytren's disease in 85 patients with Peyronie's disease, and Viljanto reported nine in 100 patients.

The association of Dupuytren's disease with Peyronie's disease and ear plaques is known as the Gallizia's triad (Gallizia, 1964).

Other lesions

Numerous other ectopic lesions associated with Dupuytren's disease have been reported in the literature, but many did not receive histologic confirmation of the fibromatous origin of the lesion. Matev (1990) reported bilateral involvement of the auricular conchae in a 40-year-old male epileptic patient's ear, with Dupuytren's disease affecting both hands and feet. The lesion involved hard, elastic subcutaneous nodules, adherent to the skin, located in the upper half of the conchae between helix and anthelix. Allen et al. (1955) reported bilateral nodules developing on the superficial aspect of the tensor fascia latae in a patient with plantar lesions. Lettin (1964) noted several nodes of the upper gums, which were hypertrophied in a 24-year-old epileptic woman with bilateral hand and feet involvement. Involvement of the Achilles tendons has also been reported (Hueston, 1977). Wheeler and Meals (1981) described involvement of the popliteal space in the form of a 1 cm mass fixed to deep tissue in a 55-year-old male with involvement of both hands and feet. Histology of the mass was consistent with Dupuytren's disease. Bunnell (1944) mentioned a patient with a subcutaneous band over the anterior shoulder and arm, which was associated with Dupuytren's disease.

References

Allen RA, Woolner LB, Ghormley RK (1955) Soft tissue tumors of the sole – with special reference to plantar fibromatosis. *J Bone Joint Surg* **37A**: 14–26.

Anderson W (1891) Lectures on contracture of the fingers and toes. *Lancet* **ii**: 1.

Andrew JG (1987) Calcification in Dupuytren's disease: a report of two cases. *J Hand Surg* **12B**: 277–78.

Aviles E, Arlen E, Miller T (1971) Plantar fibromatosis. *Surgery* **69**: 117–20.

Boyes JH (1954) Dupuytren's contracture: notes on the age at onset and the relationship to handedness. *Am J Surg* **88**: 147–54.

Boyes JH, Jones FE (1968) Dupuytren's disease involving the volar aspect of the wrist. *Plast Reconstr Surg* **41**: 204–207.

Brouet JP (1986) Etude de 1000 dossiers de maladie de Dupuytren. In: Tubiana R, Hueston JT, eds, *La Maladie de Dupuytren*, 98–105. L'Expansion Scientifique Française, Paris.

Bruner JM (1970) The dynamics of Dupuytren's disease. *Hand* **2**: 172–77.

Bunnell (1944) *Surgery of the Hand.* Lippincott, Philadelphia.

Classen DA, Hurst LN (1992) Plantar fibromatosis and bilateral flexion contractures: a review of the literature. *Ann Plast Surg* **28**: 475–78.

Cleland H, Morisson WA (1986) Dupuytren's disease in the thumb: two cases of a central cord. *J Hand Surg* **11B**: 68–70.

De la Caffinière JY (1986) Travail manuel et maladie de Dupuytren. In: Tubiana R, Hueston JT, eds, *La Maladie de Dupuytren*, 3rd edn, 92–97. L'Expansion Scientifique Française, Paris.

Donato RR, Morrison WA (1996). Dupuytren's disease in the feet causing flexion contractures in the toes. *J Hand Surg* **21B**: 364–66.

Dupuytren G (1832) Rétraction permanente des doigts. In: Dupuytren G, *Leçons orales de clinique chirurgicale faites à l'Hôtel-Dieu de Paris*, 2–24. Germer Baillière, Paris.

Early PF (1962) Population studies in Dupuytren's contracture. *J Bone Joint Surg* **44B**: 602–13.

Fisk G (1985) The relationship of manual labour and specific injury to Dupuytren's disease. In: Hueston JT, Tubiana R, eds, *Dupuytren's Disease*, 2nd edn, 104–105. Churchill Livingstone, Edinburgh.

Gallizia F (1964) A collagen triad: la Peyronie's disease, Dupuytren's disease and fibrosis of the auricular cartilage. *J Urol Nephrol* **70**: 424.

Garrod AE (1893) On an unusual form of nodule upon the joints of the fingers. *St Bartholomew's Hospital Report* **29**: 157–61.

Gordon SD (1964) Dupuytren's contracture: plantar involvement. *Br J Plast Surg* **17**: 421–23.

Haedicke GJ, Sturim HS (1989) Plantar fibromatosis: an isolated disease. *Plast Reconstr Surg* **83**: 296–300.

Hoet F, Boxho J, Decoster E et al. (1983) Dupuytren's contracture – review of 326 operated patients. *Ann Chir Main* **7**: 251–55 (in French, English summary).

Hueston JT (1963) *Dupuytren's Contracture*. Churchill Livingstone, Edinburgh.

Hueston JT (1965) Dupuytren's contracture: the trend to conservatism. *Ann Roy Coll Surg Engl* **36**: 134–51.

Hueston JT (1974) The management of ectopic lesions in Dupuytren's contracture. In: Hueston JT, Tubiana R, (eds), *Dupuytren's Disease* 145–48. Churchill Livingstone, Edinburgh.

Hueston JT (1977) Dupuytren's contracture. In: Converse JM, ed., *Reconstructive Plastic Surgery*, Vol. 6, 3403–27. WB Saunders, Philadelphia.

Hueston JT (1982) Dorsal Dupuytren's disease. *J Hand Surg* **7A**: 384–87.

Hueston JT (1984) Some observations on knuckle pads. *J Hand Surg* **9B**: 75–78.

Hueston JT, Wilson WF (1973) Knuckle pads. *Aust N Z J Surg* **42**: 274.

Iselin F, Cardenas-Baron L, Gouget-Audry I, Peze W (1988) Dorsal Dupuytren's disease. *Ann Chir Main* **7**: 247–50 (in French, English summary).

James JIP, Tubiana R (1952) La maladie de Dupuytren. *Rev Chir Orthop* **38**: 352–406.

Johnson HA (1980) The Hugh Johnson Sign of early Dupuytren's contracture. *Plast Reconstr Surg* **65**: 697.

Kirby J (1849) On an unusual affection of the penis. *Dublin Med Press* **22**: 209–10.

Ledderhose G (1897) Zur Pathologie der Aponevrose des Fusses und der Hand. *Arch Klin Chir* **55**: 694.

Lennox IA, Murali SR, Porter R (1993) A study of the repeatability of the diagnosis of Dupuytren's contracture and its prevalence in the Grampian region. *J Hand Surg* **18B**: 258–61.

Lettin A (1964) Dupuytren's diathesis. *J Bone Joint Surg* **46B**: 220–25.

Ling RSM (1963) The genetic factor in Dupuytren's disease. *J Bone Joint Surg* **45B**: 709–18.

Madelung OW (1875) Die Aetiologie und die operative Behandlung der Dupuytren'schen Fingerver-krümmung. *Berlin-Klin Wochenschr* **12**: 191.

Matev I (1990) Dupuytren's contracture with associated changes in the plantar aponevroses and in the auricular conchae. *Ann Hand Surg* **9**: 379–80.

Mawhinney I, de Frenne H, Tubiana R (1999) Historical, anatomical and clinical aspects of Dupuytren's disease. In: Tubiana R, ed., *The Hand*, 431–83, Vol. V. WB Saunders, Philadelphia.

McFarlane RM (1974) Patterns of diseased fascia in the fingers in Dupuytren's contracture. *Plast Reconstr Surg* **54**: 31.

McFarlane RM (1985) Some observations on the epidemiology of Dupuytren's disease. In: Hueston JT, Tubiana R, eds, *Dupuytren's Disease*, 2nd edn, 122–26. Churchill Livingstone, Edinburgh.

McGrouther DA (1982) The microanatomy of Dupuytren's contracture. *Hand* **14**: 215–36.

McGrouther DA (1986) Anatomie microscopique de la maladie de Dupuytren. In: Tubiana R, Hueston JT, eds, *La Maladie de Dupuytren*, 3rd edn, 32–48. L'Expansion Scientifique Française, Paris.

McIndoe AH, Beare RLB (1958) The surgical management of Dupuytren's contracture. *Am J Surg* **95**: 197–203.

Mikkelsen OA (1977) Knuckle pads in Dupuytren's disease. *Hand* **9**: 301–305.

Mikkelsen OA (1990) Epidemiology of a Norwegian population. In: McFarlane RM, McGrouther DA, Flint MH, eds, *Dupuytren's Disease*, 2nd edn, 191–200. Churchill Livingstone, Edinburgh.

Millesi H (1985) The clinical and morphological course of Dupuytren's disease. In: Hueston JT, Tubiana R, eds, *Dupuytren's Disease*, 2nd edn, 114–21. Churchill Livingstone, Edinburgh.

Pentland AP, Anderson TF (1985) Plantar fibromatosis responds to intralesional steroids. *J Am Acad Dermatol* **12**: 212–14.

Pickren JW, Smith AG, Stevenson TWJ, Stout AP (1951) Fibromatosis of the plantar fascia. *Cancer* **4**: 846.

Reynolds JW, Bostram CF (1975) Plantar fibromatosis: an unusual location. *J Ann Podiatr Assoc* **65**: 154.

Simons AW, Srivastava S, Nancarrow JD (1996) Dupuytren's disease affecting the wrist. *J Hand Surg* **21B**: 367–68.

Short WH, Watson HK (1982) Prediction of the spiral nerve in Dupuytren's contracture. *J Hand Surg* **7A**: 84–86.

Skoog T (1948) Dupuytren's contraction, with special reference to aetiology and improved surgical treatment. *Acta Chirug Scand* **96** (suppl 139): 1.

Touraine A, Ruel H (1945) La polyfibromatose héréditaire. *Ann Dermatol Syphiligr* **5**: 1–5.

Tubiana R (1999) Dupuytren's disease of the radial side of the hand. *Hand Clin* **15**: 149–59.

Tubiana R, Simmons B, de Frenne H (1982) Location of Dupuytren's disease on the radial aspect of the hand. *Clin Orthop* **168**: 222–29.

Viljanto JA (1973) Dupuytren's contracture: a review. *Semin Arthritis Rheum* **3**: 155–76.

Vorstman B, Grossman JA, Gilbert DA et al. (1986) Maladie de La Peyronie. In: Tubiana R, Hueston JT, eds, *La Maladie de Dupuytren*, 3rd edn, 221–25. L'Expansion Scientifique, Paris.

Wheeler ES, Meals RA (1981) Dupuytren's diathesis: a broad-spectrum disease. *Plast Reconstr Surg* **68**: 781–83.

Wylock P, Vansteenland H (1989) Infection associated with a palmar skin pit in recurrent Dupuytren's disease. *J Hand Surg* **14A**: 518–20.

Zachariae L (1971) Dupuytren's contracture. The aetiological role of trauma. *Scand J Plast Reconstr Surg* **5**: 116–19.

ASSESSMENT OF LESIONS

Raoul Tubiana

In recording lesions in Dupuytren's disease, many clinicians use a diagrammatic representation, with nodules being represented by a swirl, and the cords by a series of linear marks. This gives little indication in itself of the extent of contracture and is difficult to put into computerized or typed records.

An objective assessment of the lesions in Dupuytren's disease seems essential for the establishment of a prognosis and the subsequent evaluation of the results of surgery. There have been various scoring systems, but most appear to be based simply on the total angle of contracture (Tonkin et al., 1984). This gives little information on non-contractile disease, the presence of other deformities, recurrence, and an indication of the actual site of the disease. The scoring system developed by Tubiana and Michon (1961) and tested and refined in a series of publications (Tubiana et al., 1967, 1968, 1986; Tubiana, 1996, 1998) attempts to overcome most of these problems. It produces an overall score indicating severity, and indicates not only the degree of individual digital deformity but also the distribution of lesions throughout the hand.

The preoperative assessment described below is very simple and practical and may be used effectively by all physicians and physiotherapists who are presented with Dupuytren's disease. Supplementary indications given later provide further precision, which may help to determine the prognosis and permit objective judgement of operative results. They are especially useful to surgeons.

Preoperative assessment

The hand is divided into five segments, each consisting of a digit and corresponding palmar zone, which includes the pretendinous band of the palmar aponeurosis in the four medial fingers and its adjacent segment of the palmar aponeurosis. The fascia of the thenar eminence and the first web space are part of the thumb segment. For each of these five segments, the distal and palmar aponeurotic lesions are allocated a number corresponding to a certain stage of the disease. Each stage thus represented corresponds to a progression of 45° of the total extension loss of each digit (Tubiana and Michon, 1961).

The finger rays

These total deformities are measured by adding together the individual flexion deformities (deficiency of extension) of the MP, PIP and DIP joints. When there is hyperextension of the DIP, the degree of hyperextension is added to the total flexion deformity of the other joints.

Theoretically, for each finger the range of deformity is from 0° (complete extension) to 200° (contracture of the finger in the palm). Thus six stages can be distinguished for the four fingers (Figure 5.20):

Stage 0 = no lesion;
Stage N = palmar or digital nodule without established flexion deformity;
Stage 1 = total flexion deformity between 0° and 45°;
Stage 2 = total flexion deformity between 45° and 90°;
Stage 3 = total flexion deformity between 90° and 135°;
Stage 4 = total flexion deformity exceeding 135°.

The thumb ray

The fascia of the thenar eminence and the first web space are part of the thumb segment. Thus the thumb score includes both MP and

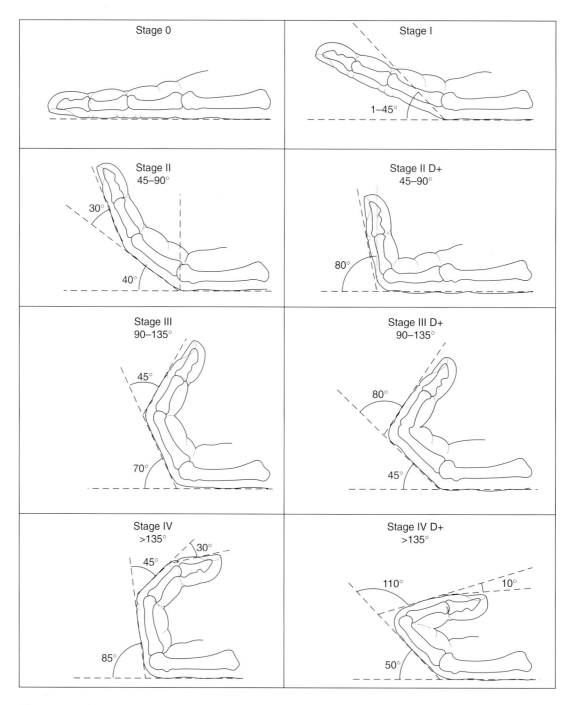

Figure 5.20 Schematic drawing of the different stages of long finger deformity in Dupuytren's disease. Each stage corresponds to a progression of 45° of the total deformation of all the joints of each finger, which may consist of different combinations. D+ indicates a PIP joint contracture of more than 70°.

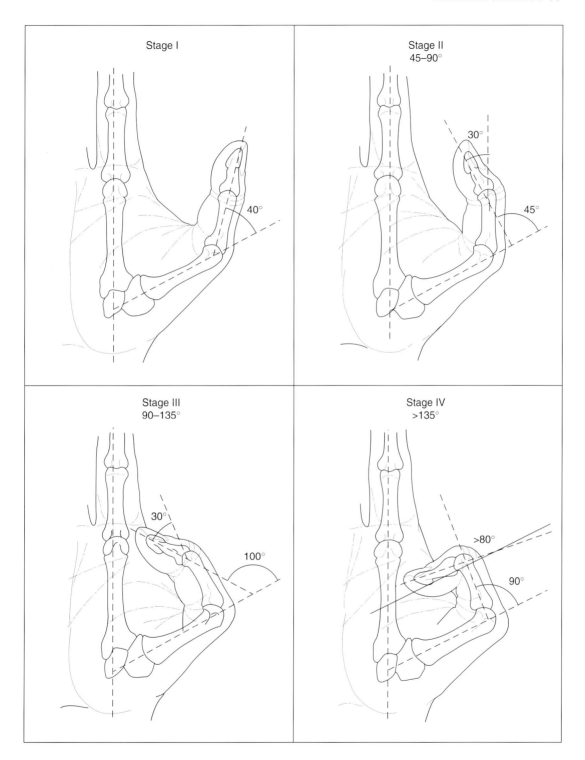

Figure 5.21 Assessment of the range of deformity of the first ray.

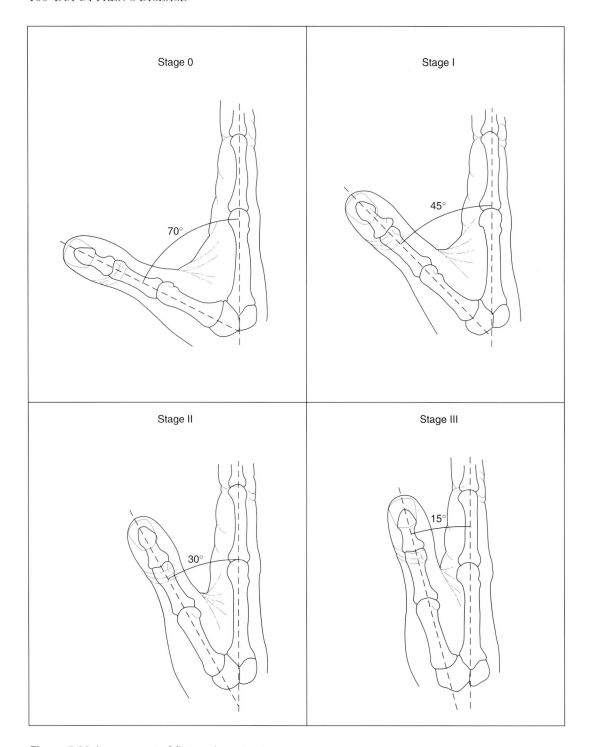

Figure 5.22 Assessment of first web contracture.

interphalangeal (IP) joint contracture and contracture of the thumb web space. MP and IP joint contracture follows the same pattern of increasing stage for each 45° loss of extension (Figure 5.21). Contracture of the thumb web space is assessed by measuring the angle formed by the axes of the first and second metacarpals. When fully separated normally the angle exceeds 45°. Four stages can be distinguished, with each stage corresponding to a loss of 15° (Figure 5.22). Theoretically the thumb's range of deformity is from 0° to 160° for the MP and IP joints, and from 0° to more than 45° at the level of the web. Thus lesions of the thumb ray, which have particular functional consequences, are evaluated by two numbers.

Both hands are systematically coded each time they are examined. The numbered assessment of each gives an accurate clinical record of the disease. Among other advantages, this scoring method also encourages a full examination of each hand and reveals lesions of the radial part of the hand, which often go undetected.

Each ray is individually examined, starting with the thumb. Palmar lesions are identified using the letter P, and digital lesions by D. The letter H indicates fixed hyperextension of the DIP joint. Each of the five rays is represented in turn by a number (or an N) indicating the stage, followed by the appropriate letters. The rays without aponeurotic lesions are indicated by zero. Thus, one can appreciate in a few minutes the number of rays affected, the localization and the severity of the lesion (Figures 5.23 and 5.24). Since the five elements (the five rays) of this evaluation express the spread of the disease and each number signifying the stage expresses the extent of the contracture, it becomes possible to indicate the total state by adding the numbers of each ray. It is necessary to assign a value to nodules without contracture, so the stage N is evaluated at 0.5. The highest possible score is then 23 for each hand, i.e. four fingers and the thumb contracted into the palm (scoring 4 each) and the

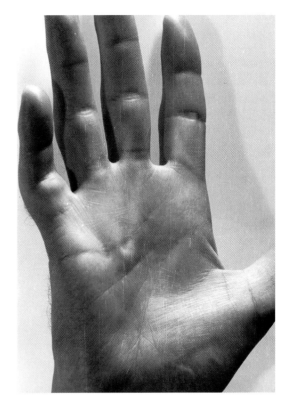

Figure 5.23 RH: OP-OD, O,O, NP, 1D = 1.5. This translates as follows: RH: right hand; OP-OD: no lesion in the thumb ray and in the thumb web; O,O: no lesion in the index and long finger rays; NP: palmar nodule without deformity in the ring finger's segment; 1D: contracture of the little finger, less than 45°; total evaluation: 1 + 0.5 (for the nodule) = 1.5.

thumb web space retracted to the radial side of the palm scoring 3.

Supplementary indications for surgeons

Further indications may be obtained using this method of assessment and these are useful for determining the preoperative prognosis and for evaluating the postoperative results. The author recommends that these more complex supplementary indications only be used by

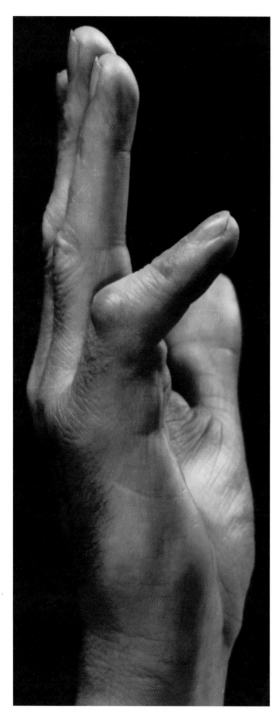

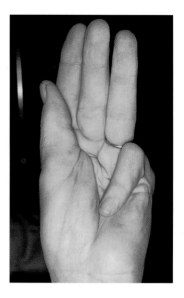

Figure 5.25 LH: 3P-ND,O,O,O, 4PD + H = 7.5. LH: left hand; 3P: contracture of the first web; the angle between the axes of first and second metacarpals is less than 15° (stage 3); ND: no deformity contracture at the MP and IP joints of the thumb, but fibrous tissue lesions (N); O,O,O: no lesions on the second, third and fourth rays; 4PD + H: palmar and digital lesions on the fifth ray; 4: total deformity of all joints of the little finger (MP 70° + IPP 110° + 10° hyperextension of the PID = 190°). D + indicates flexion deformity of more than 70° at the PIP joint. H indicates hyperextension of the PID joint.

people already familiar with this method of preoperative assessment.

It is well known that the presence of a PIP joint contracture has a more severe prognostic importance than a flexion joint contracture at the MP joint, which is easily corrected. The presence of a PIP joint contracture of greater than 70°, with obvious prognostic significance, is indicated by the symbol + after the digital letter (D+) (Figure 5.25).

In addition to the letters P, D, H, N already mentioned, other letters are used for the assessment of an operated hand:

Figure 5.24 RH: OP-OD, O,O,O, 2PD = 2. 2PD: total deformity of all joints of the little finger (MP 20° + IPP 50° = 70° = stage 2).

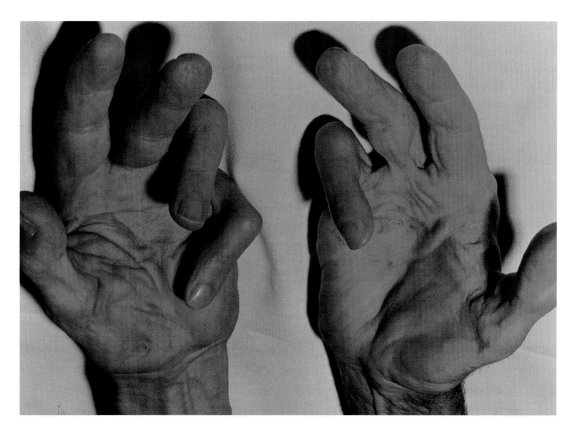

Figure 5.26 LH: 2P-1DG, O, 1D, 3PD+ H, 4PD + H = 11.
2P: contracture first web (35°); 1DG: contracture IP joint (30°); G: skin graft on the thumb proximal phalanx; 0: no lesion on index finger; 1D: contracture proximal phalanx on the long finger (35°); 3PD + H: total deformity of all joints of the ring finger 120° (MP 20° + IPP 90° + IPD 10° hyperextension H); 4PD + H: total deformity of all joints of the little finger 190° (MP 90° + IPP 80° = IPD 20° hyperextension). D+ indicates flexion deformity of more than 70° at the PIP joint of the ring and little fingers.
   RH: OPG - 1DG, 1PDR, 1PDR, 3PD+, A = 10.
OPG: no contracture at the level of the first web, which has been grafted; 1D: 25° contracture at the thumb IP joint; G: proximal phalanx of the thumb has been grafted; 1PDR: 30° contracture on the index finger (R: recurrence); PR: recurrence of the disease in the palm that has been previously operated on; 1PDR: 40° contracture on the long finger (R: recurrence); 3PD: total deformity of all joints of the ring finger 130° (MP 40° + IPP 90°); A: amputation of the little finger (four points).

G   = a skin graft;
R   = a recurrence of the disease in a previously operated area;
E   = an extension of the disease in a non-operated area;
A   = a finger amputation;
AZ = an arthrodesis;
F   = a postoperative limitation of joint flexion (the location and degree should be given precisely in the clinical record).

Finally, using this staging system it is possible to produce a single score for each finger, and for the hand as a whole. Each stage is given a score. A nodule without retraction, N, is given 0.5; a digital amputation, A, = 4; a joint arthrodesis, AZ, = 3 (Figure 5.26).

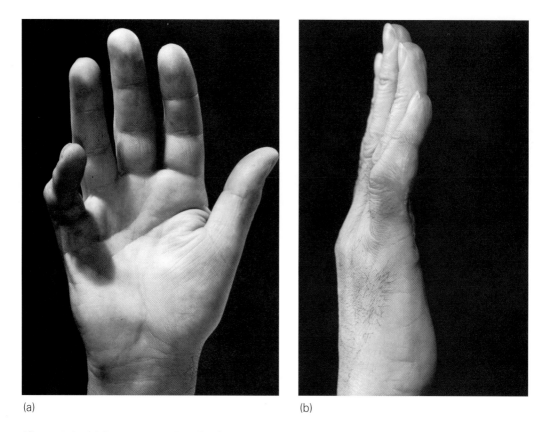

(a)   (b)

Figure 5.27 (a) Preoperative: RH: OP-OD, O,O,O, 3PD + = 3. 3PD +: total deformity of all joints of the little finger 100° (MP 25° + IPP 75°). (b) Postoperative: RH: OP-OD, O,O,O, 1DR = 1, where 1DR means 1:30° IPP contracture and DR is digital recurrence. The operative gain is of 2 points.

After operation, the evaluation is recalculated, giving evidence of the benefits for each finger (Figures 5.27 and 5.28). A new summary is obtained by adding the figures of the new formula. Both hands are routinely scored at each clinic attendance and before and after any surgical intervention. This allows the surgeon to have an accurate clinical record of the disease, to follow the progression of the disease (Figures 5.29 and 5.30) and evaluate the results of any operation. By comparing the pre- and postoperative values, an objective evaluation of the gain in extension can be easily obtained.

The system is practical to use, once one is familiar with it, despite the initial apparent complexity, and is recorded in two short formulae. For statistical purposes, it is the author's practice to classify under the heading 'severe' (S), either those cases with a total preoperative score of 8 or more, or those with a score of less than 8 but with a single ray scoring D+.

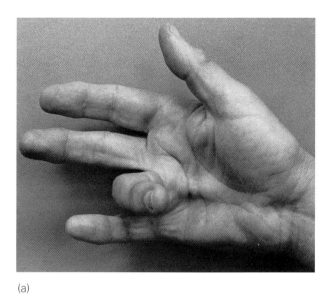

(a)

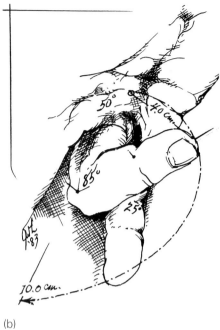

(b)

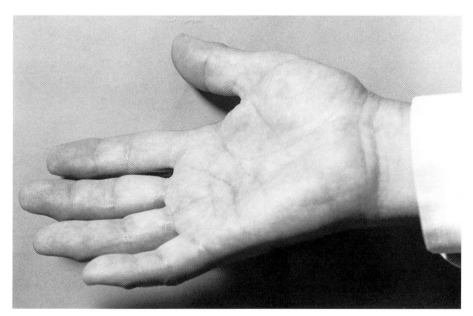

(c)

Figure 5.28 Dr Littler's patient.
(a) Preoperative: RH: OP-OD, O,O, 4PD +, 1 = 5. (b) Littler's drawing showing the joint's contracture:
4PD +: total deformity of all joints of the ring finger: 135° (MP 50° + IPP 85°): PD: lesions are palmar
and digital; D +: flexion deformity of more than 70° at the PIP joint. 1: 25° contracture on the 5th ray.
(c) Five years later: RH: OP-OD, O,O,O,O = O. The improvement is of 5 points.

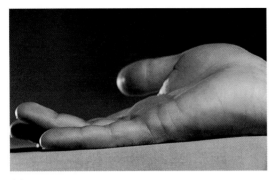

(a)

Figure 5.29 Evolution of a rare form of the disease involving only the digits.
(a) RH: OP-OD, O,O, 1D, O = 1. (b) Seven years later: RH: OP, ND, O, 1D, 2D, 3D = 6.5.
OP-ND: no contracture of the first web, a nodule at the base of the thumb without contracture of the thumb's joints (0.5); O: no lesion on the index ray; 1D: contracture of the long finger, less than 45°; 2D: contracture of the ring finger, less than 90°; 3D: total deformity of all joints of little finger ray = 110° (PIP 70° = PID 40°).

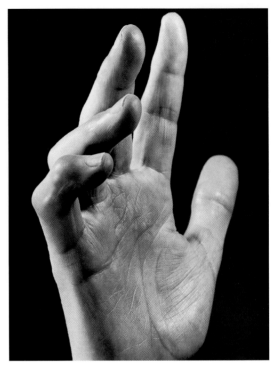

(b)

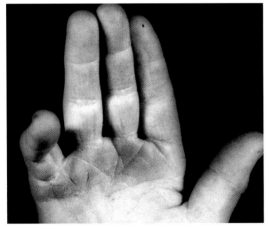

(a)

Figure 5.30 (a) Preoperative view: RH: OP-OD, O, O, O, 3PD = 3. (b) Seven years later: RH: 3PE-2DE, O, O, 1DR = 6.
3PE - 2DE: severe contracture on the radial aspect of the hand; 1DR: recurrence on the little finger with moderate contracture at the PIP joint. Contracture increase of 3 points.

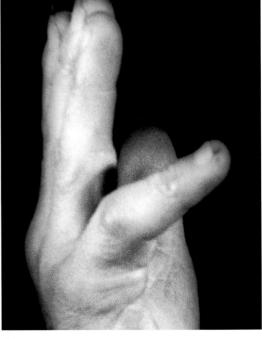

(b)

References

Tonkin MA, Burke FD, Varian JPW (1984) Dupuytren's contracture: a comparative study of fasciectomy and dermofasciectomy in 100 patients. *J Hand Surg* **9B**: 156–62.

Tubiana R (1986) Evaluation des déformations dans la maladie de Dupuytren. In: Tubiana R, Hueston JT, eds, *La Maladie de Dupuytren*, 3rd edn, 111–14. L'Expansion Scientifique Française, Paris.

Tubiana R (1996) Evaluation des lésions dans la maladie de Dupuytren. *Main* **1**, 3–11.

Tubiana R (1998) Dupuytren's disease. Surgical treatment. In: Tubiana R, ed., *The Hand*, Vol. 5, 442–48. WB Saunders, Philadelphia.

Tubiana R, Michon J (1961) Classification de la maladie de Dupuytren. *Mem Acad Chir* **87**: 886–87.

Tubiana R, Thomine J-M, Brown S (1967) Complications in surgery of Dupuytren's contracture. *Plast Reconstr Surg* **39**: 603–12.

Tubiana R, Michon J, Thomine J-M (1968) Scheme for the assessment of deformities in Dupuytren's disease. *Surg Clin North Am* **48**, 979.

Tubiana R, Thomine J-M, Mackin E (1996) *Examination of the Hand and Wrist*. Martin Dunitz, London.

ASSOCIATED CONDITIONS

Caroline Leclercq

Diabetes mellitus

As suggested simultaneously by two French authors as early as 1883 (Cayla, 1883; Viger, 1883), there is a prevalence of diabetes mellitus in Dupuytren's disease and, reciprocally, there is a prevalence of Dupuytren's disease in diabetes mellitus. It is difficult, however, to ascertain an accurate rate for each of these, as figures vary greatly in the literature. For instance, if one looks at diabetic populations in the literature, incidence of Dupuytren's disease in these populations varies from 2–63%. This may be explained by the frequency of mild cases of Dupuytren's disease in diabetes, limited to palmar nodules, which may be overlooked when examined by non-specialist physicians.

Large series of patients with diabetes who were specifically examined for Dupuytren's symptoms have revealed incidences of 17.5% (Merle, 1970; 200 patients); 18% (Quintana Guitian, 1988; 200 patients); 21.5% (Montenero et al., 1965; 1816 patients); 24.4% (von Paeslack, 1962; 475 patients); and 32% (Schneider, 1964; 716 patients). Table 5.2 gives a breakdown of these figures according to gender, which demonstrates higher rates for men. Finally a large survey of the literature by Fossati et al. (1982) has shown an incidence of 21% in 3534 patients with diabetes.

These figures, when compared with the global prevalence of Dupuytren's disease in today's Caucasian population, which is estimated at between 3 and 6%, show that Dupuytren's disease occurs three to four times more frequently in patients with diabetes.

The most accurate figures, however, come from those series in which the authors have compared groups of patients with and without diabetes, who were matched for age and sex (von Paeslack, 1962; Merle, 1970; Chammas et al., 1995). These series tend to demonstrate that the incidence of Dupuytren's disease is four times larger in patients with diabetes than in the general population, except for von Paeslack's series, where the incidence is only twice as great, but his series is probably biased by the fact that he included only patients aged 45 and over.

Similarly, if one looks at Dupuytren's disease populations, the incidence of diabetes mellitus also varies considerably from series to series. This is partly due to the diagnostic criteria of diabetes: only clinical diabetes was included in some studies, while in others a 2-hour glucose loading test was performed systematically, and 'pre-diabetic' patients were included. Wegmann (1966), who studied 268 Dupuytren's patients, found that 12.8% had diabetes, and Quintana Guitian (1988, 398 patients) found 5%, whereas Merle (1970), who performed glucose-loading tests on 61 Dupuytren's patients found 19.6% had diabetes. McFarlane, in his multicenter study (1985), found only 8% had diabetes, but states

Table 5.2 Incidence of Dupuytren's disease in diabetic patients.

Author	No. diabetic patients	Total patients with DD (%)	Men with DD (%)	Women with DD (%)
Merle, 1970	200	17.5	24.7	6.3
Montenero et al., 1965	1 816	21.5	25.5	18.7
Quintana Guitian, 1988	200	18.0	38.0	3.4
Von Paeslack, 1962	475	24.4	36.0	19.5

DD: Dupuytren's disease.

that this figure is questionable as the incidence of both Dupuytren's disease and diabetes varies greatly around the world, and as the diagnosis of diabetes was based on history only.

Dupuytren's disease in patients with diabetes is usually mild, non-progressive and limited to palmar nodules. The fingers most commonly involved are the long and ring fingers, rather than ring and little as in the general population (Fossati et al., 1982; Noble et al., 1984; Chammas et al., 1995). Some authors have stressed that occurrence in the little finger, and in women, although less frequent, is often more severe. The prevalence of Dupuytren's disease is significantly correlated to increasing age of the patient, and duration of diabetes (Figure 5.31), but it is not correlated with the type of diabetes (insulin dependent or non-insulin dependent). There is often a co-existing limitation of finger joint motion unrelated to contracted aponeurotic tissues (Lawson et al., 1983; Jennings et al., 1989; Chammas et al., 1995) and a modification of thickness and texture of the skin described as 'thick waxy palmar skin' by Hurst and Badalamente (1990). Skin biopsies from these tissues have shown increased non-enzymatic glycosylation compared with controls (Knowles, 1981) but more recent studies have shown this increase to be present in patients with diabetes even without limited joint mobility. As a result of this finding, it has been suggested that limited joint mobility may be a 'vascular related phenomenon of aging' (Larkin and Frier, 1986). Interestingly, it has also been demonstrated that fibroblasts from people with diabetes show characteristics of accelerated aging (Rowe et al., 1977).

Merle and Merle (1986) stress the high incidence of complications after surgery in patients with diabetes (hematoma, skin slough, delayed healing) and report a postoperative incidence of reflex sympathetic dystrophy eight times larger in women when they have diabetes.

The reason why Dupuytren's disease is more frequent in patients with diabetes is not

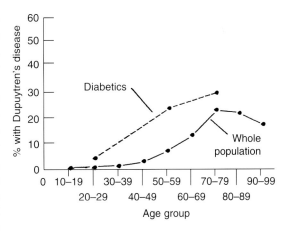

Figure 5.31 Incidence (%) of Dupuytren's disease versus age in the diabetic population. Data from several authors and a general (normal) population. (Mikkelsen, 1979; reproduced with permission from Hurst and Badalamente, 1990.)

yet known. A combined genetic predisposition has been suggested (von Paeslack, 1962; Noble et al., 1984). Others have discussed the possibility that the metabolic and biochemical changes of diabetes, such as diabetic microangiopathy, cause or promote the onset of Dupuytren's disease (Hurst and Badalamente, 1990), and Montenero et al. (1965) have noted an increased incidence of Dupuytren's disease related to the vascular complications of diabetes and diabetic neuropathy.

Epilepsy

In 1941, Lund had noted that epilepsy and Dupuytren's disease were often associated. Skoog (1948), studying 207 patients with epilepsy treated in a specialized center, found a very high incidence of Dupuytren's disease of 42%. Although this association was later denied by Gordon (1954) and Arieff and Bell (1956), it was later confirmed by Early (1962). In 1960, Hueston examined 124 patients with epilepsy in an institution, and 35% had evidence of Dupuytren's disease, with a high incidence in both sexes under 40 years of age (men 43%, women 18%). In a similar institution Quintana Guitian (1988) found a percentage of Dupuytren's disease of only 11% in 82 patients with epilepsy, but his report seems to indicate that he reviewed only the charts, not the patients. Winslow and Suk (unpublished data, reported by Pojer et al., 1972), in a study of 1934 epileptics, found an incidence of Dupuytren's disease of approximately 20%, and Pojer et al. (1972) found an incidence of 55% in 65 patients with epilepsy of long standing.

The incidence of epilepsy in Dupuytren's patients is 2–3% in most series (James, 1985; McFarlane, 1985; Murrell and Hueston, 1990; Quintana Guitian, 1988), whereas it is reported to be 0.8% (McFarlane, 1985) to 1.8% (Fairfield, 1954) in the general population. A much higher incidence has been reported in a single work by Thieme (reported by James, 1974), who examined 131 Dupuytren's patients and their first-degree relatives in Edinburgh, with a total of 371 patients involved, and who found an incidence of epilepsy of 8.6%. This may be related to the familial recruitment of the patients.

The incidence of Dupuytren's disease in patients with epilepsy is not correlated with the frequency or severity of the seizures, nor with the age of onset of epilepsy, type of electroencephalogram (EEG) changes or the type of drug therapy. It is, however, correlated with age and duration of epilepsy (Hurst and Badalamente, 1990) (Figure 5.32).

The correlation between epilepsy and Dupuytren's disease is statistically significant (Brenner et al., 1994), suggesting a linkage or causative relationship between the two diseases. This is further supported by the work of Zachariae et al. (1970) reporting that EEGs of Danish patients with Dupuytren's disease but without epilepsy were abnormal in 50% of the patients (which is higher than in a normal control group).

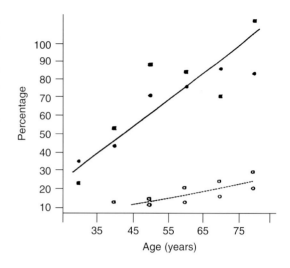

Figure 5.32 Incidence (%) of Dupuytren's disease versus age in a population with epilepsy (unbroken line) and a general (normal) population for comparison (dashed line). (Reproduced with permission from Hurst and Badalamente, 1990.)

Also, Stuhler et al. (1977) demonstrated in the region of Lower Saxony (Germany) that Dupuytren's disease is more common in idiopathic than in post-traumatic epilepsy. However, population studies did not show a prevalence of epilepsy in first-degree relatives of Dupuytren's disease patients, nor a prevalence of Dupuytren's disease in first-degree relatives of patients with epilepsy. Therefore it seems that there is no genetic linkage between these two conditions (Thieme, quoted by James, 1985; Hurst and Badalamente, 1990).

Arafa et al. (1992) also questioned this correlation, which they showed to be positive only in patients over 50 years. They did not find a higher incidence of the disease in patients with epilepsy, but found the disease to be more severe in those *with* rather than those *without* epilepsy.

Phenobarbital has also been incriminated in the occurrence of Dupuytren's disease

(Lund, 1941; Skoog, 1948; Fröscher and Hoffmann, 1983), and Critchley et al. (1976) have suggested that phenobarbital may cause the release of peripheral growth factors, which may affect the myofibroblasts. However, the matter remains controversial (Pojer et al., 1972; James, 1985; Brenner et al., 1994).

Dupuytren's disease in patients with epilepsy is usually bilateral and roughly symmetrical. It follows a course similar to the usual picture (Skoog, 1948; Stuhler et al., 1977).

Alcoholism

The relationship between Dupuytren's disease and alcoholism was outlined in 1938 by Shaunann. Examination of patients with liver disease by Wolfe et al. (1956), Hueston (1960), Pojer (Pojer and Jedlickova, 1970; Pojer et al., 1972), and Aron (1977) have shown a high incidence of Dupuytren's disease, from 25% to 66%, and Hueston (1960) showed that incidence of Dupuytren's disease in patients with liver disease from alcoholism was significantly higher (44%) than in those with a non-alcoholic liver disease (18.8%).

Attali et al. (1987) performed a prospective study of 432 consecutive patients hospitalized in a gastroenterology unit, with a control group of 174, to establish the prevalence and possible relationship of Dupuytren's disease with alcohol consumption and chronic liver disease. They concluded that Dupuytren's disease is not correlated with chronic liver disease, but found a positive correlation between the severity of Dupuytren's disease and total alcohol consumption. This confirms previous work by Bradlow and Mowat (1986) who found a positive correlation between Dupuytren's disease in men and heavy drinking but state that the mechanism of this correlation remains unknown.

Pojer and Jedlickova (1970) wondered if there were some liver disturbance in Dupuytren's patients. They selected two groups of patients: a group of 90, randomly selected from 750 patients operated on for Dupuytren's disease, and a group of 35, hospitalized for different reasons, in which Dupuytren's disease was found at random (usually in the form merely of a palmar nodule). They performed laboratory investigations and found in both groups a significant increase of leucine aminopeptidase (LAP) and glutamyl transpeptidase (GGTP), along with a frequent but non-significant increase in alkaline phosphatase. These results indicate a conspicuous disturbance of enzymes, suggesting a latent liver injury in Dupuytren's disease patients, independently of alcohol consumption, which is in contradiction to the results of the two studies mentioned above.

Searching for a pathogenic linkage between Dupuytren's disease and alcoholism, Aron (1977) has looked for HLA groups, but failed to find any difference from a control group. This would indicate absence of a genetic link between these two conditions.

Dupuytren's disease and trauma

Occupation

It has long been debated whether Dupuytren's disease is linked to heavy manual labor. Dupuytren himself attributed the palmar lump to pressure in those who, in their activity, make the palm a 'point d'appui'. This has even gained a certain medicolegal stature in the theory of aggravation or acceleration on the basis of occupation (Moorhead, 1953).

Skoog, in 1948, observed at the margin of nodules microscopic ruptures of the collagen fibers of the palmar fascia and hemosiderin deposits within the cellular areas, which, he believed, were evidence of previous small hemorrhages. He suggested that longitudinal stretching of the palmar aponeurosis could produce traumatic microruptures of the longitudinal fibers, which would, in turn, stimulate hypertrophic repair of the aponeurosis, with development of a contracture.

Larsen et al. (1960) reproduced Skoog's microscopic examination of Dupuytren's specimens, and found abrupt termination of collagen fibers at the edge of areas of cellular proliferation, suggestive of microruptures. However, this is in contrast with the work of Nezelof and Tubiana (1958), whose specimens were sectioned and prepared in the same manner, and who did not find any fiber interruption.

Furthermore, Larsen et al. (1960) produced experimental scarification of the palmar and plantar fascia of monkeys, and found that the proliferative reaction observed in the first 3 months resembled Dupuytren's disease both macroscopically and microscopically. However, by the ninth month, the lesion resembled a mature scar, with a decrease in vascularity and hemosiderin pigments, and the authors had no assurance that the lesion would progress to the formation of a contracture, even if the lesion were reproduced repeatedly over a long period of time.

More recently, MacKenney (1983) lent further support to this microtraumatic theory as he found a positive correlation between repeated stretching of the palmar fascia and the presence of Dupuytren's disease in a group of 36 Dupuytren's patients within a population of 919 patients examined in a rural area. However, this correlation was significant only in those patients whose disease was confined to the palm, and the authors failed to explain why it was not significant in the more severe palmodigital forms.

Two studies, by Flint and McGrouther (1990), and by Bergenudd et al. (1993) have recently demonstrated a reduction of subcutaneous fat tissue, including in the palm, in Dupuytren's patients, and they state that the risk of damaging the palmar fascia with repeated trauma is probably increased in these subjects.

Hueston (1987), who does not support this traumatic theory, correctly stresses that any study of correlation of Dupuytren's disease with manual labor should include a break-down of age, sex and race in the affected workers, together with the prevalence of the condition in a non-manual population, all of which do not appear in any of the above mentioned series.

Fisk (1974) also questions this theory because of the bilaterality of the disease without evidence of a more frequent involvement of the dominant hand, and because of the ectopic lesions, which this theory does not account for.

Moorhead (1953) also stresses that Dupuytren's disease usually affects the ulnar border of the hand, whereas it is the thumb, index and middle fingers that most often participate in manual effort.

Finally, studies of large population groups have generally failed to find any difference between the prevalence of Dupuytren's disease in manual laborers and clerical workers (Hueston, 1960; Early, 1962; Zachariae, 1971; Fisk, 1974; Quintana Guitian, 1988; Bergenudd et al., 1993) with the exception of two surveys. One, by Mikkelsen (1976), who examined 11 000 inhabitants of a small Norwegian town, concluded that Dupuytren's disease was commoner in manual workers (but his study was severely criticized by Hueston (1988) for excluding part of the town's population, and moreover for excluding patients with a specific injury to the hand). Another survey, by de la Caffinière et al. (1983) of 5206 ironworkers reported a positive correlation between long-duration heavy manual work (25 years or more) and the occurrence of the disease (but these long-duration manual workers were also aging men, which is the target group for Dupuytren's disease, and there was no control group in the study).

Trauma

A single episode of injury can be followed, within weeks or months, by the appearance of Dupuytren's disease. This injury is not necessarily a penetrating wound in the palm or fingers, but can equally be a fracture around the wrist or hand, a burn, a crush injury, or a more proximal trauma (shoulder dislocation) or even elective surgery of the upper limb (Wroblewski, 1973). Hueston (1987) underlines the role of edema, and reports a study by Plewes (1956) of chronically swollen hands, from many different causes, that shows a high incidence of Dupuytren's disease.

This precipitating or aggravating role of trauma has been recognized for a long time (James and Tubiana, 1952; Clarkson, 1961; Hueston, 1968; Fisk, 1974). Morley (quoted by Clarkson, 1961) described the most impressive evidence: out of 122 consecutive RAF pilots with Dupuytren's disease, he found a definite history of injury to the palm with an almost immediate onset of Dupuytren's disease in 25 cases.

More recently, while studying the hand complications of Colle's fractures, Stewart et al. (1985) found an incidence of Dupuytren's disease of 4% at 3 months post-trauma, and of 11% at 6 months. All cases were mild, limited to a palmar or digital nodule in more than half of the patients. When reviewed again at an average time of 20.7 months post-fracture, the disease had not progressed significantly in any patient, and had even regressed in two. This condition occurred in patients significantly older than those who did not develop it.

Miscellaneous

Many conditions have been found to be associated with Dupuytren's disease, and several have been believed to be responsible for it over the years. Although many of these associations, such as gout, rheumatism, coronary failure, tuberculosis and degenerative conditions, have later been shown to be of no significance, some are worth mentioning.

1) The presence of a palmaris longus tendon has been shown by Powell et al. (1986) to be significantly more frequent in Dupuytren's disease patients than in a control group with normal hands.

2) Men with Dupuytren's disease have significantly less subcutaneous fat tissue, as measured by a triceps skinfold index, than the general population (Flint and McGrouther, 1990; Bergenudd et al., 1993).

3) The frequency of blood group A has been reported to be higher than normal in Dupuytren's patients (von Speiser and Millesi, 1964). This has been confirmed by Medori in his thesis (1982), but not by Mikkelsen (1967) in a work specifically on Dupuytren's disease and blood groups. An earlier work, by Graubard (1954), had shown 80 patients with Dupuytren's disease to have the same Rhesus blood group.

4) Arcus cornealis senilis has been shown to be more frequent in patients with Dupuytren's disease (Hillemand et al., 1975; Caroli et al., 1992). The latter authors studied a population of 336 patients treated surgically for Dupuytren's disease, aged between 34 and 84 years (average 59.9 years) and observed a corneal arc in 77.1%. Owing to the significant correlation between corneal arc and hyperlipidemia, they tested serum cholesterol and triglycerides in all 336 patients, and this revealed a dyslipidemia in 184 patients (54.8%), 156 of whom had a corneal arc. The authors suggest that a lipid disorder may be a common etiopathogenic factor to corneal arc and Dupuytren's disease. However, their study fails to compare this group with a group of similar age not affected by Dupuytren's disease.

5) Dupuytren's disease seems to be more frequent in AIDS patients (Bower et al., 1990). No significant correlation was found either with related infections or with the type of medical treatment, or the rate of p24 antibodies. The authors

suggest that an increased release of free radicals may be involved. However, another study performed also in the UK failed to confirm any such prevalence (French et al., 1990).

6) No correlation seems to exist between Dupuytren's disease and cigarette smoking, as shown by Fraser-Moodie (1976), but this is in contradiction to a more recent work by An et al. (1988).

7) Patients with rheumatoid arthritis were found by Arafa et al. (1992) to have a statistically significant lower incidence of Dupuytren's disease than a control group matched for sex and age.

8) A recent paper by Mikkelsen et al. (1999) indicates an increased mortality in Dupuytren's patients.

References

An HS, Southworth SR, Jackson WT et al. (1988) Cigarette smoking and Dupuytren's contracture of the hand. *J Hand Surg* **13A**: 872–74.

Arafa L, Noble J, Royle SG et al. (1992) Dupuytren's and epilepsy revisited. *J Hand Surg* **17B**: 221–24.

Arieff AJ, Bell J (1956) Epilepsy and Dupuytren's contracture. *Neurology* **6**: 115–17.

Aron E (1977) Maladie de Dupuytren et alcoolisme chronique – recherche d'un lien pathogenique groupes HLA. *Sem Hop Paris* **53**: 139.

Attali P, Ink O, Pelletier G et al. (1987) Dupuytren's contracture, alcohol consumption, and chronic liver disease. *Arch Int Med* **147**: 1065–67.

Bergenudd H, Lindgarde F, Nilson BE (1993) Prevalence of Dupuytren's contracture and its correlation with degenerative changes of the hands and feet and with criteria of general health. *J Hand Surg* **18B**: 254–57.

Bower M, Nelson M, Gazzard BG (1990) Dupuytren's contracture in patients infected with HIV. *BMJ* **300**: 164–65.

Bradlow A, Mowat AG (1986) Dupuytren's contracture and alcohol. *Ann Rheum Dis* **45**: 304–307.

Brenner P, Mailänder P, Berger A (1994) Epidemiology of Dupuytren's disease. In: Berger A et al., eds, *Dupuytren's Disease*, 244–54. Springer Verlag, Berlin.

Caroli A, Marcuzzi A, Pasquali-Ronchetti I et al. (1992) Correlation between Dupuytren's disease and arcus cornealis senilis: is dyslipidaemia a common aetiopathogenic factor? *Ann Chir Main* **11**: 314–19 (in French, English summary).

Cayla A (1883) Diabète et rétraction de l'aponévrose palmaire. *J Hebdo Med* **20**: 770.

Chammas M, Bousquet P, Renard E et al. (1995) Dupuytren's disease, carpal tunnel syndrome, trigger finger, and diabetes mellitus. *J Hand Surg* **20**: 109–14.

Clarkson P (1961) The aetiology of Dupuytren's disease. *Guy Hosp Rep* **110**: 52–62.

Critchley EMR, Vakil SD, Hayward HW, Owen VMH (1976) Dupuytren disease in epilepsy: result of prolonged administration of anticonvulsants. *J Neurol Neurosurg Psychiatr* **39**: 498.

De la Caffinière JY (1983) Travail manuel et maladie de Dupuytren. Résultat d'une enquête informatisée en milieu sidérurgique. *Ann Chir Main* **2**: 66–72.

Early PF (1962) Population studies in Dupuytren's contracture. *J Bone Joint Surg* **44B**: 602–13.

Fairfield L (1954) *Epilepsy*. Duckworth, London.

Fisk G (1974) The relationship of trauma to Dupuytren's contracture. In: Hueston JT, Tubiana R, eds, *Dupuytren's Disease*, 43–44. Churchill Livingstone, Edinburgh.

Flint M, McGrouther D (1990) Is Dupuytren's disease a connective tissue response? In: McFarlane R, McGrouther D, Flint M, eds, *Dupuytren's Disease. Biology and Treatment*, Vol. 5, 282–87. Churchill Livivingstone, Edinburgh.

Fossati P, Romon M, Vennin Ph (1982) Maladie de Dupuytren et diabète sucré. *Ann Chir Main* **1**: 353–54.

Fraser-Moodie A (1976) Dupuytren's contracture and cigarette smoking. *Br J Plast Surg* **29**: 214–15.

French PD, Kitchen VS, Harris JRW (1990) Prevalence of Dupuytren's contracture in patients infected with HIV. *BMJ* **301**: 967.

Fröscher W, Hoffmann F (1983) Dupuytrensche Kontraktur und Phenobarbitaleinrahme bei Epilepsie-Patienten. *Nervenarzt* **54**: 413–19.

Gordon S (1954) Dupuytren's contracture: the significance of various factors in its etiology. *Ann Surg* **140**: 683.

Graubard DJ (1954) *J Int Coll Surg* **21**: 15, cited in Hueston JT (1963) *Dupuytren's Contracture*, 15. Churchill Livingstone, Edinburgh.

Hillemand B, Joly JP, Huet P et al. (1975) Anomalies palmaires, maladie de Dupuytren et arc cornéen. *Sem Hop Paris* **51**: 2001–10.

Hueston JT (1960) The incidence of Dupuytren's contracture. *Med J Aust* **2**: 999–1002.

Hueston JT (1968) Dupuytren's contracture and specific injury. *Med J Aust* **1**: 1084.

Hueston JT (1987) Dupuytren's contracture: medicolegal aspects. *Med J Aust* **147** (suppl): S1–S11.

Hueston JT (1988) Dupuytren's contracture. *Curr Orthop* **2**: 173–78.

Hurst LC, Badalamente M (1990) Associated diseases. In: McFarlane RM, McGrouther DA, Flint MH, eds, *Dupuytren's Disease*, 253–60. Churchill Livingstone, Edinburgh.

James JIP (1974) The genetic pattern of Dupuytren's contracture and idiopathic epilepsy. In: Hueston JT, Tubiana R, eds, *Dupuytren's Disease*, 37–42. Churchill Livingstone, Edinburgh.

James JIP (1985) The genetic pattern of Dupuytren's contracture and idiopathic epilepsy. In: Hueston JT, Tubiana R, eds, *Dupuytren's Disease*, 94–99. Churchill Livingstone, Edinburgh.

James JIP, Tubiana R (1952) La maladie de Dupuytren. *Rev Chir Orthop* **38**: 352–406.

Jennings AM, Milner PC, Ward JD (1989) Hand abnormalities in Type II diabetes. *Diabet Med* **6**: 43–47.

Knowles HB (1981) Joint contractures, waxy skin, and control of diabetes. *N Engl J Med* **305**: 217.

Larkin JG, Frier BM (1986) Limited joint mobility and Dupuytren's contracture in diabetic, hypertensive, and normal population. *BMJ* **292**: 1494.

Larsen RD, Takagishi N, Posch JL (1960) The pathogenesis of Dupuytren's contracture. *J Bone Joint Surg* **42A**: 993–1007.

Lawson PM, Maneschi F, Fohner EM (1983) The relationship of hand abnormalities to diabetes and diabetic retinopathy. *Diabetes Care* **6**: 140–43.

Lund M (1941) Dupuytren's contracture and epilepsy. *Acta Psychiatr Neurol* **16**: 465–91.

MacKenney RP (1983) A population study of Dupuytren's contracture. *Hand* **15**: 155–61.

McFarlane R (1985) Some observations on the epidemiology of Dupuytren's disease. IN: Hueston JT, Tubiana R, eds, *Dupuytren's Disease*, 122–28. Churchill Livingstone, Edinburgh.

Medori C (1982) Résultats chirurgicaux de 80 mains atteintes de maladie de Dupuytren revues avec un recul moyen de 5 ans. Thesis, Paris.

Merle M, Merle S (1986) Maladie de Dupuytren et diabète. In: Tubiana R, Hueston JT, eds, *La Maladie de Dupuytren*, 90–91. L'Expansion Scientifique Française, Paris.

Merle S (1970) Maladie de Dupuytren et diabète. Thesis, Nancy.

Mikkelsen OA (1967) Dupuytren's disease and blood groups. *Scand J Plast Reconstr Surg* **1**: 148–49.

Mikkelsen OA (1976) Dupuytren's disease – a study of the pattern of distribution and stage of contracture in the hand. *Hand* **8**; 265–71.

Mikkelsen OA, Hoyeraal HM, Sandvik L (1999) Increased mortality in Dupuytren's disease. *J Hand Surg* **24B**: 515–18.

Montenero P, Colleti A, Fabri G (1965) *Maladie de Dupuytren et diabète*. Journées annuelles de Diabétologie de l'Hôtel-Dieu. 75–87. Flammarion, Paris.

Moorhead JJ (1953) Trauma and Dupuytren's contracture. *Am J Surg* **85**: 352–58.

Murrell GAC, Hueston JT (1990) Aetiology of Dupuytren's contracture. *Aust N Z J Surg* **60**: 247–52.

Nezelof G, Tubiana R (1958) La maladie de Dupuytren: étude histologique. *Sem Hop Paris* **34**: 1102–10.

Noble J, Heathcote JG, Cohen H (1984) Diabetes mellitus in the aetiology of Dupuytren's disease. *J Bone Joint Surg* **66B**: 322–25.

Plewes L (1956) Sudeks's atrophy in the hand. *J Bone Joint Surg* **38B**: 195.

Pojer J, Jedlickova J (1970) Enzymatic pattern of liver injury in Dupuytren's contracture. *Acta Med Scand* **187**: 101–104.

Pojer J, Radivojevic M, William TF (1972) Dupuytren's disease – its association with abnormal liver function in alcoholism and epilepsy. *Arch Intern Med* **129**: 561–66.

Powell BW, McLean NR, Jeffs JV (1986) The incidence of a palmaris longus tendon in patients with Dupuytren's disease. *J Hand Surg* **11B**: 382–84.

Quintana Guitian A (1988) Epidemiological features of Dupuytren's disease. *Ann Chir Main* **7**: 256–62 (in French).

Rowe DW, Starman BJ, Fujimoto WY, Williams RH (1977) Abnormalities in proliferation and protein synthesis in fibroblast cultures from patients with diabetes mellitus. *Diabetes* **26**: 284.

Schneider (1964) Dupuytren's contracture in diabetes mellitus. Personal communication. Vth congress of International Diabetes Federation, Toronto, Canada.

Shaunann (1938) Uber die pathogenese des lupus erythematosus. *Acta Derm Venereol* **1**: 545.

Skoog T (1948) Dupuytren's contraction, with special reference to aetiology and improved surgical treatment. *Acta Chir Scand* **96** (suppl 139): 1.

Stewart HD, Innes AR, Burke FD (1985) The hand complications of Colle's fracture. *J Hand Surg* **10B**: 103.

Stuhler T, Stankovic P, Ritter G, Schmulde E (1977) Epilepsie und Dupuytren'sche Kontraktur. *Hand Chir Mikrochir Plast Chir* **9**: 219–23.

Viger J (1883) De la rétraction de l'aponévrose palmaire chez les diabétiques. Thèse no. 1883/57, Paris.

Von Paeslack (1962) Dupuytren's contracture and diabetes mellitus. *Schweiz Med Wochenschr* **92**: 349–53.

Von Speiser P, Millesi H (1964) Hereditary serologic structure in Dupuytren's disease. *Wien Med Wschr* **114**: 756–57 (in German).

Wegmann T (1966) Dupuytren's contracture, diabetes mellitus and chronic alcoholism. *Schweiz Med Wochenschr* **96**: 852–54.

Wolfe SJ, Summerskill WHJ, Davidson CS (1956) Thickening and contraction of the palmar fascia (Dupuytren's contracture), associated with alcoholism and hepatic cirrhosis. *New Engl J Med* **255**: 559–63.

Wroblewski BM (1973) Carpal tunnel decompression and Dupuytren's contracture. *Hand* **5**:69–70.

Zachariae L (1971) Dupuytren's contracture. The aetiological role of trauma. *Scand J Plast Reconstr Surg Hand Surg* **5**: 116–19.

Zachariae L, Dahlerup JV, Olesen E (1970) The electroencephalogram in patients with Dupuytren's contracture. *Scand J Plast Reconstr Surg Hand Surg* **4**: 35–40.

EVOLUTION AND RISK FACTORS

Caroline Leclercq

Evolution

The natural course of Dupuytren's disease varies greatly among individuals. Nevertheless a few stereotypical patterns have been recognized.

Usually, early changes appear in the palm. They are insidious, in the form of a nodule or a skin pit, or there is distortion of a palmar crease. Sometimes patients do not notice it until a local injury draws their attention to the palm (and the injury is then often claimed to be responsible for the disease)! Other nodules may appear with confluence of adjacent foci producing a raised plaque across which the flexor creases pass deeply and over which the dermis becomes fixed. The palmar changes then gradually become more discrete with a shrinking of the diffuse palmar nodules into denser bodies (Hueston, 1963). Flexion deformity has not been reported in the presence of palmar nodules alone; the cords are responsible for the contracture. Whether isolated or multiple, nodules evolve towards cords. Usually a fibrous thickening appears around the nodule in the line of the relevant digit and develops into a cord, usually better defined proximal than distal to the nodule at this early stage. When a cord is present it leads, with a variable delay, to finger contracture. This usually involves the MP joint first, then nodules appear within the digit, then the contracture progresses to the PIP joint.

However, in some patients the disease starts and evolves differently. Whereas no nodule can be seen or palpated, a progressive, insidious contracture appears at the PIP joint (or even at the DIP joint). At this early stage, even careful palpation may miss a subtle, deep lateral cord on one side of the joint, and so the diagnosis of Dupuytren's disease may be difficult. Then the cord becomes more apparent as the flexion contracture progresses. Palmar lesions may appear secondarily but sometimes the digital contracture remains isolated. This type of evolution is more frequent in women and in the young, and usually involves the little finger.

The natural history of Dupuytren's disease does not follow a linear progression (Millesi, 1985). Usually the changes are slow; the palmar nodules may remain unchanged for decades. Millesi (1974) observed 150 hands that initially presented with a nodule or cord without any finger contracture. After 3 to 5 years a contracture was present in 37% of patients, and after 6 to 12 years in 46.5%. When a cord is present the contracture may appear either insidiously over the years or it may progress rapidly within a few months until it reaches a plateau and then it may not evolve again for several months or years. In some patients, though, the course is much faster, leading to severe multiple contractures of the fingers within a few years.

Although the course of the disease remains subject to large individual variation, two different patient populations may be discerned:

- Those with a late onset of the disease (in their fifties or sixties) with a single palmar nodule evolving slowly to a thin cord, with late retraction of the MP joint and finally the PIP joint. These patients are prone to a limited risk of recurrence after surgery;
- Those with an early onset of the disease, with multiple palmar involvement, large nodules, massive skin adhesion, and rapid progression to finger contracture. This population also includes those with isolated involvement of the little finger. In this population, there is a high incidence of recurrence after surgery.

Dupuytren's diathesis

Although the hereditary nature of Dupuytren's disease and its possible association with knuckle pads and plantar or penile lesions had already been recognized (Skoog,

1948), it is Hueston (1963) who gathered these factors under the term 'Dupuytren's diathesis', a diathesis being (from Webster's *Dictionary*) 'a bodily condition, constitution or morbid habit which predisposes to a particular disease' (Hueston, 1963). Not only did he coin this term, which is now widely used, but he also pointed out the possible influence of the diathesis on the course of the disease. From a series of 159 personal cases followed for more than 3 years, he showed that in the group of 48 patients who had a recurrence, a family history was twice as frequent, knuckle pads three-and-a-half times and plantar lesions eight times as frequent as in the group who remained clear of the disease after surgery (Table 5.3). He also showed that the patients in the recurrence group were younger (average age 45 years versus 58 years) and that their disease was almost always bilateral (98% versus 80%).

This negative influence of the diathesis had not been detected in previous studies (Tubiana, 1955). But since Hueston described it, many authors have specifically studied the factors included in the diathesis, as well as other general factors (associated diseases) or local factors (topography of the lesions, bilaterality, severity of the contracture, and even histological type) in order to determine whether or not they were 'risk factors' (Hueston, 1974; Mikkelsen, 1977; Legge and McFarlane, 1980; Morane, 1983; McFarlane, 1985; Alnot and Morane, 1986; Leclercq and Tubiana, 1986).

Risk factors

Diathesis

The literature widely confirms Hueston's views on the prognostic value of the diathesis. A positive family history, an early age of onset, and the presence of ectopic lesions are all pejorative factors, indicating a severe course of the disease with early and marked finger contractures and a high rate of recurrence after surgery. Only the study by Mikkelsen (1977) does not support the supposition of a higher predisposition and a more aggressive disease in patients with Dupuytren's disease and knuckle pads. Bilaterality, however, is not frequently mentioned, except by McFarlane (1985) who found unilateral cases to have a lower incidence of family history, ectopic lesions and associated disease, thus indicating a better prognosis than bilateral cases.

Gender

Although Dupuytren's disease usually starts later in life and has a slower progression in women, several studies have found the results of surgery to be less satisfactory in women (Wallace, 1965), partly due to a higher incidence of reflex sympathetic dystrophy (RSD) (Zemel, 1991) and to a higher incidence of lesions in the little finger (Brouet, 1986), which are more exposed to recurrence. However, retrospective studies by Tonkin et

Table 5.3 Hueston's series of 159 patients followed for more than 3 years after surgery.			
	No recurrence	Extension	Recurrence
No. of patients (*n* = 159)	70	41	48
Average age (years)	58	55	45
Evidence of diathesis (%)			
family history	10 (12%)	4 (10%)	13 (27%)
bilateral disease	56 (80%)	39 (95%)	47 (98%)
knuckle pads	14 (20%)	17 (41.5%)	36 (75%)
plantar lesions	3 (4%)	4 (10%)	12 (25%)

al. (1984) and Zemel et al. (1987) have shown a lower recurrence rate in women.

Associated diseases

- Diabetes: Dupuytren's disease in patients with diabetes is usually mild, limited to palmar nodules, and progresses slowly. However, complications after surgery are more frequent (Merle and Merle, 1986) including hematoma, delayed healing, and RSD (especially in women), as well as the frequent pre-existing limitation of joint motion contributing to postoperative stiffness.
- Epilepsy: Although there is a significant prevalence of Dupuytren's disease in patients with epilepsy, the disease in these patients seems to follow a course similar to the usual evolution pattern (Skoog, 1948; Stuhler et al., 1977).
- Alcoholism: Although there seems to be a positive correlation between Dupuytren's disease and alcoholism, its mechanism as well as its prognostic value remain unclear (Attali et al., 1987; Pojer and Jedlickova, 1970).

Race and country

The incidence of Dupuytren's disease is much lower in non-Caucasian populations, although it is difficult from the literature to judge if there is a difference in prognosis in these different races. Whereas the disease seems to follow a milder course in Asian populations (Egawa et al., 1990; Liu and Chen, 1991) it seems to be similar in black patients as in Caucasians (Gonzalez et al., 1998; Mitra and Goldstein, 1994).

Local factors

Local factors can also greatly influence the prognosis of Dupuytren's disease. They are studied in Chapter 6, pages 219–20.

Histological factors

Some histological factors have been shown by Rombouts et al. (1989) to influence the course of the disease. These authors classified the histological aspects from Dupuytren's disease samples in a proliferative, a fibrocellular, and a paucicellular type, and found recurrences to be more frequent in patients with the proliferative type and the least frequent with the paucicellular type.

All these risk factors must be assessed carefully before deciding on an operation on Dupuytren's disease. They will influence our choice of treatment.

References

Alnot JY, Morane L (1986) Appréciation des facteurs de risque évolutif dans la maladie de Dupuytren. In: Tubiana R, Hueston JT, eds, *La Maladie de Dupuytren*, 3rd edn, 122–25. L'Expansion Scientifique Française, Paris.

Attali P, Ink O, Pelletier G et al. (1987) Dupuytren's contracture, alcohol consumption, and chronic liver disease. *Arch Intern Med* **147**: 1065–67.

Brouet JP (1986) Etude de 1000 dossiers de maladie de Dupuytren. In: Tubiana R, Hueston JT, eds, *La Maladie de Dupuytren*, 3rd edn, 98–105. L'Expansion Scientifique Française, Paris.

Egawa T, Senrui H, Horiki A, Egawa M (1990) Epidemiology of the oriental patient. In: McFarlane RM, McGrouther DA, Flint MH, eds, *Dupuytren's Disease*, 239–45. Churchill Livingstone, Edinburgh.

Gonzalez MH, Sobeski J, Grindel S et al. (1998) Dupuytren's disease in African-Americans. *J Hand Surg* **23B**: 306–307.

Hueston JT (1963) The Dupuytren's diathesis. In: Hueston JT, ed., *Dupuytren's Contracture*, 51–63. Churchill Livingstone, Edinburgh.

Hueston JT (1974) Prognosis as a guide to the timing and extent of surgery in Dupuytren's contracture. In: Hueston JT, Tubiana R, eds, *Dupuytren's Disease*, 61–62. Churchill Livingstone, Edinburgh.

Leclercq C, Tubiana R (1986) Résultats à long terme des aponévrectomies pour maladie de Dupuytren. *Chirurgie* **112**: 195.

Legge JWH, McFarlane RM (1980) Prediction of results of treatment of Dupuytren's disease. *J Hand Surg* **5**: 608–16.

Liu Y, Chen WY (1991) Dupuytren's disease among the Chinese in Taiwan. *J Hand Surg* **16A**: 779–86.

McFarlane RM (1985) Some observations on the epidemiology of Dupuytren's disease. In: Hueston JT, Tubiana R, eds, *Dupuytren's Disease*, 122–28. Churchill Livingstone, Edinburgh.

Merle M, Merle S (1986) Maladie de Dupuytren et diabète. In: Tubiana R, Hueston JT, eds, *La Maladie de Dupuytren*, 3rd edn, 90–92. L'Expansion Scientifique Française, Paris.

Mikkelsen OA (1977) Dupuytren's disease. Initial symptoms, age of onset, and spontaneous course. *Hand* **9**: 11–15.

Millesi H (1974) The clinical and morphological course of Dupuytren's disease. In: Hueston JT, Tubiana R, eds, *Dupuytren's Disease*, 49–60. Churchill Livingstone, Edinburgh.

Millesi H (1985) The clinical and morphological course of Dupuytren's disease. In: Hueston JT, Tubiana R, eds, *Dupuytren's Disease*, 2nd edn, 114–21. Churchill Livingstone, Edinburgh.

Mitra A, Goldstein RY (1994) Dupuytren's contracture in the black population: a review. *Ann Plast Surg* **32**: 619–22.

Morane L (1983) Utilisation pronostique des facteurs de risque dans la maladie de Dupuytren. Thesis, Paris.

Pojer J, Jedlickova J (1970) Enzymatic pattern of liver injury in Dupuytren's contracture. *Acta Med Scand* **187**: 101–104.

Rombouts JJ, Noel H, Legrain Y, Munting E (1989) Prediction of recurrence in the treatment of Dupuytren's disease: evaluation of a histological classification. *J Hand Surg* **14A**: 644–52.

Skoog T (1948) Dupuytren's contraction with special reference to aetiology and improved surgical treatment. *Acta Chir Scand* **96** (suppl. 139): S1.

Tonkin MA, Burke FD, Varian JPW (1984) Dupuytren's contracture: a comparative study of fasciectomy in one hundred patients. *J Hand Surg* **9B**: 156–62.

Tubiana R (1955) Prognosis and treatment of Dupuytren's contracture. *J Bone Joint Surg* **37A**: 1155–68.

Wallace AF (1965) Dupuytren's contracture in women. *Br J Plast Surg* **13**: 385–86.

Zemel NP, Balcomb TV, Stark HH, Ashworth CR et al. (1987) Dupuytren's disease in women: evaluation of long-term results after operation. *J Hand Surg* **12A**: 1012–16.

Zemel NP (1991) Dupuytren's contracture in women. *Hand Clin* **7**: 707–11.

6

Treatment

NON-SURGICAL TREATMENT

Caroline Leclercq, Lawrence C Hurst and Marie A Badalamente

Many treatments other than surgical have been attempted in Dupuytren's disease, ever since the time of Baron Dupuytren himself, who in his *Leçons orales* reports having 'employed one after the other vaporised fumigation ... plasters ... leeches, friction with resolvent ointments and calomel, alkaline, simple sulfurous and saponaceous douches at various temperatures, and all without the slightest effect' (Dupuytren, 1832).

Most of these treatments have since been abandoned, in view of their ineffectiveness or potential harm to other structures, but some of them are still popular in some countries. In their comprehensive review of all the pharmacological treatments that have been attempted, Naylor et al. (1994) state firmly that the major problem '... is the lack of objective, multicenter controlled trials of potentially beneficial drugs. Most studies have included limited numbers of patients of varying ages, different sexes, and at various stages of the disease. In addition some of the subjects used in these studies have had previously unsuccessful treatments, which may complicate interpretation of any later results ... thus it is not surprising that the usefulness of drug treatment in Dupuytren's contracture is so controversial.'

Among all the drugs that have been attempted, there has been continuing interest since the turn of the century in substances that would be able to dissolve Dupuytren's tissue. Although none has proved effective so far, a promising trial of collagenase injections is presently being conducted by Hurst and Badalamente.

Physiotherapy

Ultrasound therapy and ionization have been said to lead to a certain amount of softening of nodules, but have not been effective on cords. Stiles (1966) has studied, using the electron microscope, samples of Dupuytren's tissue that were excised a few weeks after a 2-week ultrasonic therapy. He found that ultrasonic waves produced changes in the interfibrillar cement substance of fibrous tissue, but did not find any modification of the usual aspects of Dupuytren's tissue itself, nor did he find any clinical change after the ultrasonic therapy, whether or not associated with splinting.

Splints, whether static or dynamic, might be effective in preventing worsening of a contracture if they could be applied continuously. However, this would represent a major functional impairment, which would not be accepted by patients. When applied discontinuously, splints are ineffective (James and Tubiana, 1952).

Unwitting traumatic ruptures of Dupuytren's cords have also been reported both in the ancient literature and recent medical literature (Grace et al., 1984; D'Arcangelo et al., 1995; Siratokova and Elliot, 1997).

Radiotherapy

In the early days of roentgen therapy, this technique was used experimentally for treating Dupuytren's disease (Finney, 1953), but abandoned because of a lack of evidence of any curative effect, even before the potential side-effects of X-ray therapy were identified. However, this is still debated in Germany, and a recent report by Keilholz et al. (1996) on 57 patients treated with ortho-voltage radiotherapy (total dose 30 Gy) seems to show a slowing down of evolution of the disease at 5 years' follow-up.

Nevertheless, radiotherapy is still considered by many as too dangerous for treating this benign condition (Falter et al., 1991). And another recent report by Weinzierl et al. (1993), failed to find any difference, at 7 years' follow-up, between a treated and an untreated group.

Pharmacological treatments

Vitamin E

Isolated by HM Evans in 1922, vitamin E was soon shown to have an effect on muscle (Evans and Burr, 1928) and on fibrous tissue (Le Roy Steinberg, 1941), although the mechanism remained unclear. It was subsequently advocated in the treatment of 'fibrositis', including Dupuytren's disease, and administered orally.

In the 1950s an increasing number of articles were published in the English literature, with contradictory results using this treatment. Whereas Thomson (1949), Le Roy Steinberg (1951) and others obtained satisfactory results, especially in diseases of short duration, others following King (1949) did not observe any positive results, even when high doses were being used (Parsons, 1948). It has subsequently been abandoned, although it is not clear from the literature whether this was because of its lack of efficacy or because of its potential toxicity.

Enzymatic fasciotomy

The idea of dissolving Dupuytren's tissue chemically arose early in the 1900s when fibrinolysin injections were advocated by Langemak in 1907 and Quenu in 1918 (reported by James and Tubiana, 1952). This practice was said to soften and improve the elasticity of the tissues, and was shown in vitro to convert collagen into gelatin.

Later, drugs aimed at the degradation of collagen were employed. Pepsin was first used by Hesse (1931) and Gold (1926), reported by James and Tubiana (1952), and, in 1965, Bassot reported on the use of trypsin and hyaluronidase. His technique, called 'pharmacodynamic removal' consisted of injecting a mixture of trypsin and hyaluronidase with a local anesthetic. After 15 minutes, a forcible extension was applied in order to rupture the cords; a plaster slab then maintained the correction for a few days.

Four years later Bassot (1969) published his results in 34 patients, with illustrations of impressive corrections of severe deformities (Hueston, 1971). He had by then added two other enzymes to his formula: thiomucase and alphachymotrypsin. Similar encouraging results have been published by other authors (Aron, 1968; Hueston, 1971).

However, it was generally agreed that, while full metacarpophalangeal correction was the rule, there was difficulty in obtaining rupture of the digital cords and PIP joint extension. Rupture of the overlying skin has also been reported to occur, mainly in severely flexed cases with adherent skin in the flexor creases.

These skin defects have usually healed rapidly, without the need for subsequent grafting. Swelling of the hand has also been reported after the injection, which usually subsided on rest and elevation.

But, more than these minor complications, it is the rapid recurrence of the disease that has led progressively to the abandonment of this technique. McCarthy (1992) reviewed 10 hands with an average follow-up of 6.5 years and found that the initial deformity was again present in 75% of patients at 2–3 years' follow-up. Comparison with surgical fasciotomy suggested a similar recurrence rate, but a greater potential morbidity. However, there has been continuing research in this field and recently Starkweather et al. (1996) demonstrated in vitro that collagenase may be effective in enzymatic fasciotomy of residual-stage Dupuytren's disease.

Collagenase enzymatic fasciotomy

In 1995, Hurst and Badalamente's laboratory investigated the effect of purified Clostridial collagenase (Cordase, Biospecifics Technologies, Lynbrook, NY) on the tensile strength of Dupuytren's cords obtained from surgery (Starkweather et al., 1996). In this in vitro study, Dupuytren's cords, obtained from patients who had undergone fasciectomy, were injected with 3600 units Clostridial collagenase, incubated at 37°C for 24 hours, and stretched to failure. This pilot study found a 93% decrease in the modulus of elasticity of collagenase-injected cords compared with control cords injected with buffer only. Following this pilot experiment, controlled multiple-dose injections of 150, 300, and 600 units and a control saline injection were performed on additional Dupuytren's cords obtained from surgery. The results indicated that 300 units of collagenase allowed cord rupture after injection into surgical specimens (Starkweather et al., 1996). The force applied to these cords was less than the force produced by the finger muscles during active extension.

Badalamente and Hurst (1996) examined the potential adverse extravasation of 150 and 300 units collagenase to adjacent collagen-containing tissues using an in vivo rat model. The results showed no adverse collagenase dissemination or local toxicity to any tissue structure near the tail tendon. The injected collagen of the tail tendon was disrupted by the collagenase.

An open-label Phase 2 study to evaluate the efficacy of Clostridial collagenase as a non-operative treatment for Dupuytren's disease was carried out under an investigational new drug number (IND) from the US Food and Drug Administration. To date, there are 35 patients in this ongoing study, with an average age of 64.8 years. There are 32 men and 3 women in the study. The first 6 patients were part of a dose escalation analysis, with the first patient receiving only 300 units and the sixth patient receiving 9600 units. These initial patients all had MP joint contractures. There was no clinical effect of collagenase injection in these 6 patients.

After the dose escalation analysis, an additional 29 patients were treated with 10 000 units. More than 90% of the MP joint contractures were corrected to full extension. Six of 9 PIP joint contractures were fully corrected. Seven patients had more than one joint contracture corrected by a single injection. MP and PIP joint contractures in the same digit were corrected simultaneously in 4 patients. For example, MP joint contractures in the fourth and fifth digits, caused by a combined central and natatory cord, were also corrected by a single injection at the point of juncture of the two cords. Side effects have been limited to pain at the injection site, minimal swelling, and hematoma. No serum IgE (immune) abnormalities of significance have occurred and there have been no clinical adverse reactions.

Technique

The authors' collagenase percutaneous fasciotomies have been performed under sterile technique with a 0.5 ml insulin syringe and 28-gauge (0.36 mm × 13 mm) insulin needle. 10 000 units of collagenase were delivered in 0.25 ml of sterile diluent for MP joint contractures and in 0.2 ml of diluent for PIP joint contractures (Hurst and Badalamente, 1999). The diluent consists of sodium chloride containing calcium chloride.

Prior to each injection, the finger and palm were studied with ultrasonographic imaging to determine the depth of the underlying flexor tendons. The authors' studies show that the average distance between the skin and the flexor tendon sheath at the point of injection averages 7.4 ± 3.9 mm (range 4–16 mm) in patients with MP joint contractures. In patients with PIP joint contractures, the average skin-to-tendon sheath distance is 4.7 ± 1.6 mm (range 3–7 mm). The safe zone thereafter is defined as the distance from the skin to a point approximately 4–6 mm below the skin in patients with MP contractures, and approximately 3–4 mm below the skin in patients with PIP contractures.

The ultrasonographic images do not show the depth of the Dupuytren's cord but do show the distance from the skin to the flexor tendon motion segment in the sagittal image. By staying superficial to the measured tendon depth, the injection remains in the safe tendon-free zone where the Dupuytren's cord is located.

After preparing the skin with a suitable antiseptic, the insulin needle is placed through the skin and into the cord (Figure 6.1); the gristly scar-like structure of the cord is easily palpated with the end of the needle. A small amount of gentle passive motion at the distal interphalangeal joint also helps to confirm that the needle is in the Dupuytren's cord and not in the flexor tendons. If any paresthesias are noted by the patient, the needle is repositioned to avoid any direct neural injections, especially if the patient has a spiral cord. Once the needle is in the middle of the cord, a portion of the 0.25 ml is injected (Figure 6.2a). Next, the needle is partially withdrawn

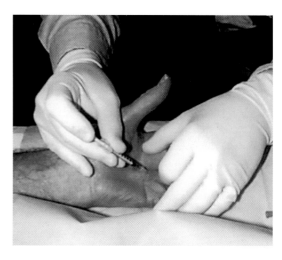

Figure 6.1 Collagenase injection into a cord causing an MP joint contracture. (Reproduced with permission from Hurst and Badalamente, 1999.)

and replaced in a slightly more distal position in the pathologic cord material and another portion (approximately one-third) is injected into the middle of the cord. Finally, the needle is repositioned again, this time proximal to the initial injection, and the final portion of the collagenase is injected. When the skin is severely deformed or the contracture interferes with positioning, the first portion is injected, the needle withdrawn completely and a second injection site located 1–2 mm more distally on the cord is used for the second portion of the injection. The third and final portion is injected 1–2 mm proximal to the first site (Figure 6.2b). A single injection into the apex of a central and natatory cord can result in the correction of contractures in two adjacent fingers (Figure 6.3).

After injection, patients are instructed to hold their hand steady, with elevation, and the finger and hand are placed in a bulky dressing. The patient is told to remove the dressing the same evening. All patients are discharged on the day of injection; no overnight stay has been necessary. The following day, patients

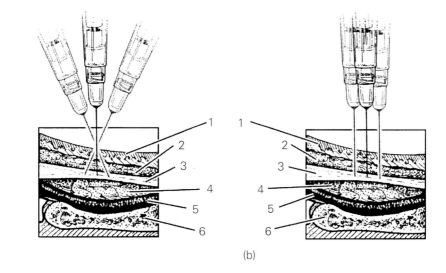

(a)   (b)

Figure 6.2 (a, b) Two different needle techniques used to place the three portions of the single 0.25 ml dose within the cord while keeping all the portions close to each other. This technique spreads the dose over a segment of the cord and reduces the risk of extravasation of the collagenase out of the Dupuytren's cord and into the superficial or deep fat: (1) skin; (2) subcutaneous fat; (3) Dupuytren's cord; (4) deep fat; (5) flexor tendon; (6) metacarpal. (Reproduced with permission from Hurst and Badalamente, 1999.)

are followed in the outpatient hand center. Many patients experience 'popping' of their cords by the next morning. At the hand center, gentle manipulation of the finger often provides immediate, complete correction of the contracture. By the end of the first week, the degree of correction is observable and complete (Figures 6.4 and 6.5).

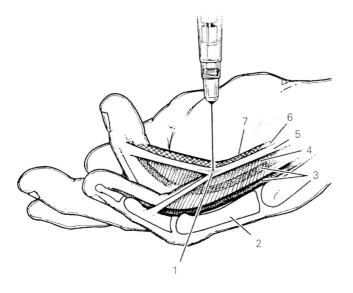

Figure 6.3 Single injection into the apex of a combined central cord and natatory cord can result in the correction of more than one contracture in the two adjacent fingers: (1) collagenase and diluent; (2) metacarpal; (3) flexor tendons; (4) deep fat; (5) Dupuytren's cord; (6) subcutaneous fat; (7) skin. (Reproduced with permission from Hurst and Badalamente, 1999.)

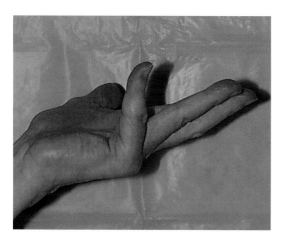

Figure 6.4 Patient with MP joint contractures in the left little and ring fingers.

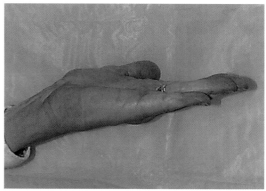

Figure 6.5 The same patient as in Figure 6.4 after collagenase injection. Both contracted fingers were corrected with a single 10 000 unit injection.

Steroid injections

Steroids were known to have a restraining effect on the formation of fibrous tissue, and proved effective in the treatment of other fibromatoses such as Peyronie's disease. Their local use in Dupuytren's contracture was first advocated by Baxter et al. in 1952, but these authors restricted its use to the postoperative period.

Despite initial optimism, the results for hydrocortisone (Zachariae and Zachariae, 1955) and later more powerful derivates such as 6-methyl prednisolone were disappointing (Kaufhold, 1962). The drugs appeared to have little effect on the contracture, and did not cause a regression of the disease.

More recently, the use of dimethylsulphoxide (DMSO), which was said to dissolve new pathological collagen but leave normal collagen intact (Vuopala and Kaipainen, 1971) proved to be of questionable effectiveness.

Steroids are still used by several authors, however, and recently Ketchum (1996) has reported a complete resolution of the nodule in 25 solitary nodules with a follow-up over 3.5 years, following injection of triamcinolone.

Complications of these injections include dermal atrophy and skin depigmentation, and flexor tendon ruptures have been reported in cases where injections have been repeated at short intervals (Ketchum, 1996). The author restricts their use to painful solitary nodules.

Other drugs

- Procarbazine was incidentally noted by Aron (1968) to improve not only a patient's Hodgkin disease, but also his Dupuytren's disease. This led to clinical trials, but the incidence of side-effects and questionable effectiveness precluded its widespread use (Morgan and Pryor, 1978).
- The lathyrogens are designed to inhibit the formation of collagen. Several clinical trials have been reported (Bray and Galeazzi, 1980; Cimmino et al., 1982), but their effect on Dupuytren's disease is yet to be fully determined.
- Allopurinol has, incidentally, also been noted by Murrell et al. (1986) to improve Dupuytren's disease in some patients. This

later led to the development of a hypothesis of pathogenesis (Murrell et al., 1987), suggesting that agents that decrease oxygen free radical release may inhibit or prevent Dupuytren's contracture. However, a personal clinical trial by Hueston (1990) has failed to confirm this hypothesis.

• Recent studies (Naylor et al., 1994) have shown that some prostaglandins inhibit myofibroblast contractility, but the authors are not aware of their clinical effect on Dupuytren's disease.

• Gamma-interferon has also been tried by Pittet et al. (1994), who observed a decrease in the symptoms and size of the lesion in a limited number of cases.

Needle fasciotomy

Local injection of steroids combined with a forceful extension of the finger(s) and followed by a corrective night splint was advocated by French rheumatologists de Seze and

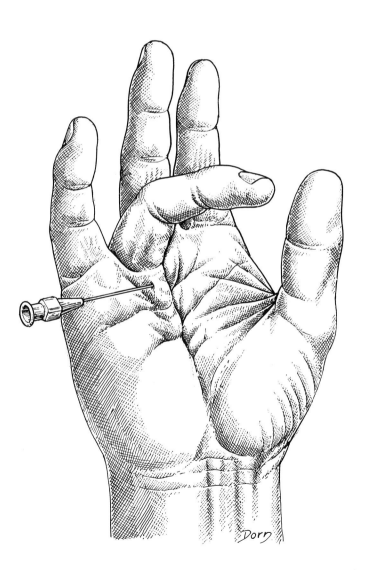

Figure 6.6 Needle fasciotomy: the needle is inserted sideways perpendicular to the cord.

Debeyre in 1957. The authors reported excellent results in 135 cases with this technique (Debeyre, 1958). However, this method required repeated injections for up to 1 year or several years. In order to obtain a quicker improvement, their team has progressively modified the technique by breaking the nodules or the cords subcutaneously with the injection needle (Figure 6.6). This has led to the current technique of 'needle fasciotomy', which has gained local popularity in some countries such as France.

The technique, as described by Lermusiaux and Debeyre in 1980 consists of injecting a mixture of prednisolone and lignocaine in and under the nodule/cord, then 'internally dissecting' the nodule by back and forth movements of the needle, then forcefully extending the finger. It takes approximately two to four injections at 1-week intervals to obtain, during forceful extension, an audible rupture of the nodule/cord with consequent straightening of the finger.

In these authors' experience, it was necessary to break two or three nodules/cords to obtain full extension of a finger with a Stage II disease. The full length of the treatment thus lasted approximately 4 months. In a recent update of the technique (Badois et al., 1993), it was reported that an average of 6 weeks was required to obtain full extension, probably because of a more aggressive division of the nodules/cords during each session. From their experience with 123 hands, Badois et al. (1993) report only minor complications:

- 16% skin breakages, which healed in 1–2 weeks;
- 2% dysesthesiae related to a trauma of a collateral nerve by the needle, 'almost always transient';
- 2% local infections, which always healed with antibiotics.

However, more severe complications have been observed by surgeons to whom patients came as a second referral:

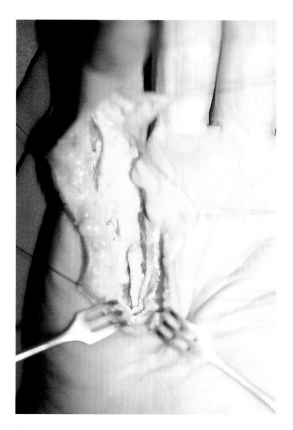

Figure 6.7 Rupture of both flexor tendons in the palm after needle fasciotomy.

- Traumatic division of the flexor tendons usually involves both tendons, usually in the 'No Man's Land', sometimes in the palm (Figure 6.7). It results from the tendons being mistaken for a cord by the operator, and thoroughly divided using the needle. The rupture occurs either immediately during the forceful extension maneuver, or secondarily during a forceful grip (incomplete division). Secondary repair of these dilacerated tendons is always difficult, and hampered by the surrounding Dupuytren's and scar tissue consecutive to the previous needle fasciotomies.

- Nerve lesions are in some cases permanent, resulting from a traumatic section of the collateral nerve. This usually occurs during attempted fasciotomy at the digital level, where the cord can assume any position around the neurovascular bundle. Here again secondary repair of such a traumatized nerve usually leads to a mediocre result.
- Reflex sympathetic dystrophy seems as frequent as with conventional surgery.

In the report of their long-term results, Badois et al. (1993) have found recurrences to be less frequent than the usual postsurgical rates but they did not include nodular recurrences in their patients' figures. If corrected accordingly, their rates become slightly higher than surgical ones.

When treating a palmar cord with this technique, one should not expect any long-term effect on the PIP joint, as shown by a prospective study on 107 fingers by Rowley et al. (1984): even though extension of the PIP may be temporarily improved, recurrence of the deformity at this level is very quick.

This seemingly simple technique, which has gained a lot of popularity with patients because of its non-surgical aspect, is indeed not that simple, and has definite potential dangers. It must be restricted to the palmar level, where the neurovascular bundles are deeper than the cords, and to well-delineated cords, covered by supple skin. It should not be used at the digital level. Moreover, it should be utilized only by physicians fully aware of the normal anatomy of the hand and of the pathoanatomy of Dupuytren's nodules and cords.

More recently, Foucher (pers. comm., 1999) has reported his experience on 241 needle fasciectomies in 198 hands of 171 patients. He uses a somewhat different technique. After local anesthesia and skin preparation, a forearm tourniquet is inflated and a 19-gauge needle is used to section the cords; no steroid injection is performed. Two preoperative tests are useful: a positive 'fasciodese' test with full

PIP extension in MP flexion is a good prediction of extension after fasciotomy; and the Short–Watson test (1982; pages 42–43), which is useful to predict a spiral cord. Fasciotomies are performed in one stage at multiple levels and beginning in the finger as the digital cord is frequently difficult to palpate after proximal palmar fasciotomy. Palmar cords are cut clearly whereas at the digital level the needle is used to weaken the cords slowly until a cracking can be heard during attempted extension, and the finger straightens. However, Foucher states that he does not proceed further at the digital level when the neurovascular bundle is at risk, even if the extension of the finger remains incomplete. Fasciotomy was performed in the palm alone in 154 cases, in the palm and digit in 82 cases, and in the finger only in 5 cases. He reports an extremely low rate of complications: 3 transient paresthesiae and 2 positive Tinel's signs, also transient. He stresses the difficulty in assessing recurrence due to the persistence of diseased tissue, but reports that on 65 hands reviewed at an average 2.5 years, 35 had a recurrent lack of extension (54%). In the whole series, 21 hands (11%) necessitated a second surgical procedure for recurring contracture. From his experience, Foucher states that the best indications for this technique are visible cords adhering to the skin (such as palmar pretendinous cords and digital central cords), whereas retrovascular cords are too dangerous to deal with using this technique. He advises using the technique in the early stages of the disease (where one would usually advise the patient to wait for an aggravation of the contracture before performing a fasciectomy), in women (because of the increased risk of RSD with fasciectomy), and in old or unhealthy patients. Besides local contraindications, such as retrovascular cords, he advises against the use of this technique in recurrences after surgery (where the anatomical relationships of the neurovascular bundles may have been greatly modified) and in severe forms in young adults where dermofasciectomy is best indicated.

References

Aron E (1968) Le traitement médical de la maladie de Dupuytren par agent cytostatique (methyl-hydrazine). *Presse Med* **76**: 1956–58.

Badalamente MA, Hurst LC (1996) Enzyme injection as a non-operative treatment for Dupuytren's disease. *Drug Delivery* **3**: 33–40.

Badois FJ, Lermusiaux JL, Masse C, Kuntz D (1993) Traitement non chirurgical de la maladie de Dupuytren par aponévrotomie à l'aiguille. *Rev Rhum* **60**: 808–13.

Bassot J (1965) Traitement de la maladie de Dupuytren par exérèse pharmaco-dynamique isolée ou complétée par un temps plastique uniquement cutané. *Lille Chirurg* **20**: 1

Bassot J (1969) Traitement de la maladie de Dupuytren par exérèse pharmaco-dynamique: bases physio-biologiques; technique. *Gazette Hop* 557.

Baxter H, Schiller C, Johnson LH et al. (1952) Cortisone therapy in Dupuytren's contracture. *Plast Reconstr Surg* **9**: 261–73.

Bray E, Galeazzi M (1980) First results in the treatment of Dupuytren's disease. *Arthritis Rheum* **23**: 1408.

Cimmino MA, Cutolo M, Beltrame F (1982) Local injections of tiopronin in Dupuytren's contracture. *Arthritis Rheum* **25**: 1505.

D'Arcangelo M, Maffulli N, Kolhe S (1995) Traumatic release of Dupuytren's contracture. *Acta Orthop Belg* **61**: 53–54.

Debeyre N (1958) Traitement de la maladie de Dupuytren par l'hydrocortisone locale associée aux manoeuvres de redressement (135 cas traités). *Sem Hôp Paris (Thér)* **34**: 728–30.

De Seze S, Debeyre N (1957) Traitement de la maladie de Dupuytren par l'hydrocortisone locale associée aux manoeuvres de redressement (70 cas traités). *Rev Rhum* **24**: 540–50.

Dupuytren G (1832) *Leçons Orales de Clinique Chirurgicale Faites à l'Hôtel-Dieu.* Ballière, Paris.

Evans HM, Burr GO (1928) Development of paralysis in the suckling young of mothers deprived of vitamin E. *J Biol Chem* **76**: 273–97.

Falter E, Herndl E, Muhlbauer W (1991) Dupuytren's contracture. When operate? Conservative preliminary treatment? *Fortschr Med* **109**: 223–26.

Finney R (1953) Dupuytren's contracture. A radiotherapeutic approach. *Lancet* **2**: 1064–66.

Foucher G (1998) Quoi de neuf dans le traitement de la maladie de Dupuytren? *Ann Chir Plast Esthet* **43**: 593–99.

Grace DL, McGrouther DA, Phillips H (1984) Traumatic correction of Dupuytren's contracture. *J Hand Surg* **9B**: 59–60.

Hesse (1931) Zur Behandlung der Dupuytren'schen Krankheit. *Zentralbl Chir* **24**: 1532–33.

Hueston JT (1971) Enzymatic fasciotomy. *Hand* **3**: 38–40.

Hueston JT (1990) Historical review-addendum. *Curr Orthop* **4**: 286.

Hurst LC, Badalamente MA (1999) Non-operative treatment of Dupuytren's disease. *Hand Clin* **15**: 97–107.

James J, Tubiana R (1952) La maladie de Dupuytren. *Rev Chir Orthop* **38**: 352–406.

Kaufhold N (1962) Die örtliche Behandlung mit 6-methyl-prednisolon (Urbason). *MMW* **104**: 2252–53.

Keilholz L, Seegenschmiedt M, Sauer R (1996) Radiotherapy for prevention of disease progression in early stage Dupuytren's contracture: initial and long-term results. *Int J Radiat Oncol Biol Phys* **36**: 891–97.

Ketchum LD (1996) Dupuytren's contracture: triamcinolone injection. *Correspondence Newsletter, ASSH No. 131.*

King RA (1949) Vitamin E therapy in Dupuytren's contracture. *J Bone Joint Surg* **31B**: 43.

Langemak (1907) Zur Thiosinaminbehandlung der Dupuytren'schen Fascienkontraktur. *Münchener Mediz Wochenscr* **54**: 1380.

Lermusiaux JL, Debeyre N (1980) Le traitement médical de la maladie de Dupuytren. In: de Seze S, Rickewaert A, Kahn MF, Guerin C, eds, *L'Actualité Rhumatologique 1979*, 238–43. L'Expansion Scientifique Française, Paris.

Le Roy Steinberg C (1941) Vitamin E in the treatment of primary fibrositis. *Am J Med Sci* **201**: 347–49.

Le Roy Steinberg C (1951) Tocopherols in the treatment of primary fibrositis. *Arch Surg* **63**: 824–33.

McCarthy DM (1992) The long-term results of enzymatic fasciotomy. *J Hand Surg* **17B**: 356.

Morgan RJ, Pryor JP (1978) Porcarbazine (Natulan) in the treatment of Peyronie's disease. *Br J Urol* **50**: 111–13.

Murrell GAC, Murrell TGC, Pilowski E (1987) A hypothesis for the resolution of Dupuytren's contracture with allopurinal. *Specul Sci Technol* **10**: 107–12.

Murrell TGC, Murrell GAC, Pilowski E (1986) Resolution of Dupuytren's contracture with allopurinol. *Proceedings of the 10th Fed Europ Connective Tissue Societies, Manchester,* July/August 1986.

Naylor IL, Coleman DJ, Coleman RA et al. (1994) Reactivity of nodular cells in vitro: a guide to the pharmacological treatment of Dupuytren's contracture. In: Berger A, Delbruck A, Brenner P, Hinzman R, eds, *Dupuytren's Disease*, 139–50. Springer Verlag, Berlin.

Parsons AR (1948) Dupuytren's contracture treatment by massive doses of vitamin E. *Ir J Med Sci* **270**: 272–75.

Pittet B, Rubbia-Brandt L, Desmoulière A et al. (1994) Effect of gamma-interferon on the clinical and biologic evolution of hypertrophic scars and Dupuytren's disease: an open pilot study. *Plast Reconstr Surg* **93**: 1224–35.

Quenu (1918) Société de Chirurgie séance du 24 juin 1918. In: Palmer RG (1933) Maladie de Dupuytren: rétraction de l'aponévrose palmaire. *Gazette Hop* **106**: 1369.

Rowley DI, Couch M, Cheesney RB, Norris SH (1984) Assessment of percutaneous fasciotomy in the management of Dupuytren's contracture. *J Hand Surg* **9B**: 163–64.

Short WH, Watson HK (1982) Prediction of the spiral nerve in Dupuytren's contracture. *J Hand Surg* **7A**: 84–86.

Siratokova H, Elliot D (1997) A historical record of traumatic rupture of Dupuytren's contracture. *J Hand Surg* **22B**: 198–200.

Starkweather KD, Lattuga S, Hurst LC et al. (1996) Collagenase in the treatment of Dupuytren's disease: an in vitro study. *J Hand Surg* **21A**: 490–95.

Stiles PJ (1966) Ultrasonic therapy in Dupuytren's contracture. *J Bone Joint Surg* **48B**: 452–54.

Thomson GR (1949) Treatment of Dupuytren's contracture with vitamin E. *BMJ* **17**: 1382–83.

Vuopala LU, Kaipainen WJ (1971) DMSO in the treatment of Dupuytren's contracture – a therapeutic experiment. *Acta Rheum Scand* **17**: 61–62.

Weinzierl G, Flugel M, Geldmacher J (1993) Lack of effectiveness of alternative nonsurgical treatment procedures of Dupuytren's contracture. *Chirurg* **64**: 492–94.

Zachariae L, Zachariae F (1955) Hydrocortisone acetate in the treatment of Dupuytren's contracture and allied conditions. *Acta Chir Scand* **109**: 421–31.

FASCIOTOMY

Caroline Leclercq

Fasciotomy (also termed aponeurotomy) consists of merely sectioning Dupuytren's cords, without any excision. Sir Astley Cooper is widely referred to as the first to describe this technique, in 1822. However, Henry Cline has been credited with describing the disease in 1808 and stating that the treatment '...consists in cutting through the aponeurosis with a common knife' (Windsor, 1834; McGrouther, 1988). Adams (1878) subsequently popularized subcutaneous fasciotomy, but since the turn of the century it has been progressively abandoned in favor of fasciectomy, probably because of its inefficiency on digital contracture, and of the frequency of recurrence.

Fasciectomy steadily increased in popularity during the first half of the 20th Century, with a trend towards 'radical' or 'extensive' procedures. Nevertheless, the rate of complications increased drastically, while the rate of recurrence did not decrease. In 1952, Hamlin reported that a more limited excision led to a sharp decrease in complications and in patients taking time off work. Then, in 1959, Luck introduced a new pathogenic concept based on the evolutionary stage of the nodules (see page 133), which led him to reintroduce subcutaneous fasciotomy, isolated or associated with excision of the nodules in the early phases of the disease.

Since then it has become accepted as one of the methods available for treatment of Dupuytren's disease, and reports are regularly published on indications and results of this technique (Rodrigo et al., 1976; Colville, 1983; Rowley et al., 1984; Bryan and Ghorbal, 1988).

Technique

Apart from needle fasciotomy, which is performed during clinical sessions by some physicians (see non-surgical treatment, pages 127–29), surgical fasciotomy may be performed either subcutaneously or openly. The controversy is not new: in the early days of Dupuytren's surgery some advocated a closed technique to prevent the entry of air, which was thought to provoke infection, while others preferred the open technique, hoping for drainage to prevent suppuration (McGrouther, 1988).

Subcutaneous fasciotomy (Figure 6.8)

A skin stab incision is performed on one side of the cord. The preferred incision is longitudinal as the palmar tension produced by straightening the skin will tend to close the wound (Hueston, 1963). Surgeons have used either a regular Morton no. 11 blade, or a modified blade (Colville, 1983), a tenotome, or a 'fasciatome' (designed by Luck, 1959). When there is adhesion between the skin and the nodules and cords, the blade is introduced horizontally to dissect the skin away from the surface of the cord in order to allow subsequent separation of the divided segments after the fasciotomy. The blade is then turned perpendicular to the cord. Hueston (1963) advises firm pressure by a finger of the surgeon's other hand to force the blade into the cord so it is less likely to slip suddenly through the cord into the neurovascular bundles or the flexor tendons. Resistance to further progression ceases when the cord has been divided, and Luck (1959) states that the feeling one experiences then is 'as though the blade were pressing against sponge rubber.' The finger is then extended, until the skin becomes the limiting factor (Colville, 1983).

When there is a deep crease, or dimple, Luck (1959) advises dividing the cord first,

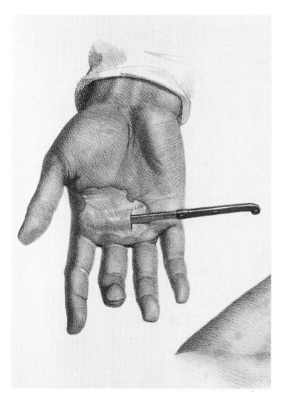

Figure 6.8 Subcutaneous fasciotomy: reproduced with permission from Bourgery and Jacob (1832) who called it the Astley Cooper procedure.

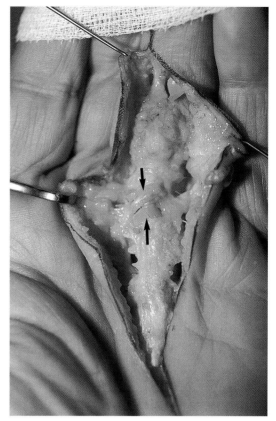

Figure 6.9 Preoperative view (fasciectomy) showing the neurovascular bundle (arrows) overlying the cord at the level of the distal palmar crease.

then undermining the skin so as to sever the apex of the crease.

After the fasciotomy has been completed, Luck (1959) removes the nodules when they are at an early stage ('proliferative' and 'involutional' according to his theory) through a separate transverse incision in either the distal or the proximal palmar crease.

Owing to the unpredictable relationship between the cord and neurovascular bundles at the digital level, most authors restrict this procedure to the palm, where it is performed simultaneously at multiple levels, from the distal palmar crease (DPC) up. The palmar area distal to the DPC is also at risk, because the

cord can displace the bundles to a superficial position, between skin and cord (Figure 6.9). Some authors (such as Colville, 1983), however, perform it also at the PIP joint level 'if necessary', provided that the cord is well defined and bow stringing. In his experience with 95 patients, Colville reports some tingling of fingers, which invariably ceased but with no permanent damage to digital nerves. Such an attitude is not shared by many of his colleagues (Luck, 1959; Tubiana, 1974; Burge, 1994).

After the procedure has been completed some authors apply an extension splint for a few days or weeks, and a night splint for a further few months. Colville (1983) insists that this is an essential adjunct to the operation. His patients have gained an average 14° of improvement with the splint between the immediate postoperative measurement and 3 months later. Active exercises are usually advocated as soon as the skin is healed.

Specific complications of this technique include skin tears, which have been experienced in most series, and which seem more frequent when the skin has been left adherent to the cord (Colville, 1983). This is regarded as a minor, 'accepted' complication, which heals in a few days with an appropriate dressing.

Temporary nerve dysfunction has also been reported, even when the fasciotomy was limited to the palmar level. It has been attributed to overstretching of the finger(s) after a severe flexion contracture, but Luck (1959) reports that five of his eight cases of 'hypalgesia' did not improve with time. However, he used a different approach, which may have put the nerves at a higher risk: he performed all fasciotomies through a single approach along the medial border of the palm. In other series, when the incision was along the side of the cord, no neurovascular complications were reported (Bryan and Ghorbal, 1988; Rowley et al., 1984).

Luck (1959) also reports cases of pain and itching, which resolved in 2–10 weeks.

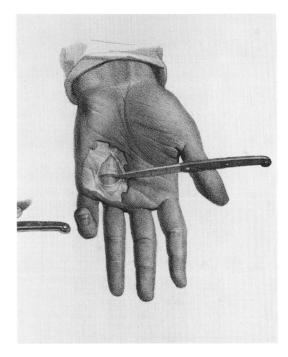

Figure 6.10 Open fasciotomy: reproduced with permission from Bourgery and Jacob (1832) who called it the Goyrand procedure.

Open fasciotomy (Figure 6.10)

In view of some incomplete results with the subcutaneous technique, the deep fibers (which cannot be severed subcutaneously) were incriminated. Some surgeons also felt uneasy with this 'blind' procedure.

In the open technique, transection of the cord is performed under direct vision. A skin incision measuring 2 cm at the least is necessary to obtain a clear vision. It is best performed longitudinally, along one side of the cord. If it is transverse, a skin graft may be necessary after correction of the contracture.

The cord is dissected proximally and distally under direct vision; then it is accurately divided in its entirety, including its deeper

fibers, while preserving the neurovascular bundles. The skin is then closed with a few interrupted sutures.

Several variants of this technique have been described:

- Z-plasties of the skin and underlying cord have been performed by Watson (1984), McGregor (1985) and Thurston (1987). The skin flaps are raised together with the divided cord and transposed as a single unit into a Z-plasty. There is no removal of any part of the cord. Thurston (1987), who performed this technique on 38 hands, reports no complications but states that it is technically difficult to perform at the finger level, and on adjacent rays in the palm. Of 16 patients reviewed at 2 years only one had a recurrence at the operated site.

- Skin-grafting had been advocated in Dupuytren's disease by Gordon (1948, 1963) to replace a devascularized zone. Later, Hueston (1969) used it as a radical treatment of excision and skin-grafting in order to prevent recurrences. In fasciotomies, Gonzalez was the first to use it, mainly at the digital level (Gonzalez, 1971, 1974). The incision runs from one mid-lateral side of the finger to the other. After visualization of the neurovascular bundles, the diseased fascia is completely transected, then a full-thickness skin graft harvested from the groin is applied. The finger is then immobilized for 10 days. Of 100 patients operated on using this technique, Gonzalez experienced no complication except for one graft necrosis with infection and consecutive necrosis of the flexor tendons. At 3 years' review, he noted only one case of recurrence at the PIP joint level. McGregor (1985), who experienced several cases of recurrence under or at the edge of the graft, modified the technique so as to create a rectangular defect instead of the initial triangular one (Figure 6.11). This is achieved by dissection of the fascial fibers on each side of the fasciotomy including the deep fibers, so that the cord retracts on both sides. He also performs larger incisions on each side of the actual area of contracture, ending up in some cases with a complete transection of the palm in palmar contractures. When the contracture involves both the MP and PIP joints, he usually favors fasciotomy at the PIP level, which he finds more effective. From experience based on 153 patients he noted that recurrence occurred only in cases where the graft had partially necrosed.

    Ebelin et al. (1991) have applied this technique to recurrences of Dupuytren's disease at digital level in 25 patients. At 28 months' follow-up they noticed no recurrence under the graft.

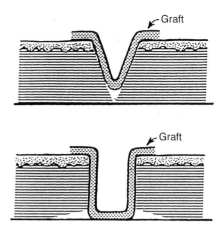

Figure 6.11 The initial triangular defect is changed to a rectangular one by dissection of the fascial fibers on each side of the fasciotomy. (Reproduced with permission from McGregor, 1985.)

- Tenotomy of the palmaris longus at the wrist, associated with a limited excision of the palmar fascia through the same approach has been described by Le Chuiton (1957) but there seems to be no further record of this technique.

Results

Several authors have studied the results of fasciotomy, especially the subcutaneous type. They all agree that, despite the absence of any fascial excision, the remaining cord softens after the fasciotomy, and eventually disappears. Hueston (1992) stresses that the resolution of the proximal segment may take up to 6 months, and that the distal segment may never disappear, and may even later progress if its digital attachments remain. Thurston (1987) measured skin compliance after the operation and found a striking reduction in the stiffness of the skin associated with softening of the underlying cord.

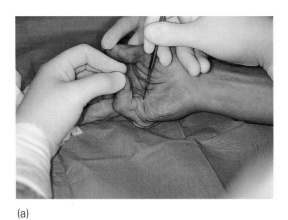
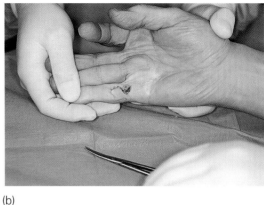

(a)   (b)

Figure 6.12 (a) Dupuytren's disease with contracture of both MP and PIP joints; (b) Immediate postoperative view, after subcutaneous fasciotomy at the distal palmar crease, and open fasciotomy (through a Z-plasty approach) at the finger level.

For most authors, who restrict fasciotomy to the palmar level, this procedure is not suited for contractures predominant at the PIP joint level, as this joint will remain contracted after a palmar fasciotomy (Rodrigo et al., 1976; Rowley et al., 1984; Bryan and Ghorbal, 1988). This has been specifically measured by Rowley et al. (1984) who showed that in MP-joint-dominant fingers (that is, those where the contracture was more important at the MP joint level) the gain in extension at 3 months was 40° (35° at MP joint level and 5° at PIP joint level), whereas in PIP joint-dominant fingers, the gain was 29° (18° at PIP joint level and 11° at MP joint level). On the whole, these results are less satisfactory than those one would expect from limited fasciectomy for correction of MP joint contractures.

Thurston (1987) states that fasciotomy does not preclude combination with other procedures to release contracted PIP joints (Figure 6.12).

In the long term, most series show some degree of recurrence of the contracture after a few months or years (Rodrigo et al., 1976: 1 year; Richards, 1954: less than 18 months). In Colville's series (1983), the average extension deficit was 102° preoperatively, had improved to 31° at 3 months but was back to 75° at 3 years. In Rowley et al.'s series (1984), MP joint-dominant hands improved from an average 46° preoperatively to 8° at 3 months but were back to 17° at 15 months. Also, in Bryan and Ghorbal's series, when patients who required a further fasciectomy are excluded, the mean MP joint contracture (26 digits), which was 36° preoperatively was back to 31° after an average of 5.3 years.

Although comparison of series is made difficult because of uncertainty that the patient groups are comparable, the evidence indicates that recurrence of MP joint contracture is more likely after fasciotomy than after limited fasciectomy (Burge, 1994).

Indications

Fasciotomy is certainly a simple and safe technique when performed at palmar level proximal to the distal palmar crease. It is also quick and therefore used to be advocated for elderly

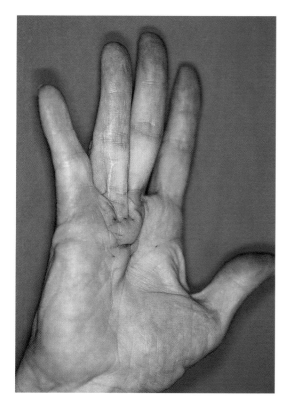

Figure 6.13 Massive palmar skin involvement contraindicating fasciotomy.

people and 'those whose general health precludes longer and more sophisticated surgery' (Bryan and Ghorbal, 1988). The availability of safe local anesthesia has diminished the importance of such indications.

Fasciotomy is also best suited for well-defined and bow-stringing cords. However, those cases are also managed in a quite straightforward way by fasciectomy (Burge, 1994). Therefore indications for this technique are nowadays ill defined. However, some specific contraindications remain:

- Massive skin involvement overlying the cord will prevent separation of the two fascial segments when the cord has been divided (Figure 6.13).

- Digital cords, because of the unpredictable course of the neurovascular bundles with respect to the cord, cannot be treated by subcutaneous fasciotomy and require previous localization of the bundles through an open approach.

Fasciotomy should certainly not be discarded from the surgeon's armory in treating Dupuytren's disease. Its use will depend upon the surgeon's experience and the patient's needs. It may be considered, in the presence of a well-defined palmar cord, for a patient requiring a quick short-term result, and aware that the long-term result will be less satisfactory and recurrence more likely than with some other techniques.

References

Adams W (1878) Contraction of the fingers (Dupuytren's contraction) and its successful treatment by subcutaneous divisions of the palmar fascia and immediate extension. *BMJ* 1: 928.

Bourgery JM, Jacob NA (1832) *Traité complet de l'anatomie de l'homme comprenant la médecine opératoire, 134–35 (Plate 23).* CA Delaunay, Paris.

Bryan AS, Ghorbal MS (1988) The long-term results of closed palmar fasciotomy in the management of Dupuytren's contracture. *J Hand Surg* **13B**: 254–56.

Burge P (1994) Fasciotomy and the open palm technique. In: Berger A, Delbrück A, Brenner P, Hinzmann R, eds, *Dupuytren's Disease: Pathobiochemistry and Clinical Management,* 264–66. Springer Verlag, Berlin.

Colville J (1983) Dupuytren's contracture. The role of fasciotomy. *Hand* **15**: 162–66.

Cooper A (1822) *A treatise on dislocations and fractures of the joints,* 1st edn, 524–25. Longman, Hurst, Rees, Orme, Brown & Cox, London.

Ebelin M, Leviet D, Auclair E et al. (1991) Traitement des récidives de la maladie de Dupuytren par incision scalaire et greffe 'coupe-feu'. *Ann Chir Plast Esthet* **36**: 26–30.

Gonzalez RI (1971) Open fasciotomy and Wolfe graft for Dupuytren's contracture. In: Hueston JT, ed., *Transactions of the Fifth International Congress of Plastic and Reconstructive Surgery, Melbourne, 1971,* 630–31. Butterworth, Melbourne.

Gonzalez RI (1974) Open fasciotomy and full-thickness skin graft in the correction of digital flexion deformity. In: Hueston JT, Tubiana R, eds, *Dupuytren's Disease*, 123–28. Churchill Livingstone, Edinburgh.

Gordon S (1948) Dupuytren's contracture. *Can Med Assoc J* **58**: 543.

Gordon S (1963) Dupuytren's contracture: the use of free skin grafts in treatment. *Transactions of the Third International Congress of Plastic Surgeons, Washington DC, 1963,* 963–67. Excerpta Medica, Amsterdam.

Hamlin EJ (1952) Limited excision of Dupuytren's contracture. *Ann Surg* **135**: 94–97.

Hueston JT (1963) *Dupuytren's Contracture.* Churchill Livingstone, Edinburgh.

Hueston JT (1969) The control of recurrent Dupuytren's contracture by skin replacement. *Br J Plast Surg* **22**: 152–56.

Hueston JT (1992) Regression of Dupuytren's contracture. *J Hand Surg* **17B**: 453–57.

Le Chuiton M (1957) Traitement de la maladie de Dupuytren par téno-aponévrectomie antibrachiale du petit palmaire. *Mem Acad Chir* **83**: 29–30.

Luck JV (1959) Dupuytren's contracture: a new concept of the pathogenesis correlated with surgical management. *J Bone Joint Surg* **41A**: 635–64.

McGregor IA (1985) Fasciotomy and graft in the management of Dupuytren's contracture. In: Hueston JT, Tubiana R, eds, *Dupuytren's Disease*, 2nd edn, 164–71. Churchill Livingstone, Edinburgh.

McGrouther DA (1988) La maladie de Dupuytren. To incise or to excise? *J Hand Surg* **13B**: 368–70.

Richards HJ (1954) Dupuytren's contracture: surgical treatment. *J Bone Joint Surg* **36B**: 90–94.

Rodrigo JJ, Niebauer JJ, Brown RL, Doyle JR (1976) Treatment of Dupuytren's contracture: long-time results after fasciotomy and fascial excision. *J Bone Joint Surg* **58A**: 380–87.

Rowley DI, Couch M, Chesney RB, Norris SH (1984) Assessment of percutaneous fasciotomy in the management of Dupuytren's contracture. *J Hand Surg* **9B**: 163–64.

Thurston AJ (1987) Conservative surgery for Dupuytren's contracture. *J Hand Surg* **12B**: 329–34.

Tubiana R (1964) Limited and extensive operations in Dupuytren's contracture. *Surg Clin N Am* **44**: 1071–80.

Tubiana R (1974) Surgical treatment of Dupuytren's contracture: technique of fasciotomy and fasciectomy. In: Hueston JT and Tubiana R, eds, *Dupuytren's Disease*, 85–92. Churchill Livingstone, Edinburgh.

Watson JD (1984) Fasciotomy and Z-plasty in the management of Dupuytren's contracture. *Br J Plast Surg* **37**: 27–30.

Windsor J (1834) Permanent contraction of the fingers. *Lancet* **ii**: 501–502.

FASCIECTOMY

Raoul Tubiana

History

Goyrand (1833) was probably the first to mention excision of fibrous tissue in Dupuytren's disease: '...many loose ends of the fascia within the wound after straightening the fingers should be excised.' He was followed by Velpeau (1835) who believed that nodules should be excised. In most of the surgical procedures used before the discovery of general anesthesia in 1842, the contracted fascia was divided transversally by subcutaneous methods (Cline, 1777; Cooper; 1822; Adams, 1878) or by open methods (Dupuytren, 1831) (Figure 6.14), (Goyrand, 1833) (Figure 6.15). Without anesthesia, surgery had to be carried out with great speed.

Fergusson (1842), in London, for the first time carried out an extensive fasciectomy of a finger under anaesthesia. Partial excision of the bands was recommended in Germany by Gersuny (1884) and by Kocher (1887) using a longitudinal incision. The disadvantage of longitudinal incisions on the palmar aspect of the hand is their tendency to contract. Russ (1908) performed partial excision of the fascia through multiple small incisions. Routier (1908) used a V incision in the palm and practiced a localized fasciectomy (Figure 6.16).

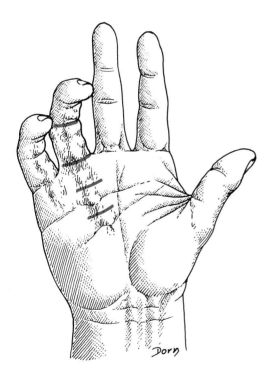

Figure 6.14 Skin incisions used by Dupuytren. Dupuytren originally used one or two incisions but, according to Sanson (1834), he finally adopted four.

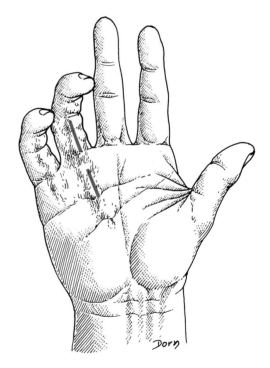

Figure 6.15 Goyrand (1833) recommended longitudinal incision of the skin to avoid causing the wound to gape when straightening the finger.

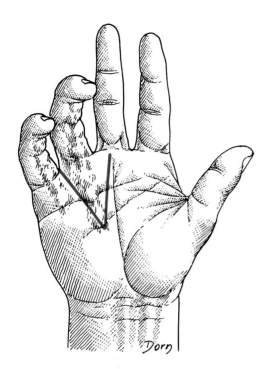

Figure 6.16 Busch, according to Madelung (1875) and Routier (1908), used a V incision for local resection.

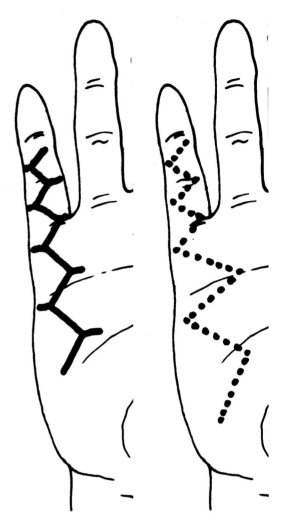

Figure 6.17 Palmen's Y–V incisions (1932).

The disappointing results of these partial fasciectomies were shown by Davis and Finesilver (1932): in a follow-up study of 31 cases after an average of 3 years, 38% were cured, 32% showed partial and 10% complete return of the contracture, and 20% were worse.

Lexer in 1931 published his results of 200 patients operated on over 30 years using a 'Complete excision of the palmar aponeurosis, including its digital extension and the fascia of the thenar region as well as the part of the skin involved' (see ahead to Figures 6.66 and 6.67, pages 186–87). The skin defect was covered by full-thickness skin grafts. Lexer stated that he had seen very few relapses.

In spite of Goyrand's dissections (1833) and detailed descriptions showing that the fingers were held in flexion by bands of fibrous tissue, little attention was paid to the disease localized to the fingers. Palmen (1932) was the first

to use a series of Y–V incisions (Figure 6.17). Bunnell (1944) performed palmar fasciectomies preceded in certain cases by a subcutaneous fasciotomy in order to lengthen the skin and allow better preoperative skin cleansing.

McIndoe's operation for Dupuytren's disease was described first by Skoog in his thesis of 1948. It consists of radical excision of the palmar aponeurosis and its extensions, including both the normal and pathological

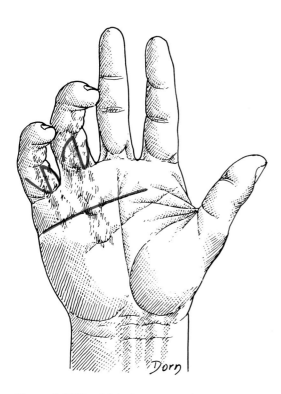

Figure 6.18 The McIndoe approach.

areas. The incision in the palm is made transversally in the distal palmar crease. A **Z**-plasty is made over the proximal phalange of each contracted finger (Figure 6.18). This procedure was the standard operation when the author started to become interested in Dupuytren's disease (James and Tubiana, 1952). As Hueston (1981) diplomatically wrote, 'It was his [McIndoe's] superlative technique that allowed radical fasciectomy to become established as the accepted treatment of Dupuytren's contracture, but in lesser hands the complications of this extensive dissection have since led to it being more restricted in its application.' Even if McIndoe's radical fasciectomy (McIndoe and Beare, 1958) provided good results for McIndoe (Hakstian, 1966), for Skoog and other experienced surgeons the fear of complications led them to look for

more constructive operative procedures (Clarkson, 1963).

Definitions

Fasciectomies, or aponeurectomies, consist of a more or less extensive resection of the diseased Dupuytren's tissue. The aim is to regain as much extension as possible *while preserving full flexion of the digital joints.* The extent of excision of the diseased fibrous tissue varies considerably according to the techniques and biologic theories of each surgeon. Thus Luck (1959) recommended a 'nodulectomy' as, for him, 'the nodule is the essential lesion . . . and it is not necessary to do a radical excision of all the palmar fascia and associated fibrous cords.' Other surgeons practice '*segmental fibrous excision*' of the cords using multiple staged incisions in the palm and fingers. This procedure was described by Russ (1908) who began his operation on the contracted fingers instead of the palm, then by Heyse (1960; local resection method), Freehafer and Strong (1963; partial fasciectomy), and by Vilain and Michon (1977) who used short longitudinal incisions for Dupuytren's disease operated on for the first time, and transverse horizontal incisions – which they called *scalaires* (as in the rungs of a ladder) – for recurrence (Djermag, 1983; Ebelin et al., 1987). Moermans (1991) uses small, curved, longitudinal incisions (Figure 6.19). These segmental fasciectomies avoid major palmar complications (such as skin devascularization and hematomas) but dissection of neurovascular bundles is more hazardous. Some surgeons practice a limited fibrous excision in the palm but an extensive fasciectomy in the finger (McGrouther, 1998).

Usually 'aponeurectomy' indicates an excision of abnormal fibrous tissue, which follows the anatomy of the palmar aponeurosis.

Extensive or '*radical fasciectomies*' (or aponeurectomy) consist of the excision of the

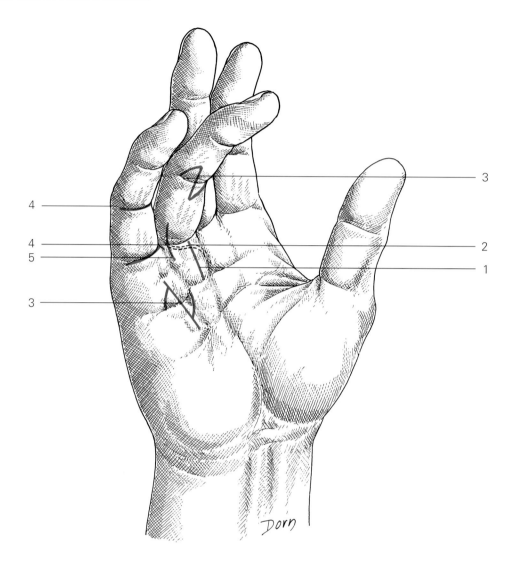

Figure 6.19

Incisions for fasciotomies and segmental fasciectomies: (1) Longitudinal incision; (2) a neurovascular bundle may be pushed superficially by the contracture of a longitudinal cord at the base of the finger; (3) longitudinal incision converted into a Z-plasty; (4) staged transverse incisions; (5) curved longitudinal incision (Moermans, 1991).

diseased palmar fascia extended to the apparently normal aponeurosis, in the hope of preventing extension or recurrence of the lesions. The excision of the fibrous structures in the fingers is always elective. The excision does not extend into apparently normal fingers and a 'total' fasciectomy is never performed. When Clarkson (1963) asked Moberg if he still did a radical fasciectomy, he replied 'What do you mean, a radical fasciectomy? Amputation at the wrist?'.

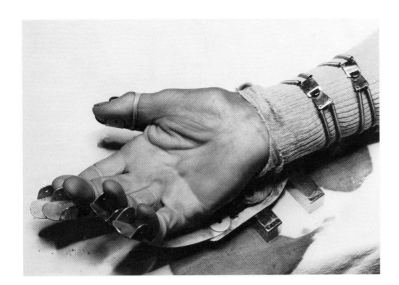

Figure 6.20 Operative malleable splint (Tubiana's design).

Partial or *regional fasciectomies* consist of the excision of macroscopically abnormal fibrous tissue. The extent of the aponeurotic excision in these limited fasciectomies has been variously assessed by different authors (Hamelin, 1952; Tubiana, 1955; Hueston, 1961).

The so-called radical aponeurectomy extending into apparently healthy areas has been shown to have no real prophylactic effect on recurrence. It has been abandoned by the majority of surgeons in favor of partial fasciectomies.

Anesthesia and operative set-up

The author prefers to operate on such patients using regional anesthesia from a transaxillary brachial plexus block. This allows a rapid postoperative mobilization, and the sympathetic action has a beneficial effect on the vascular status. This method allows most patients with Dupuytren's disease to be day-case patients when the surgical center is well equipped and follow-up is ensured. However, when vascularization of the fingers is in doubt the patient should be observed in hospital for at least 24 hours.

The operation is performed using a pneumatic tourniquet; it is inflated, generally without using an Esmarch bandage (except in well-developed muscular arms), after simple elevation of the arm. This allows a small amount of blood to remain in the vascular lumen, facilitating the dissection and hemostasis. The tourniquet is placed high on the upper arm, leaving ready access to the medial aspect of the arm for a skin graft if required. Some surgeons prefer to use only a regional anesthesia of the hand at the wrist level.

The patient is placed supine, and the arm rests on an arm board attached solidly to the operating table. After adequate preparation of the skin and nails, the hand is held in place, fingers spread out and maximally extended using a malleable splint (Figure 6.20).

Exposure

The skin incisions are the first operative stage. The marking of the incisions should not be improvised. In those cases with severe finger flexion, it is preferable to consider different markings before the inflation of the tourniquet.

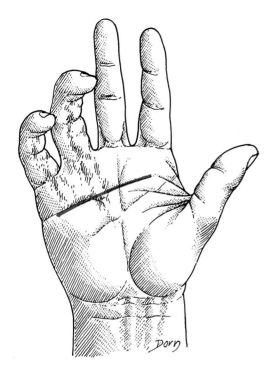
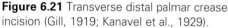

Figure 6.21 Transverse distal palmar crease incision (Gill, 1919; Kanavel et al., 1929).

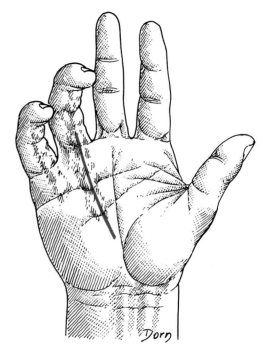

Figure 6.22 Longitudinal incision (Kocher, 1887).

The older authors, for whom palmar fasciectomy was the standard operation, recommended well-defined incisions in the palm. There were those who used transverse distal palmar crease incisions (Gill, 1919; Kanavel et al., 1929) (Figure 6.21) or longitudinal ones (Kocher, 1887) (Figure 6.22). Others, however, designed an L-shaped flap (Lotheissen, 1900 (Figure 6.23); Bunnell, 1944 (Figure 6.24)) or T (von Stapelmohr, 1947) (Figure 6.25), V (Routier, 1908 (see Figure 6.16); Iversen, 1909) or Z incision (Meyerding, 1936) (Figure 6.26) or multiple incisions (Desplas and Meillière, 1932 (Figure 6.27); Moure, 1932; Davis and Finesilver, 1932 (Figure 6.28)).

The digital incision was often neglected. In the finger, midlateral incisions (Figure 6.29), Z-plasty and zig-zag incisions (Bruner, 1951) were used later under the influence of plastic surgeons.

Most surgeons now do not use a routine incision, but adapt the shape of the incision to the given clinical condition, with the following aims:

• To achieve an adequate exposure for dissection of the neurovascular bundles under direct vision and to permit the desired excision of the diseased tissue in the palm and digits;

• To reduce the risk of skin necrosis; no flap should be elevated where a cord crosses its bases, or where a nodule sits. One should remember that the central area of the palm, which is proximal to the distal palmar crease and bordered by the thenar and hypothenar regions, has a relative paucity of arterial supply (Conway and Stark, 1954). Extensive undermining in this central area should be avoided;

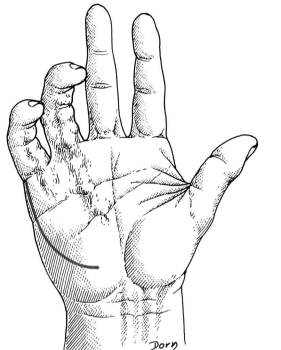

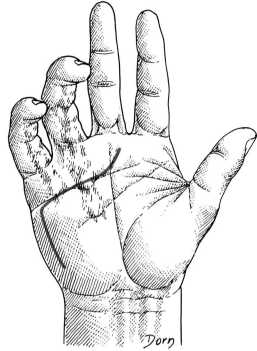

Figure 6.23 Incision used by Lotheissen (1900).

Figure 6.24 Bunnell's palmar incision (1944).

- To permit a rapid postoperative mobilization;
- To avoid contractile scars;
- To permit, if possible, a lengthening of the skin at closure.

Transverse incisions

Transverse incisions do not cause scar contracture. However, they do necessitate extensive undermining of the skin for adequate exposure (Figure 6.30). Moreover, a subcutaneous tunnel is left between the palmar and digital incisions in an area where the dissection is more difficult. Also, the extension of the fingers tends to enlarge the wound. The classical incision in the distal transverse palmar crease is still used by many surgeons when

more than two fingers rays are involved (McCash (1964); see section on the open palm technique, pages 180–85).

Digitopalmar incisions

These offer considerable advantages: an incomparable view, allowing the fibrous cord and neurovascular bundles to be followed in continuity, and the possibility of extension of the exposure to permit adequate excision. Several types of digitopalmar incisions are used:

- Straight, longitudinal incision along the axis of the finger, extending into the palm, followed by a series of Z-plasties (Figure 6.31). These flaps prevent scar

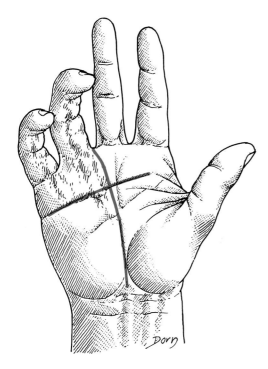

Figure 6.25 Incision used by von Stapelmohr (1947).

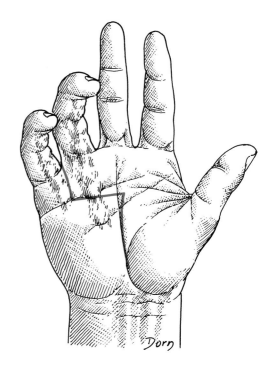

Figure 6.26 Meyerding's (1936) Z incision.

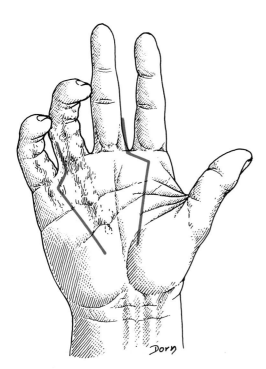

Figure 6.27 Desplas and Meillière's (1932) double palmar incision.

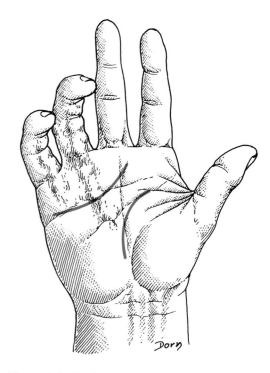

Figure 6.28 Davis and Finesilver's (1932) incisions.

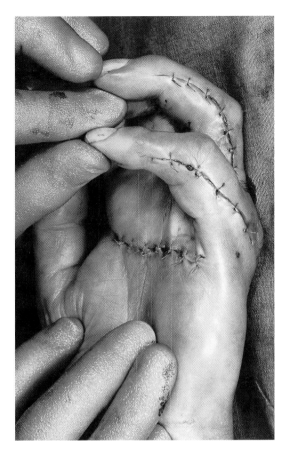

Figure 6.29 Midlateral finger incisions associated with a transverse palmar incision. (Reproduced from James and Tubiana, 1952.)

- Zig-zag digitopalmar incisions (Bruner, 1951, 1974) are the author's favored approach (Figure 6.33a). They allow effective skin lengthening by increasing the number of angles: a V–Y-plasty may be performed at each angle. Bedeschi's 'honeycomb' incision (1990) incorporates a Bruner approach, with lateral darts.

The zones of adherence between the skin and the underlying fibrous tissue are defined. The incision is then drawn in ink and should preferably pass through the middle of these adherent zones, thus avoiding the need for extensive skin devascularization (Figure 6.33b), just as nodule formations are preferably approached through an incision placed over their center. Incisions in the finger are performed only after partially releasing the palm because, as the finger straightens out, it becomes more clear where to safely make the incisions in the finger (Hurst, 1996).

Ideally, the angles of the incision should be the skin flexion creases, but often a W-shaped (hemi-Bruner) incision on the side of the proximal phalanx is used in order to increase the number of angles (Figures 6.33c and d). The incision on the middle phalanx extending to the distal finger crease is always required when the PIP joint is contracted. Each angle is about 90°. If it is too acute, there is a risk of necrosis; if it is too open, there is a tendency to create a longitudinal scar, which could become contractile (see Figure 6.33d). Foucher (1992) has described a useful modification of Bruner's zig-zag incision in order to avoid the centralization of the scar at the level of the proximal finger crease, the incision should follow the transverse crease (Figure 6.33e).

There should be just one long digitopalmar incision running from the most affected finger on to the palm. Other digital incisions may pass for 2–3 cm onto the distal palm. Two adjacent digitopalmar incisions, however, may be joined in the distal part of the palm (Skoog, 1985). Proximally to the distal palmar crease, there is

contracture at the level of flexion creases and permit a lengthening of the skin. The flaps must not be too wide, because they produce a risk of constriction in the fingers and of skin necrosis of the tips, particularly marked in the center of the palm, which is normally poorly vascularized;

- Sinuous, longitudinal incision produces an excellent view, but the gain of length permitted by mobilizing the edges of the flaps is quite limited (Figure 6.32);

only one incision, which ends at approximately the level of the superficial palmar arch.

Hurst (1996) uses a 'three-part incision' for the zig-zag-plasty fasciectomy for pretendinous central cords involving both the ring and small fingers (Figure 6.34).

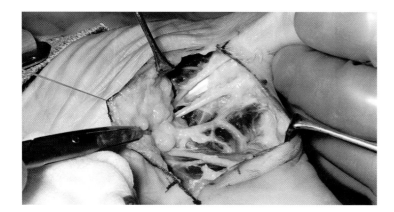

Figure 6.30 Transverse palmar approach.

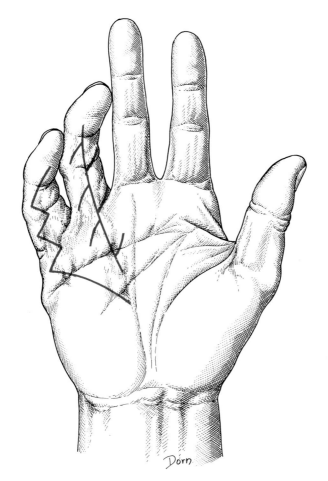

Figure 6.31 On the ring finger a longitudinal digitopalmar incision with Z-plasties at the level of the skin creases. On the little finger a zig-zag Bruner-type incision.

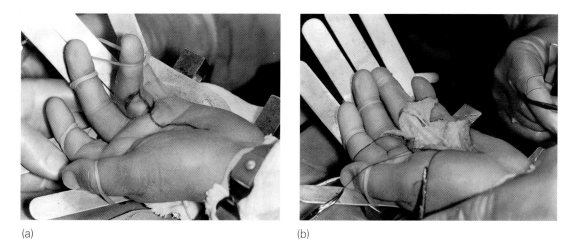

(a)   (b)

Figure 6.32 (a and b) Sinuous longitudinal palmar incision associated with a Z-plasty on the ring finger.

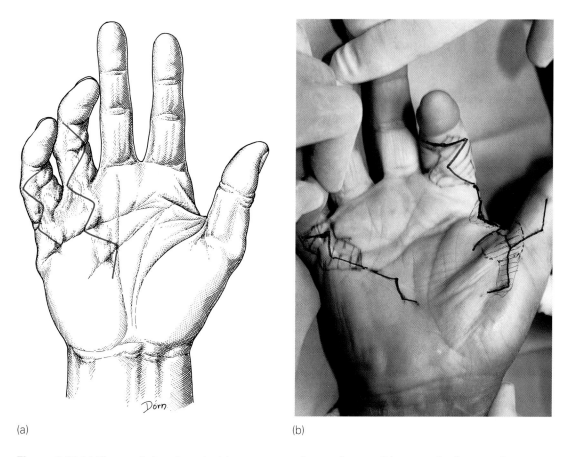

(a)   (b)

Figure 6.33 (a) Zig-zag digitopalmar incisions on two adjacent fingers; (b) zones of adherence between the skin and the underlying fibrous tissue.　　　　　　*Continued*

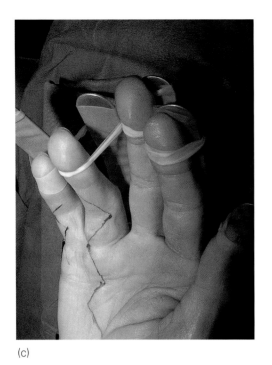

(c)

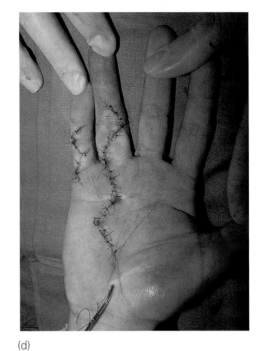

(d)

Figure 6.33 *Continued* (c) Clinical example before surgery; (d) clinical example after surgery. The angle at the base of the finger is too open, risking the creation of a longitudinal scar; (e) Foucher's modification of Bruner's zig-zag incision, which avoids the centralization of the scar.

(e)

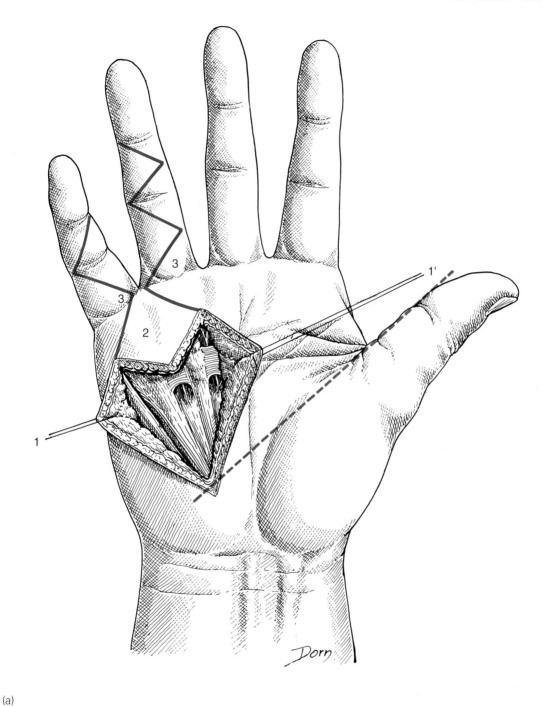

(a)

Figure 6.34 Hurst's 'three-part' incision for fasciectomy. (a) Zig-zag-plasty incisions for fasciectomy involving the right ring and little fingers. 1–1': palmar flaps are open and retracted; 2: web-based distal palmar flap; 3: triangular flaps of the ring and little fingers.   *Continued*

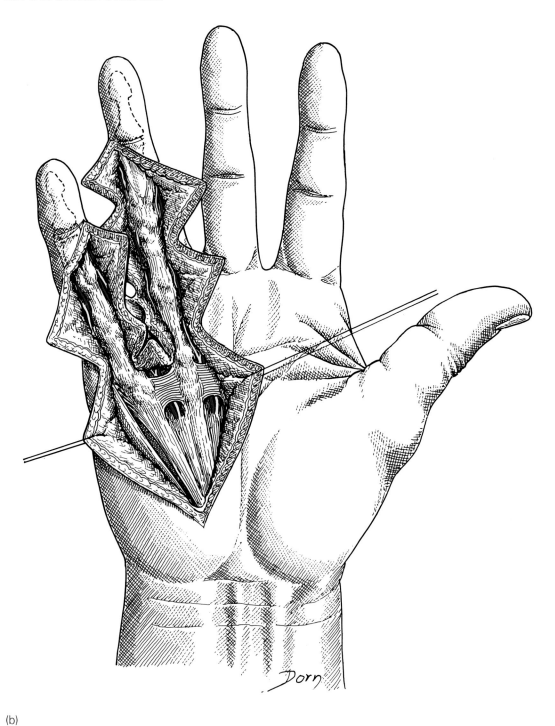

(b)

Figure 6.34 *Continued* (b) Zig-zag-plasty incisions open and two pretendinous central cords exposed. (Reproduced with permission from Hurst, 1996.)

Excision of the palmar fibrous tissue

Familiarity with the palmodigital fibrous structures and the location of the neurovascular bundles are essential for successful surgical treatment.

There are important variations in the extent of palmar fasciectomy according to the extension of the resection of the palmar dis-

eased tissue. In the so-called partial fasciectomy, surgeons differ in the proximal extent and depth of the palmar fasciectomy. There is a tendency to limit the extent of the palmar excision for four reasons:

1) Limited distal palmar fasciectomy can release MP joint contractures but even an extensive palmar fasciectomy does not

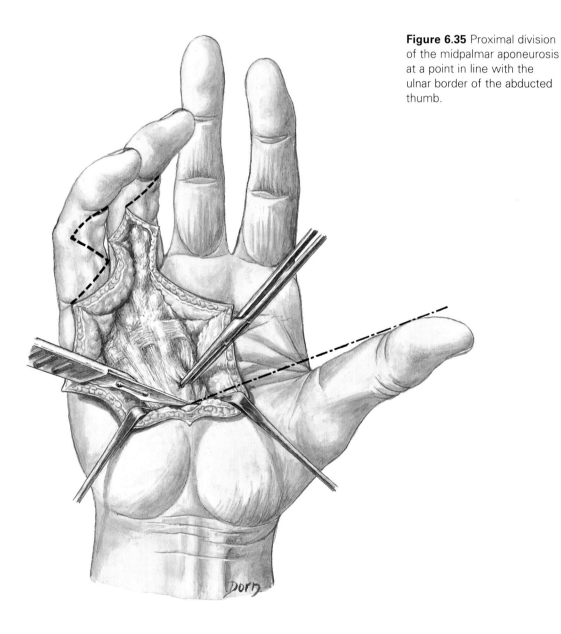

Figure 6.35 Proximal division of the midpalmar aponeurosis at a point in line with the ulnar border of the abducted thumb.

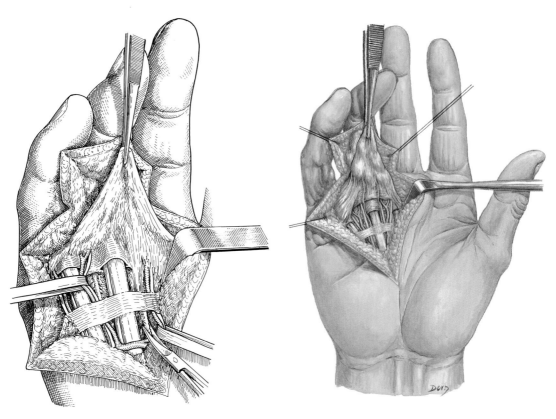

Figure 6.36 Division of the vertical septae.

Figure 6.37 Excision of the fibrous pathological tissue in the palm. The proximal (superficial) transverse ligament is preserved.

correct the interphalangeal joint contracture;

2) Extensive palmar fasciectomy does not seem to have much influence on prevention of recurrence, although according to Millesi (1974) extensive fasciectomy may contribute to an improvement in the long-term result;

3) Recurrences in the proximal part of the palm are rare. They are much more frequent in the distal part of the palm and in the fingers;

4) Complications are more common after extended palmar fasciectomies than after limited operations. As a general rule, one should limit subcutaneous undermining, which encourages hematomas and skin necrosis.

The skin should be dissected from the entire area overlying the aponeurotic excision. Essentially, this is determined by the extent of the lesions, the quality and nature of the tissue and the age of the patient. According to the extent of the disease, one may have to perform an aponeurectomy on one or more rays. When the contractures are severe and extend to all the digits, due to the duration of the operative procedure and the difficulty of the dissection, one may stage the surgery, performing the ulnar and radial aspects of the hand at separate sittings.

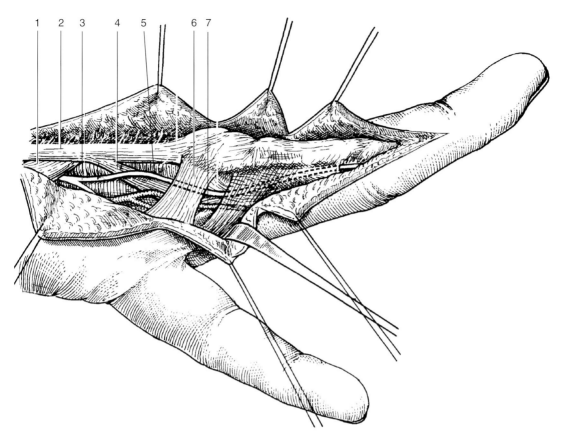

Figure 6.38 Operative aspect of a central cord: (1) proximal transverse ligament (superficial transverse); (2) pretendinous band invaded by Dupuytren's fibrous tissue adherent to the dermis; (3) digital collateral nerve; (4) distal bifurcation of the pretendinous band passing deep to the neurovascular bundle; (5) proximal pulley (A₁) of the flexor tendon sheath; (6) natatory ligament; (7) collateral digital artery.

To avoid extensive palmar skin devascularization, the normal subcutaneous fat should be left intact rather than dissecting in a plane between dermis and fat. If possible, some perforating vessels to the skin are preserved.

The neurovascular bundles only become subcutaneous distal to Skoog's superficial transverse ligament. They are separated from the skin by the palmar aponeurosis in the proximal part of the palm. The dissection of the aponeurosis for many surgeons starts proximally in the palm at a point in line with the ulnar border of the abducted thumb (Kaplan's cardinal line). The two edges of the superficial palmar aponeurosis are freed with blunt-tipped scissors and, with forceps lifting the aponeurosis, may be divided transversely under direct vision (Figure 6.35). Excision is more conservative in older patients or those with vascular problems and may start more distally, at the level of Skoog's superficial transverse ligament (which is shown in Figure 6.42 on page 159).

On the deep aspect of the middle palmar aponeurosis are vertical septa or partitions that separate the channels for both the tendons

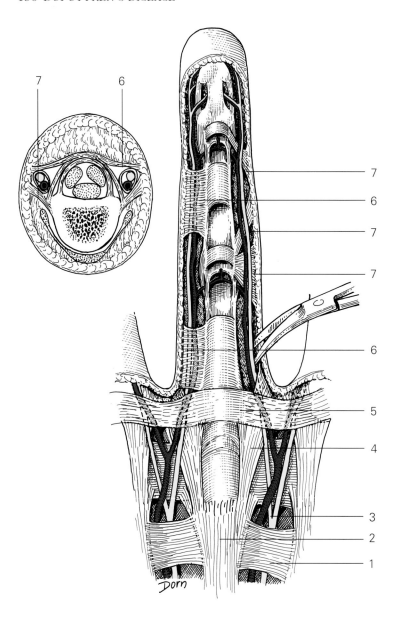

Figure 6.39 Scissors demonstrate that the skin does not adhere to the underlying fibrous structures at the lateral aspect of the web:
(1) Skoog's superficial transverse ligament or proximal transverse ligament;
(2) pretendinous band;
(3) neurovascular bundle;
(4) origin of the spiral band;
(5) natatory ligament;
(6) Grayson's ligament;
(7) Cleland's ligament.

and neurovascular bundles plus the lumbrical muscles. If they are thickened, it is preferable to section them longitudinally with small scissors, after visualizing the digital nerves and arteries (Figure 6.36). The pretendinous longitudinal bands pass superficially in relation to the proximal transverse ligament (Skoog's lig-ament), which is not invaded by the fibrosis and which may be preserved. Its removal makes the dissection easier, but it is preferable to keep it in part; it will be used to place several sutures between the ligament and the dermis (see 'Prevention of vascular complications', page 162, and Figure 6.37).

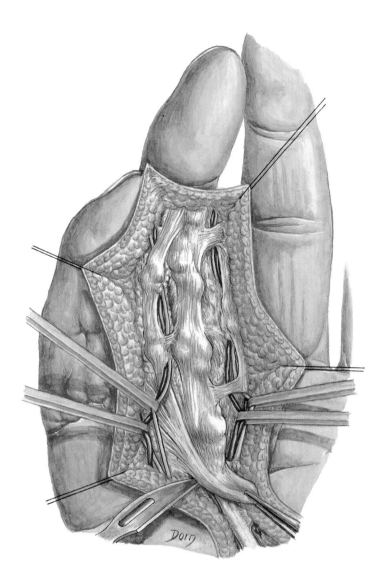

Figure 6.40 At the digitopalmar junction and in the finger, pathological tissue is often very thick. It is necessary to identify the arteries and nerves at the level of the finger

Distal to the proximal transverse ligament, the diseased tissue becomes more adherent to the dermis and must be separated by sharp dissection using magnification. The dissection is centered on the neurovascular bundles, which are no longer protected by the palmar fascia and become subcutaneous. Both nerves and arteries should be identified. This must be performed carefully; it must be remembered that the nerves divide more proximally than the arteries. At the web space, the fingers are abducted to place the natatory ligament under tension (Figure 6.38). At the distal part of the palm, pathological fibrous tissue is usually very thick. The pretendinous cords for each finger are separated with a scalpel, which splits distal transverse formations. Each pathologic cord will be dissected separately. The natatory ligament, which crosses the tendons and neurovascular bundles superficially, is usually very adherent to the skin and should be excised to allow spreading of the fingers.

There are several converging bands at the digitopalmar junction, underneath the natatory ligament, all susceptible to invasion. These include the spiral bands on one part of the MP joints, and fibrous prolongations of the septae and of the deep palmar aponeurosis. The natatory ligament has distal ramifications in the fingers extending longitudinally laterally and dorsally to the vascular bundles, contributing to the retrovascular fibrous cords (Figure 6.39).

The diseased palmar fascia is removed with the neurovascular bundles in view. This allows for correction of MP joint flexion and facilitates the dissection of the finger.

Excision of the pathologic digital fibrous tissue

This is the most delicate part of the operation. The collateral neurovascular bundles are surrounded by a fibrous envelope having a different thickness in each case, thus producing an occasionally unpredictable path for the neurovascular bundles. It is necessary to identify the arteries and nerves at the base of the finger (Figure 6.40), protect them using silicone loops and follow them step by step. In addition to an understanding of the various forms of digital cords (Figure 6.41; see also Chapter 2, 'Relationship between the palmodigital aponeurosis and Dupuytren's disease', pages 38–51), some anatomic considerations help in this process:

- At the base of the fingers, the skin does not adhere to the underlying fibrous tissues at the lateral aspect of the web. This is a useful starting point in the elevation of the skin flaps (see Figure 6.39);
- Displacement of the neurovascular bundles can occur at any point between the palmar longitudinal compartments of Legueu and Juvara, which constitute a proximal fixed position, and the base of the middle phalanx. Hueston used to say

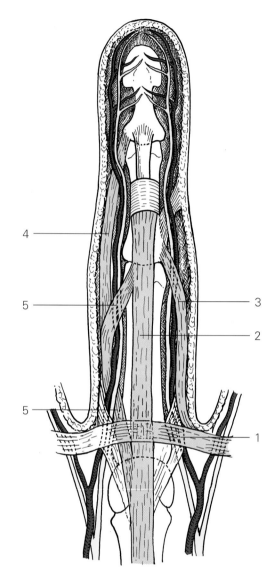

Figure 6.41 Digital cords: (1) natatory ligament; (2) midline cord; (3) lateral cords; (4) retrovascular cords; (5) spiral cords.

'distal to Skoog's ligament anything can happen.'
- Spiral cords may bring the digital neurovascular bundle into the immediate subcutaneous area (see Figure 2.30, page 43). This displacement is often heralded by a

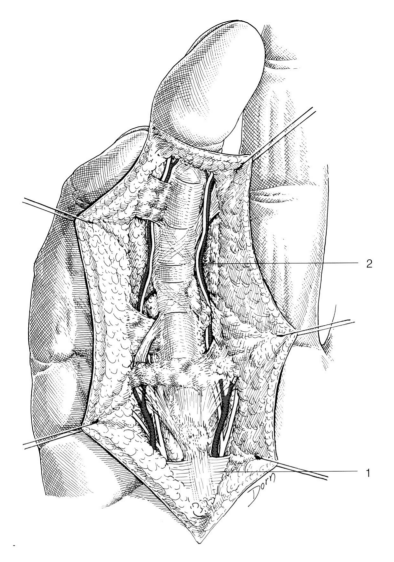

2

1

Figure 6.42 Distal partial palmar fasciectomy associated with digital fasciectomy. This limited palmar procedure reflects the actual tendency of avoiding proximal palmar fasciectomy. In the finger, the path of the neurovascular bundles depends on the contracture of different types of cords and is rather unpredictable, except at the level of the PIP joint, where the bundles are superficial on either side of the joint (2). (1) Proximal palmar transverse ligament (superficial), which may be preserved.

circular, soft, pulpy prominence to either side of the pretendinous cord at the level of the MP joint (Short and Watson, 1982). This sign is a reliable predictor of malposition of the bundle.

Regardless of the path that the collateral bundles take over the proximal phalanx, the nerves and arteries will usually be found on either side of the PIP joint coming to lie just under the skin (Figure 6.42).

It is here that the retrovascular fibrous formations adhere to the capsule and insert into the base of the middle phalanx. In the case of severe contracture of the PIP joint, it may be easiest to find the bundles at the distal finger crease and to follow them proximally.

- At the PIP joint, adherence to the middle part of the flexor tendon sheath is usual, and this sometimes requires opening of the sheath during excision of the retracted tissue. Occasionally, the artery and the nerve are separated by a sheet of fibrous tissue and must be followed separately. Retrovascular cords should be looked for systematically; they may flex the interphalangeal joints without displacing nerves and arteries. All of the thickened and retracted digital fibrous structures are excised so far as the distal phalanx, which usually allows a correction of the contraction. Sometimes, despite this excision, the extension of the IP joints remains restricted, and other procedures are required.

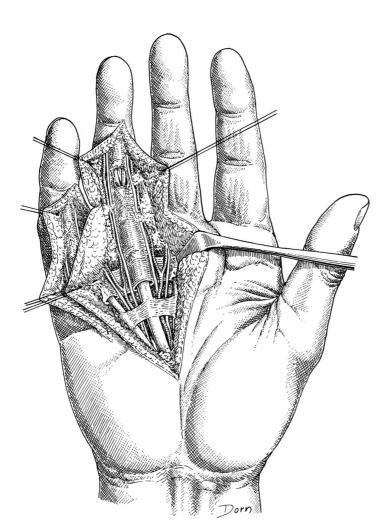

Figure 6.43 Opening of the fibrous tendon sheath at the level of the PIP joint.

Extra-aponeurotic contractures

Contracture of the fibrous sheath of the flexor tendon

The contracture of the fibrous sheath of the flexor tendon should be dealt with first. The sheath is opened transversally at the PIP joint, which often gains a few degrees of extension. This can proceed by stages, with the sheath opened proximally to the joint in the region of the C_1 pulley, which allows access to the proximal attachments of the volar plate (Figure 6.43).

Proximal interphalangeal joint contracture

If, despite opening the sheath, there still is incomplete extension of the PIP joint, the two proximal attachments of the volar plate are resected.

This option of freeing the volar plate without opening the joint was suggested by

Hueston in 1963. The technique and the good results frequently obtained were the subject of a publication by Watson and co-workers in 1979. In fact, the central part of the proximal end of the volar plate has no bony insertion. There is an arch-shaped opening filled by synovium and vessels. The proximal insertion of the plate is made by the intermediate of two ligaments (called 'check-reins' by Eaton, 1971) that are attached at each side of the neck and the distal one-third of the diaphysis of the proximal phalanx. The transverse arterial branches pass under these ligaments, coming from the palmar collateral arteries, and are destined for the long vincula of the flexor digitorum superficialis and profundus. These branches must be protected. The fibrous sheath is opened on both sides of the finger at the C_1 pulley. The small arterial branch will be seen passing toward the midline, under the superficial pillar of the ligament. Using magnification, the pillar is divided distally from the artery (Figure 6.44); then the insertion of this pillar is resected over

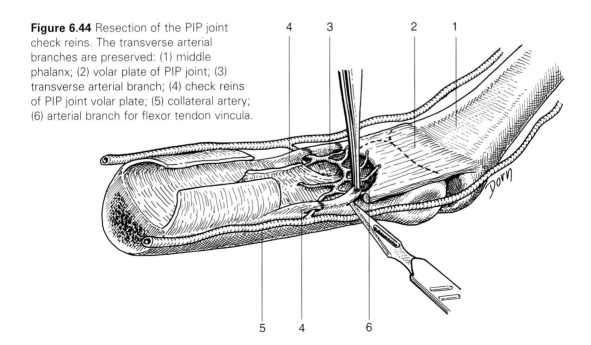

Figure 6.44 Resection of the PIP joint check reins. The transverse arterial branches are preserved: (1) middle phalanx; (2) volar plate of PIP joint; (3) transverse arterial branch; (4) check reins of PIP joint volar plate; (5) collateral artery; (6) arterial branch for flexor tendon vincula.

several millimeters in such a way as to free totally the proximal edge of the volar plate. Gentle passive manipulation of the PIP joint into extension, with the MP joint flexed, then allows the joint to be straightened in the majority of cases, especially if it is the first operation for Dupuytren's disease. For Breed and Smith (1996), 'manipulation alone, sustained for up to two minutes, ruptures periarticular adhesions and gives better results than more aggressive surgical intervention.'

If there is still an extension deficit in the PIP joint, some ambitious surgeons perform a resection of the accessory collateral ligaments inserted on the volar plate and an arthrolysis as recommended by Curtis (1974) (see Chapter 7). In a comparative study between combined fasciectomy with capsuloligamentous release versus fasciectomy alone. Weinzweig et al. (1996) did not find any advantage to capsuloligamentous release despite the immediate intraoperative gain, as the surgical assault to the capsule causes further scarring and contracture.

Other techniques have been used to correct severe PIP joint contractures; they are described in Chapter 7.

In practice, we have found that it is not exceptional – after fasciectomy and freeing the volar plate simply by check reins resection and gentle passive mobilization without arthrolysis – to be able to correct contractures of the PIP joint of greater than 90°.

Three problems then persist: skin contracture may limit the extension but this is easily corrected; tension in the neurovascular bundles; and secondary changes within flexor muscles and the extensor mechanism produce problems that are more difficult to solve.

Prevention of vascular complications

Excessive tension in the vascular bundles must be avoided, as this may lead to digital necrosis. In those cases with a severe contracture, the author occasionally uses an oblique Kirschner wire across the PIP joint to maintain the extension. It is essential after the deflation of the tourniquet to check the circulation in the finger. The MP joint may be flexed to 80° to reduce the tension in the vessels. If the circulation is not adequate after several minutes, the wire is removed, and the PIP joint is flexed until a satisfactory circulation is established. A dynamic extension splint, using progressive elastic traction, is used over the next few days. If, however, the circulation becomes adequate, it is preferable to leave the wire and to use a dorsal splint to keep the MP joints flexed to relax the neurovascular structures. One must struggle against the contracture of the flexor tendons after that. The wire is removed after seven days and a PIP joint extension splint is applied, associated with careful re-education.

Secondary changes within flexor muscles and the extensor mechanism

The correction of PIP joint contracture, which is frequently obtained at the time of operation, does not mean that full extension of the joint will be possible postoperatively. Relapse of PIP joint extension deficit is frequent after long-standing flexion contracture for two main reasons: secondary changes in elasticity within flexor muscles and secondary changes in the extensor mechanism.

Smith and Breed (1994) stressed the importance of central slip attenuation in Dupuytren's PIP joint contracture. Smith and Ross (1994) described a 'central slip tenodesis test' for early diagnosis of potential boutonnière deformities: with the wrist maintained in full flexion, the examiner places a finger on the dorsum of the proximal phalanx of the finger and flexes the MP joint. With an intact central slip, this causes passive extension of the PIP joint because of the tenodesis effect. When the central slip is deficient, this maneuver elicits an extensor lag. In such a case, the 'PIP joint should be

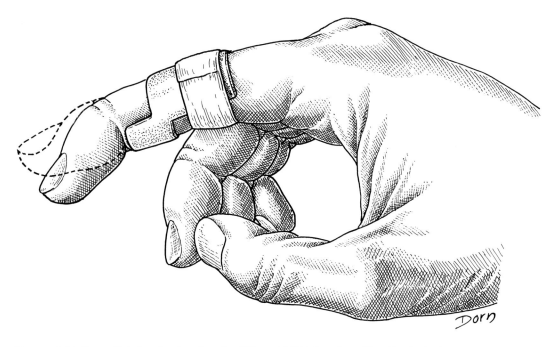

Figure 6.45 Short digital splint, leaving the DIP and MP joints free (Stack's design).

immobilized in a static splint for 3 weeks (the distal joint is left free and mobilized) [Figure 6.45] then mobilized for a further 3 weeks in a Capener splint. Failure to do this will lead to immediate recurrence of flexion deformity due to absence of extensor tone' (Breed and Smith, 1996). A long postoperative re-education, associated with splinting is necessary for 4 to 6 months (Rives et al., 1992).

Hemostasis

A careful hemostasis is performed throughout the dissection, using a bipolar coagulation about 2 mm away from the main vessel. Before deflating the tourniquet, warm saline-soaked sponges are applied to the wound. In the author's practice, the tourniquet is deflated before the skin closure. The preservation of

the proximal transverse palmar ligament allows the use of several sutures to close the potential dead space between the ligament and the skin and to reduce the risk of hematomata (Figure 6.46). A drain can be useful, but this should not be used instead of careful hemostasis.

Fasciectomy in the little finger

It is in the forms involving only the little finger that the contracture is often the most severe (Figure 6.47). Fasciectomies in the little finger are often difficult because of the small size of the digit and the abundance of fibrous tissue. In the little finger different types of cords may coexist (see Figure 2.33, page 46). The ulnar retrovascular cord, inserted on the abductor digiti minimi tendon is nearly always present

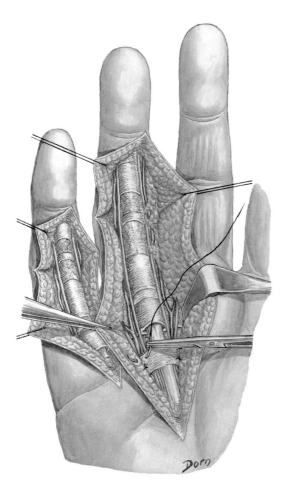

Figure 6.46 Closure of the potential dead space in the palm, between the proximal transverse ligament and the dermis.

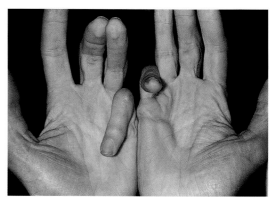

Figure 6.47 Bilateral severe little finger contracture.

and the ulnar neurovascular bundle is pushed toward the midline at the base of the finger by the fibrous formation. When dissecting the abductor digiti minimi cord, the ulnar neurovascular bundle must be carefully protected. The cord arises as a prolongation of the common tendon of insertion of the intrinsic abductor and flexor muscles. There is no clear plane of dissection between tendon and cord. The cord bridges the PIP joint and inserts into the fibrous tendon sheath and extensor mechanism (Littler, 1974) (Figure 6.48). The cord at its origin lies ulnar and dorsal to the ulnar digital nerve.

Sometimes the nerve may spiral dorsal to the ADM cord or spiral through it. Also the terminal portion of the dorsal ulnar sensory nerve may be closely applied to the dorsolateral aspects of this cord (Hurst, 1996) (see Figure 2.18, page 33).

It is in the little finger that recurrences are most frequent and that salvage procedures, including dermofasciectomies, arthrodesis and amputations, are performed most frequently (see Chapter 7) (see Figures 7.15 and 7.16, pages 234–35). It is also in the little finger that *hyperextension of the distal phalanx* may be seen, usually associated with a severe PIP joint flexion contracture. Rarely, a plaque of Dupuytren's tissue may be found beneath the extensor tendon over the middle phalanx (Iselin et al., 1988). Sometimes, the release of the PIP contracture may correct the DIP hyperextension deformity. If not, an oblique 'chevron' tenotomy on the dorsal aspect of the middle phalanx is necessary if the DIP joint is not stiff (Figure 6.51). The oblique dorsal incision should be left open if there is any skin contracture.

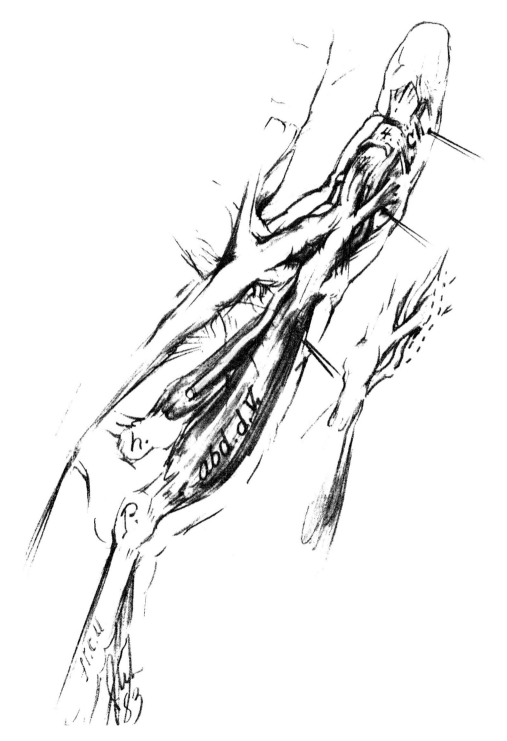

Figure 6.48 The abductor digiti mini (ADM) cord. p: pisiform; h: hamate; 4: pulley A$_4$. (Reproduced with permission from Littler, 1974.)

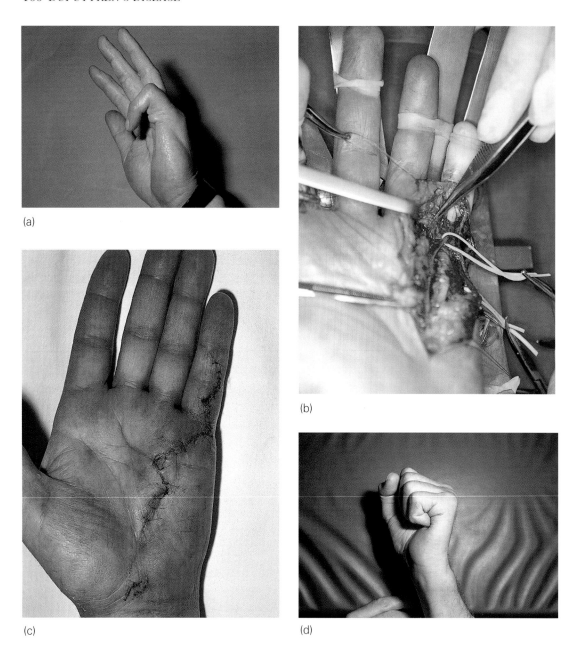

Figure 6.49 Severe Dupuytren's contracture in the little finger: (a) preoperative view; (b) digitopalmar fasciectomy with resection of the PIP joint check reins; (c and d) complete correction of the contracture.

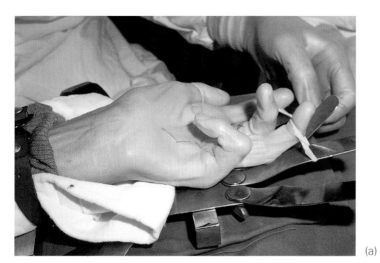

(a)

Figure 6.50 (a) Another example of severe contracture of the little finger; (b) fasciectomy; (c) a skin graft has been applied at the base of the finger.

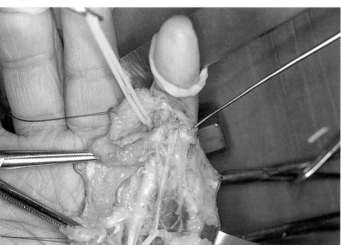

(b)

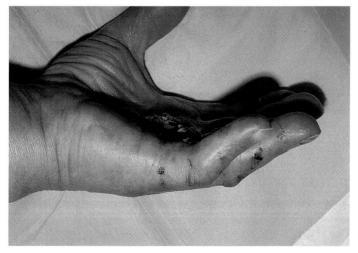

(c)

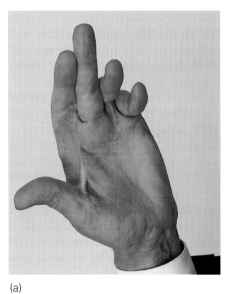

(a)

Figure 6.51 (a) Boutonnière-type deformity on the ring and little fingers; (b) oblique tenotomy of the lateral exterior tendons at the middle phalanx; (c) the obliqueness of the division allows lengthening of the distal extensor apparatus and flexion of the distal joint.

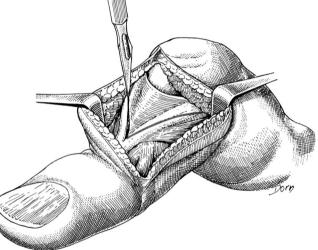

(b)

(c)

Fasciectomy in the radial side of the hand

Disease affecting the thumb was reported for the first time by Guérin (1833), one of Dupuytren's trainees.

Most of the Dupuytren's disease affecting the radial side of the hand is seen in elderly patients and produces only minimal contractures, usually associated with the more common contractures affecting the ulnar side. The radial-side lesions seldom cause the patient much trouble; surgery is rarely necessary for removing radial-side lesions, and is used in association with fasciectomy of ulnar-side lesions when there is surgical indication to treat contractures affecting the ulnar fingers (Figure 6.52a and b). Moderate contracture of the web space can be corrected by Z-plasties or by the use of combinations of V–Y- and Z-plasties. Sometimes, isolated cords at the level of the radial side of the thenar eminence and of the thumb (Figure 6.53) or a commissural cord (Figure 6.54) should be removed.

The problem is quite different in the aggressive form of radial-side lesions, which occur in young people before the age of 40 years in about 10% of cases. The severe radial involvement affecting all the fascial structures (Figure 6.55) is almost always accompanied by ulnar contractures, which occur early in the disease process. Patients with these types of radial involvement fit most of the criteria of Hueston's 'Dupuytren's diasthesis': positive family history, bilateral disease with diffuse involvement of the palm and digits, rapid cutaneous invasion, and frequent association with ectopic foci. The prognosis is severe, with a high incidence of postoperative extension and recurrence. Some of the author's patients had more than 10 operations on the two hands. These severe diffuse forms cannot be treated safely in one operative session. The ulnar and radial sides are treated in two separate operations. Contracture affecting the radial side requires a special approach (Figure 6.56) and the use of skin grafts (Tubiana et al., 1982).

The aim of surgery at the radial side of the hand is to open the thumb web space. This aim is usually achieved after the excision of the diseased tissue (see Figure 2.36, page 49). However, if the contracture is long-standing, the dorsal elements of the web space may also be contracted. The dorsal aponeurosis of the

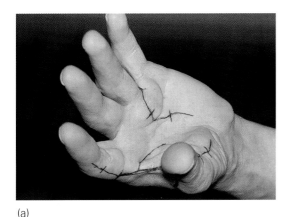

(a)

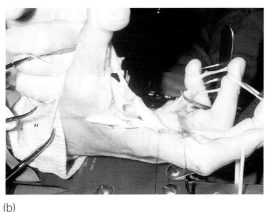

(b)

Figure 6.52 (a) Moderate Dupuytren's contractures affecting the radial and ulnar sides of the hand. Associated fasciectomies are performed at the same operation; (b) Z-plasty at the thumb web space.

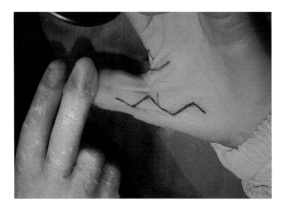

Figure 6.53 The thenar cord.

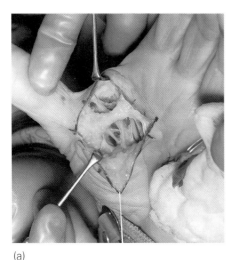

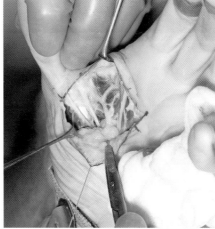

Figure 6.54 (a and b) Proximal commissural cord.

(a)   (b)

commissure as well as the dorsal skin should be divided. The medial limb of the Z is situated on the edge of the web; the radial limb should be palmar and the ulnar limb, dorsal (reverse Z-plasty because, normally, the palmar limb is ulnar in the opposition crease of the thumb). At each end of the web space, the incision may be extended on the radial side of the index finger or ulnar side of the thumb. On the index finger, the incision follows the same guidelines as on the other fin-

gers. When there is a severe fibrous lesion, a transverse skin incision at the thumb MP joint joins the radial thumb incision to the web space incision, and facilitates the dissection of the skin flaps. The excision of the diseased tissue is facilitated by a thorough knowledge of the anatomy and its relationship to the fibrous structures. It is important to start by isolating and protecting the neurovascular bundles of the thumb and index finger before dissecting the cords. The thumb's

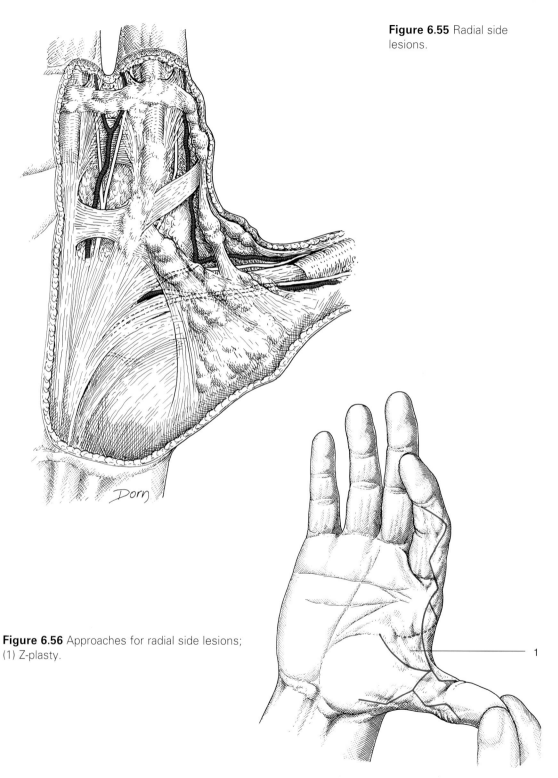

Figure 6.55 Radial side lesions.

Figure 6.56 Approaches for radial side lesions; (1) Z-plasty.

1

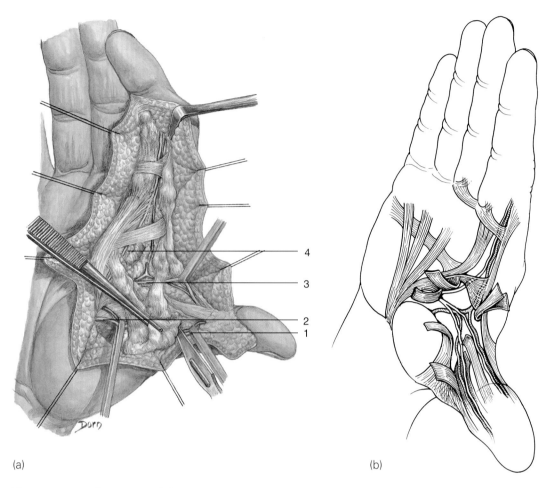

(a)   (b)

Figure 6.57 (a) Dissection of the neurovascular bundles of the first web space. The ulnar neurovascular bundle (3) is found at the base of the thumb. The radial collateral nerve of the thumb is found in the thenar eminence (2) and is followed superficially across the flexor pollicis longus tendon and only passes to the radial side of the thumb at the middle of the proximal phalanx (1). The radial collateral nerve of the index finger (4) is found at the obtuse angle made by the radial edge of the proximal transverse commissural ligament and the longitudinal pretendinous band of the index finger; (b) neurovascular bundles are isolated.

ulnar neurovascular bundle, the most important in the hand, is easily found at the base of the thumb, at the division of Grapow's ligament, where the two terminal expansions go to either side of the thumb (Grapow, 1887) (Figure 6.57). The *radial bundle* is more difficult to find at the base of the thumb since it is covered by a criss-crossing fibrous tissue at the MP joint. It is wiser to look for it more proximally in the palm, just in the thenar eminence. The nerve passes superficially across the tendon of flexor pollicis longus, medially to laterally at the metacarpal head. It stays adherent to the tendon sheath, and only passes to the radial side of the thumb distally at about the middle of the proximal phalanx. The *radial collateral nerve of the index finger* is found at the obtuse angle made by the radial edge of the proximal transverse commissural ligament and the longitudinal pretendinous band of the index finger. It is important to remember that the artery may be as much as 8 mm lateral to the nerve at this point (Coleman and Anson, 1961). The two parts of the bundle are found together at the base of the index finger. Once the neurovascular bundles are isolated and protected, it is sufficient to follow them by separating them from the surrounding fibrous tissue as is performed for ulnar-sided fingers affected by Dupuytren's disease (Figure 6.58).

The use of skin grafts on the radial side of the hand poses particular problems (Tubiana, 1999) (see within the section on skin grafts, pages 195–97). Complications are rare and minor; on the radial side of the hand the danger of hematoma and skin necrosis is less than after extensive palmar dissections.

Closure

The choice of skin closure is an important step of the operation. There are several possibilities:

- Simple skin suture;
- Skin-lengthening procedures;
- Skin flaps;
- Skin grafts;
- Open palm.

Skin sutures

We believe, and our practice has shown, that at the end of a fasciectomy, it is better to suture the skin in the absence of tension, after a perfect hemostasis. There will be healing of the wound within about 2 weeks.

One of the merits of McCash's work (1964) was that he showed that a suture under tension is much more dangerous than no suture. If there is the slightest tension, it is wiser to leave the skin edges separated by a few millimeters. This does not prevent early physiotherapy and only slightly slows wound healing. Often, the tension in the skin can be reduced by various skin-lengthening procedures.

Skin-lengthening procedures

These procedures are not planned until the tourniquet has been released.

When a Bruner-type zig-zag incision has been performed, V–Y-plasties repeated at each angle of the incision (Figure 6.59) will produce significant lengthening. If the tension complicates tips advancement, the transverse limbs of the V–Y can be left open. V–Y corrections may be inferior to those obtained by a series of Z-plasties, but these require supple and well-vascularized tissues, which are rarely found when there are severe contractures.

Z-plasties are mostly used when a straight longitudinal incision crosses a digital transverse crease. They are designed at the end of the fascial dissection. The flaps of the Z-plasty must not be too large, no more than 1.5 cm in length, since their crossing over tends to constrict the finger.

Skin flaps and skin grafts

In addition to the lengthening flaps, other local flaps can be used to cover significant skin defects. These are described later in the sections on skin flaps, skin grafts, and dermofasciectomy (pages 186–203). Flaps taken from a distance are contraindicated by their required long postoperative treatment; they are only considered if the local vascular supply is compromised. On the contrary, skin grafts are now widely used.

Figure 6.58 Radial fasciectomy with skin grafts.
(a) Dupuytren's disease affecting the radial and
ulnar sides of the hand; (b) incisions in the first
web space; (c) proximal and distal commissural
cords; (d) dissection of the neurovascular
bundles; (e) fasciectomy of the thumb and index
finger. *Continued*

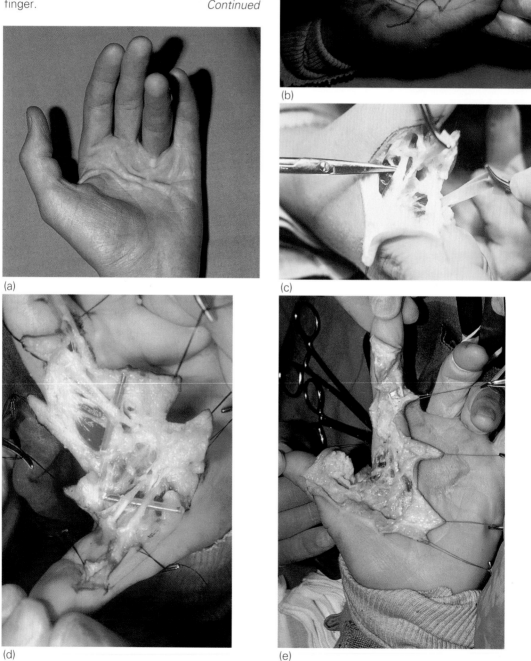

(a)

(b)

(c)

(d)

(e)

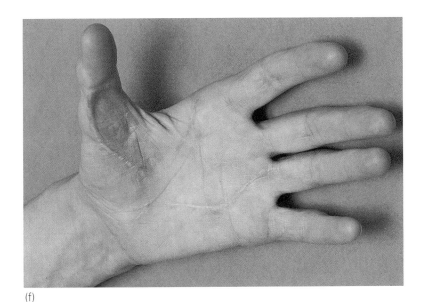

(f)

Figure 6.58 *Continued*
(f, g) Radial fasciectomy
with skin grafts.

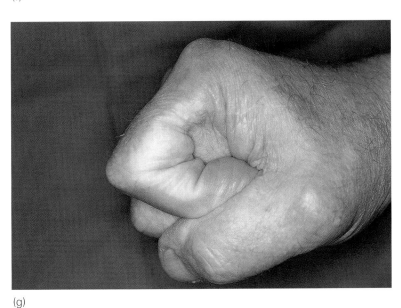

(g)

Open palm technique

Many surgeons routinely use McCash's (1964) open palm technique or one of its variations (Figure 6.60) in order to minimize the risk of complications. This procedure is fully described on pages 180–85 and our indications

of this popular technique are shown in 'Surgical indications' on pages 218–22.

Postoperative care

A mildly compressive bandage is applied, including the wrist but leaving the fingertips

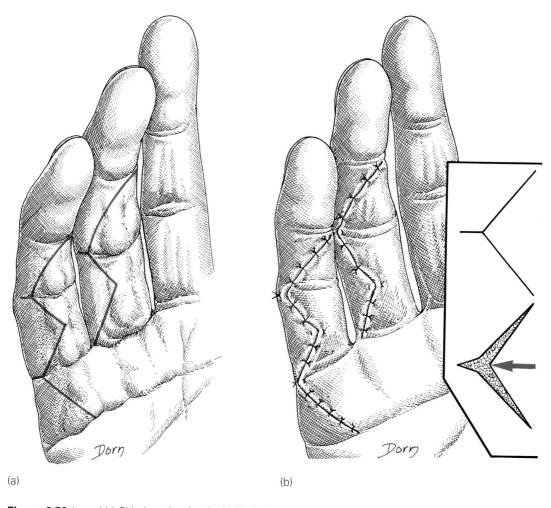

(a) (b)

Figure 6.59 (a and b) Skin lengthening by V–Y plasty.

exposed. A light dorsal splint is applied with the wrist in extension, the MP joint flexed to about 50°, and the IP joints left as free as possible. Many patients are allowed to go home the same day, after a few hours of rest with the hand kept in elevation, and once the effects of the anesthetic have worn off. The surgeon has previously inspected the vascularity and sensation at the tips of the fingers, the absence of pain and the state of the dressing. Older patients with significant medical problems or

patients living long distances away are hospitalized for 48 hours (Robbins, 1981). There should be only moderate pain. If severe pain should occur, a wound inspection is necessary. The first change of the dressing is normally performed 48 hours postoperatively by the surgeon. The wound is inspected, any drains that were thought necessary are removed, and physiotherapy is started on the third day. If a skin graft has been used, the first dressing is opened on the 7th day.

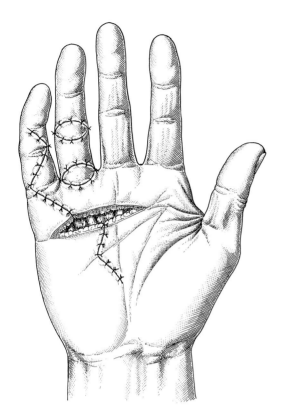

Figure 6.60 Open palm technique. McCash (1964) recommended a fasciectomy performed using transverse incisions. The incision at the distal palmar crease is left open and acts as a perfect drainage. This principle is currently used with different combinations of digitopalmar incisions and skin grafts. There are two 'fire-break' grafts on the ring finger.

Postoperative rehabilitation

In the immediate postoperative period there are two schools of thought about the best position in which to splint the hand. The author uses a dorsal splint with the wrist in extension, the MP flexed and the PIP free or extended. This position avoids tension on the soft tissues and on the sutures. In his opinion, the aim of the postoperative therapy is to regain complete finger flexion as rapidly as possible; extension will be restored progressively, taking into account the operative measures. Alternatively, the hand can be immobilized with the MP and PIP joints extended to allow maximal elongation of the wound, as is described in Chapter 9. In the author's experience, splinting with the MP and IP joints extended is contraindicated due to the risk of severe postoperative joint contracture. He prefers to splint the MP joints flexed and the IPP joints extended so as to relax the neurovascular structures while protecting surgical gains at the PIP joints. The MP joints are gradually brought out into extension. The patient should be reviewed by the surgeon at least once a week until the wounds are healed and the fingers are moving fully. Early cicatrization of the wound and return to work will improve rapid rehabilitation of the operated hand.

References

Adams W (1878) Contraction of the fingers (Dupuytren's contracture) and its successful treatment by subcutaneous divisions of the palmar fascia and immediate extension. *BMJ* 1: 928.

Bedeschi P (1990) Various views and techniques. Management of the skin. Honeycomb technique. In: McFarlane RM, McGrouther DA, Flint MH, eds, *Dupuytren's Disease: Biology and Treatment.* 311–14. Churchill Livingstone, Edinburgh.

Breed CM, Smith PJ (1996) A comparison of methods of treatment of PIP joint contractures in Dupuytren's disease. *J Hand Surg* **21B**: 246–51.

Bruner JM (1951) Incisions for plastic and reconstructive (non-septic) surgery of the hand. *Br J Plast Surg* **4**: 48.

Bruner JM (1974) Technique of selective aponeurectomy for Dupuytren's contracture. In: Hueston JT, Tubiana R, eds, *Dupuytren's Disease,* 93–94. Churchill Livingstone, Edinburgh.

Bunnell S (1944) *Surgery of the Hand.* JB Lippincott, Philadelphia.

Clarkson P (1963) The radical fasciectomy operation for Dupuytren's disease. A condemnation. *Br J Plastic Surg* **16**: 273–79.

Cline H (1777) Notes on pathology and surgery. Manuscript 28:185. St Thomas' Hospital Library, London.

Coleman SS, Anson GJ (1961) Arterial patterns in the hand based upon a study of 650 specimens. *Surg Gynecol Obstet* **113**: 409.

Conway H, Stark RB (1954) Arterial vascularization of the soft tissues of the hand. *J Bone Joint Surg* **36A**: 1238–40.

Cooper A (1822) *A Treatise on Dislocations and Fractures of the Joints*, 1st edn. Longman, Hurst, Rees, Orme, Brown & Cox, London.

Curtis RM (1974) Volar capsulectomy in the PIP joint in Dupuytren's contracture. In: Hueston JT, Tubiana R, eds, *Dupuytren's Disease*, 135. Churchill Livingstone, Edinburgh.

Davis JS, Finesilver EM (1932) Dupuytren's contracture with a note on the incidence of the contraction in diabetes. *Archives of Surgery* **24**: 933.

Desplas K, Meillière J (1932) Sur une technique opératoire concernant la maladie de Dupuytren. *Bull Mem Soc Nat Chirurg* **58**: 424 (cited by Skoog (1948)).

Djermag Y (1983) *Contribution à l'étude de la maladie de Dupuytren: A propos de 104 cas revus*. Thèse Doctorat en Médecine, Université Paris VII.

Dupuytren G (1831) Contracture permanente des doigts avec mobilité de chaque articulation et impossibilité de l'extension. *Gazette Hop*, 26 novembre.

Eaton RJ (1971) *Joint Injuries of the Hand*. Charles Thomas, Illinois.

Ebelin M, Divaris M, Leviet D, Vilain R (1987) Traitement des récidives dans la maladie de Dupuytren. *Chirurgie* **113**: 780–84.

Fergusson W (1842) *A System of Practical Surgery*. Churchill Livingstone, London.

Foucher G, Cornil C, Lenoble E (1992) Open palm technique for Dupuytren's disease. *Ann Chir Main (Ann Hand Surg)* **11**: 362–66.

Freehafer A, Strong JM (1963) The treatment of Dupuytren's contracture by partial fasciectomy. *J Bone Joint Surg* **45A**: 1207–216.

Gersuny R (1884) Operation bei Kontraktur der Palmaraponevrose. *Wien Med Wochenschr* **34**: 969.

Gill AB (1919) Dupuytren's contracture, with a description of a method of operation. *Ann Surg* **70**: 221.

Goyrand G (1833) Nouvelles recherches sur la rétraction permanente des doigts. *Mem Acad Med* **3**: 489.

Grapow M (1887) Die Anatomie and physiologische Bedeutung der Palmaraponeurose. *Arch Anat Physiol* **143**: 2–3.

Guérin G (1833) Commentaires sur la rétraction permanente des doigts. *Gaz Med Paris* **1**: 111–13.

Hakstian RW (1966) Long-term results of extensive fasciectomy. *Br J Plast Surg* **140**: 149.

Hamelin E (1952) Limited excision of Dupuytren's contracture. *Ann Surg* **135**: 94–97.

Heyse WE (1960) Dupuytren's contracture and its surgical treatment. Clinical study of a local resection method. *JAMA* **174**: 113–18.

Hueston JT (1961) Limited fasciectomy for Dupuytren's contracture. *Plast Reconstr Surg* **27**: 569–85.

Hueston JT (1963) *Dupuytren's Contracture*. E & S Livingstone, Edinburgh.

Hueston JT (1981) Historical Profiles. Archibald Hector McIndoe (1900–1960). In: Tubiana R, ed., *The Hand*, Vol. 1, WB Saunders, Philadelphia.

Hurst LC (1996) Dupuytren's fasciectomy: zig-zag-plasty technique. In: Blair WF, ed., *Techniques in Hand Surgery* 519–29. Williams and Wilkins, Baltimore.

Iselin F, Cardenas-Baron L, Gouget-Audry I, Peze W (1988) La maladie de Dupuytren dorsale. *Ann Chir Main* **7**: 247–50.

Iversen J (1909) Über die traumatische Entsehung der Dupuytrenschen Kontraktur u. deren Lokalisation am Daumen. Inaugural Dissertation, Kiel (cited by Skoog (1948)).

James JIP, Tubiana R (1952) La maladie de Dupuytren. *Rev Chir Orthop* **38**: 352–406.

Kanavel AB, Koch SL, Mason ML (1929) Dupuytren's contraction. *Surg Gynecol Obstet* **48**: 145–90.

Kocher T (1887) Behandlung der Retraktion der Palmaraponeurose. *Centralbl Chirurg* **14**: 482–87, 497–502.

Lexer E (1931) *Die gesamte Wiedererstellungschirurgie*, 2nd edn, Leipzig.

Littler JW (1974) Special points of technique in Dupuytren's contracture. In: Hueston JT, Tubiana R, eds, *Dupuytren's Disease*, 97–99. Churchill Livingstone, Edinburgh.

Lotheissen G (1900) Zur operativen Behandlung der Dupuytrenschen Kontraktur. *Zentralabl Chirurg* **27**: 761.

Luck JV (1959) Dupuytren's contracture. A new concept of the pathogenesis correlated with surgical management. *J Bone Joint Surg* **41A**: 635–64.

Madelung OW (1875) Die Aetiologie und die operative Behandlung der Dupuytren'sche Fingerverkrümmung. *Berl Klin Wochenschr* **12**: 191.

McCash CR (1964) The open palm technique in Dupuytren's contracture. *Br J Plast Surg* **17**: 271–80.

McGrouther DA (1998) Dupuytren's contracture. In: Green DP, Hotchkiss RN, Pederson WC, eds, *Green's Operative Hand Surgery*, Vol. 1, 4th edn, 563–91. Churchill Livingstone, New York.

McIndoe AH, Beare RLB (1958) The surgical management of Dupuytren's contracture. *Am J Surg* **95**: 197.

Meyerding HW, Black JR, Broders AC (1936) The etiology and pathology of Dupuytren's contracture. *Surg Gynecol Obstet* 582–90.

Millesi H (1974) The clinical and morphological course of Dupuytren's disease. In: Hueston JT, Tubiana R, eds, *Dupuytren's Disease*, 49. Churchill Livingstone, Edinburgh.

Moermans JP (1991) Segmental aponeurectomy in Dupuytren's disease. *J Hand Surg* **16B**: 243–54.

Moure P (1932) A propos de la maladie de Dupuytren. *Bull Mem Soc Nat Chir* **63**: 149.

Palmen AJ (1932) Die Sageplastik, eine unter anderen für Dupuytrensche Fingerkontraktur und Syndactylie geeignete Schnittführung. *Zentralbl Chirurg* **59**: 1377.

Razemon J (1982) Le lambeau de rotation latéro digital dans les formes graves de la maladie de Dupuytren. A propos de 141 observations. *Ann Chir Main* **1**: 199.

Rives K, Gelberman R, Smith B, Carney K (1992) Severe contractures of the proximal interphalangeal joint in Dupuytren's disease. Results of a prospective trial of operative correction and dynamic extension splinting. *J Hand Surg* **17A**: 1153.

Robbins TH (1981) Dupuytren's contracture: the deferred Z-plasty. *Ann R Coll Surg Engl* **63**: 357–58.

Routier (1908) Rétraction de l'aponévrose palmaire. Opération sans suture sans autoplastie. *Bull Mem Soc Chirurg Paris* **34**: 860.

Russ R (1908) The surgical aspects of Dupuytren's contraction. *Am J Med Sci* **135**: 856.

Sanson LJ (1834) Rapport sur le mémoire du Dr G Goyrand 'Nouvelles recherches sur la rétraction permanente des doigts' *Mem Acad R Med* **3**: 496–500.

Short WH, Watson HK (1982) Prediction of the spiral nerve in Dupuytren's contracture. *J Hand Surg* **7A**: 84–86.

Skoog T (1948) Dupuytren's contraction with special reference to aetiology and improved surgical treatment. Its occurrence in epileptics – Note on knuckle pads. *Acta Chirurg Scand* **96** (suppl 139): 1.

Skoog T (1985) Dupuytren's contracture: pathogenesis and surgical treatment. In: Hueston JT, Tubiana R, eds, *Dupuytren's Disease*, 184–92. Churchill Livingstone, Edinburgh.

Smith P, Breed C (1994) Central slip attenuation in Dupuytren's contracture. A cause of persistent flexion of the proximal interphalangeal joint. *J Hand Surg* **19A**: 840.

Smith PJ, Ross DA (1994) The central slip tenodesis test for early diagnosis of potential boutonnière deformities. *J Hand Surg* **19B**: 88.

Tubiana R (1955) Prognosis and treatment of Dupuytren's contracture. *J Bone Joint Surg* **37A**: 1155–68.

Tubiana R (1963) Les temps cutanés dans le traitement chirurgical de la maladie de Dupuytren. *Ann Chirurg Plast* **8**: 157–68.

Tubiana R (1999) Dupuytren's disease of the radial side of the hand. *Hand Clinics* **15**: 149–59.

Tubiana R, Simmons BP, de Frenne HAR (1982) Location of Dupuytren's disease on the radial aspect of the hand. *Clin Orthop Relat Res* **168**: 222–29.

Velpeau ALM (1835) Sur la rétraction des doigts. *Gaz Med Paris* **2–3**: 511.

Vilain R, Michon J (1977) *Chirurgie plastique cutanée de la main et de la pulpe*, 2nd edn. Masson, Paris.

Von Stapelmohr S (1947) Om 14 ars Dupuytrenoperatiomer à Norrköpings lasarett. *Svenska läk Tidning* **44**: 81 (cited by Skoog (1948) (in Swedish)).

Watson HK, Light TR, Johnson TR (1979) Check rein resection for flexion contracture of the middle joint. *J Hand Surg* **4**: 67–71.

Watson JD (1984) Fasciotomy and Z-plasty in the management of Dupuytren's contracture. *Br J Plast Surg* **37**: 27–30.

Weinzweig N, Culver JE, Fleegler EJ (1996) Severe contractures of the PIP joint in Dupuytren's disease: combined fasciectomy with capsuloligamentous release versus fasciectomy alone. *Plastic Reconstr Surg* **97**: 560–66.

THE OPEN PALM TECHNIQUE

Caroline Leclercq

Baron Dupuytren, in 1832, advocated treating Dupuytren's disease by transverse skin incisions over the maximum contracture and division of fascial bands; the wound was left open, healing being obtained by granulation. If the contracture was only partially corrected, he performed a second incision parallel to the first one, and if several longitudinal bands were involved, a large incision of the whole width of the palm was made, including skin and fibrous bands (Figure 6.61). The wound was then dressed with shredded linen and the hand fixed to a wooden plank until healing was obtained.

After the turn of the century this type of procedure was progressively abandoned and increasingly extensive fasciectomies performed, up to the 'radical' excisions, which attempt to remove the whole palmar fascia in the hope of eradicating recurrences. But with these changes came an increasing rate of complications, (e.g. hematoma, skin necrosis, edema and infection) (Tubiana et al., 1967; Orlando et al., 1974) which led several authors to seek other types of treatment (Luck, 1959). In 1964 McCash described the 'open palm' technique, which was not very different from that advocated by Dupuytren 132 years earlier.

Technique

The technique, as described by McCash, consisted of fasciectomy through transverse volar incisions. The first incision was in the distal palmar crease (DPC), as wide as required depending on the number of rays involved. Based on the extent of the contracture, a second incision was made in the proximal palmar crease, and further incisions in the MP and PIP digital creases. The skin was undermined, creating skin bridges under which fasciectomy was performed. McCash would not carry fasciectomy further than the PIP crease

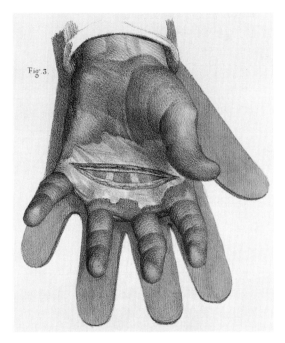

Figure 6.61 'Dupuytren's procedure' as illustrated by Bourgery and Jacob, contemporaries of Baron Dupuytren, in 1832. (Reproduced with permission from Bourgery and Jacob, 1832.)

because of the increased risk of digital nerve damage at that level. If necessary, he would carry it out distally at a later date. The proximal and distal incisions were subsequently closed with sutures, and the DPC wound left open, with a firm pressure applied to the entire hand. A volar plaster slab maintained the hand in full extension for one week, the dressings were changed at weekly intervals and the hand immobilized at night only in an extension splint, the patient being instructed to use the hand for every light duty that could be done during the day.

The principles of this technique were outlined by McCash:

- By advancing the undermined skin flaps proximally and distally, the skin shortage is accepted by the main incision in the DPC, and the other incisions close without tension;

- The central defect gives a perfect drainage so that no hematoma can occur;
- Patients are able to treat themselves at home without physiotherapy.

The latter implies good co-operation from patients, and McCash felt the procedure to be unsuitable for those not willing or able to co-operate.

The technique has subsequently undergone several modifications:

- Some authors leave all wounds open (Borden, 1974; Beltran et al., 1976) including the distal ones (Figure 6.62). The digital defects take 5–8 days longer to heal than those in the palm (Beltran et al., 1976);
- The finger incisions have been modified. Some felt that fasciectomy at the finger level could not be satisfactory through a transverse incision – due to limited exposure, limited excision, incomplete PIP correction (Beltran et al., 1976) or risk to the neurovascular bundles – and favored a longitudinal incision usually with a Z-plasty type of closure (Briedis, 1974; Noble and Harrison, 1976) at the finger level, combined with the transverse open palm incision. Some authors leave the transverse limb of the Z-plasty open (Lubahn et al., 1984);
- Allieu (1988) performs an excision of the invaded palmar skin.

However, the main criticisms of this technique were the undermining and the 'blind' fasciectomy under skin bridges. It was felt that vascularization of the distal palm, which, as shown by Conway and Stark (1954), is scarce, could be compromised, and that fasciectomy was difficult, putting the neurovascular bundles at great risk (Gelberman et al., 1982). Indeed, several reports of the technique mentioned transient (Beltran et al., 1976) or lasting hypoesthesia (Noble and Harrison, 1976) or nerve laceration (Gelberman et al., 1982). Most authors now favor longitudi-

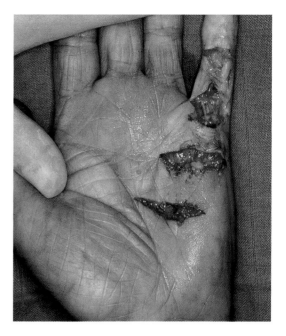

Figure 6.62 Open palm and digit: all wounds are left open.

nal (with Z-plasties) or zig-zag incisions branching distally from the transverse wound towards the involved finger(s) (Figure 6.63) (Lubahn et al., 1984; Foucher et al., 1985; Schneider et al., 1986; Allieu and Tessier, 1986);

- Some modifications to the postoperative regimen have also been carried out. Noble and Harrison (1976) put the hand in a boxing glove for 12–19 days. Beltran et al. (1976) felt that the postoperative splint was unnecessary and even harmful. Most other authors favored early active motion associated with an extension splint, which was usually permanent (Gelberman et al., 1982; Schneider et al., 1986; Lubahn, 1999) or nocturnal (Lubahn et al., 1984). Allieu and Tessier (1986) felt that the postoperative period was best managed in a rehabilitation center, with several periods of physiotherapy per day and dynamic splints as needed.

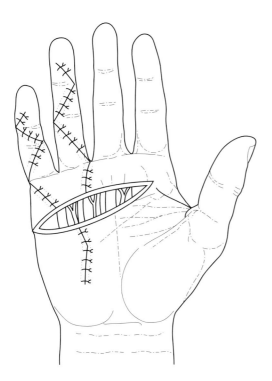

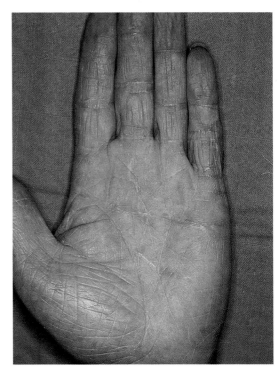

Figure 6.63 Open palm technique combined with digital zig-zag incisions. (Reproduced with permission from Allieu and Tessier, 1986.)

Figure 6.64 Same patient as in Figure 6.62. Result at 1 year: the palmar scars are linear.

Results

Wound healing

The wound dressed at weekly intervals heals in 4–8 weeks, according to the size of the skin gap, except in specific instances such as diabetes where healing may take up to 10 weeks (Noble and Harrison, 1976).

Some superficial infections have been reported that did not require antibiotics nor delayed skin healing (McCash, 1964; Noble and Harrison, 1976). Contrary to McCash's statement, it seems that the wound does not close only by granulation and epithelialization but also by a gradual flattening of the transverse skin wrinkles caused by the Dupuytren's bands, and by attraction of the skin edges (Conolly, 1974). This has been confirmed by tattooing points on either side of the transverse wound before incision: the two points, which can be as much as 2.5 cm apart after fascietomy, return to their original relationship with wound healing (Lubahn et al., 1984).

Although this is rarely mentioned (Noble and Harrison, 1976), the patient should be warned, before the operation, that the wound will be deliberately left open, and of the unsightly aspect of the hand at first dressing. The patient may otherwise become suspicious of the surgeon 'who forgot to close the wound.'

When wound healing is achieved, the scar is usually linear (Figure 6.64) and no more noticeable than after a primary closure (McCash, 1964) but skin puckering and hardening can

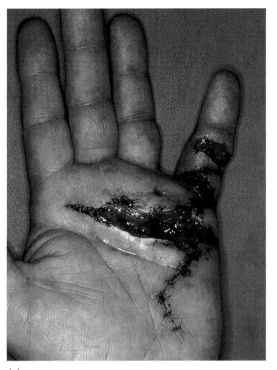 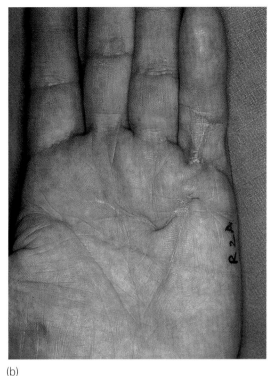

(a)   (b)

Figure 6.65 (a) Open palm: clinical aspect at 1 week; (b) result at 2 years: skin puckering on the palmar scar.

occur (Foucher et al., 1985) (Figure 6.65) Allieu (1988) insists on the necessity, once healing has been obtained, of softening the skin with massages, selective compressive dressings inside the splint and hydrotherapy, in order to avoid skin hardening, which impinges upon finger flexion.

Complications

One of the major advantages of this technique is the lack of all those complications that were so common after a Dupuytren's disease procedure in the days of McCash. This is put forward in all reports on this technique, especially in the two studies that have compared the open palm with other techniques (Gelberman et al., 1982; Lubahn et al., 1984).

The lack or paucity of postoperative pain was one of the features that struck most early reporters of this technique (who were probably accustomed to much higher levels of pain after such procedures as McIndoe's, where edema, hematoma, and the subsequent pain were common postoperative features). But even more recently the randomized prospective study of Gelberman et al. (1982) comparing three techniques, showed that the postoperative pain (assessed daily up to Day 5 then weekly up to Week 3) was significantly lower with the open palm technique than with the discontinuous Z-plasties (McGregor, 1967) or the volar zig-zag incisions (Bruner, 1974). However, this technique seems to have no influence on the occurrence of reflex sympathetic dystrophy (RSD). The 12% rate of RSD reported by Schneider et al. (1986) in his open palm series is higher than that usually reported with other techniques, whereas in Lubahn et al.'s comparative study (1984) there was no RSD in their 38 open palm cases as compared to 8 in their 115 closed wound cases (7%). The most recent open palm series mention rates of 4% to 6%.

Edema is also very infrequent. This is attributed by McCash (1964) to the importance of discharge through the wound. Most series did not report any case of persistent edema, except for Briedis (1974; 1 case), Lubahn et al. (1984; 2 cases), and Allieu (1988; 14 cases or 8.5%).

The lack of hematoma was one of the spectacular improvements with this technique as compared to other techniques used in the days of McCash. There is no reported instance of hematoma after the open palm procedure, whereas for instance Tubiana (1967) reported 15.8% hematomas after the McIndoe procedure, and Orlando et al. (1974) 9% after closed transverse palmar incision.

Skin necrosis is also very rare with this technique and has only been reported by Noble and Harrison (1976) who experienced 4 cases of necrosis of the skin edges, which all healed within 6 weeks.

Infection, as mentioned earlier, is also infrequent and limited to a mild superficial sepsis that heals spontaneously without the need for antibiotics (McCash, 1964; Noble and Harrison, 1976).

Correction of the deformity was often incomplete with the McCash technique (Beltran et al., 1976), particularly at the PIP level. This problem was solved by a better exposure of the digital lesions with the longitudinal incisions branching on the transverse one.

Loss of finger flexion has not been mentioned often but it is probably more frequent than reported. Schneider et al. (1986) report 41% flexion loss at one or more joints, especially on the ring and little fingers. Noble and Harrison (1976) report a limitation of flexion in 16 patients (21%), mainly at the DIP joint. More recently Foucher et al. (1985) noted at 3 weeks' postop a 14% rate of flexion loss,

which was treated by a dynamic flexion splint applied for a few hours daily.

Allieu (1988) noticed some degree of ulnar drift of the little finger when the incision was prolonged on the ulnar border of the palm. He treated it successfully with 'buddy taping' of the little finger to the ring finger.

Evolution

Does the open palm technique have an incidence on the long-term evolution of Dupuytren's disease, i.e. recurrence and extension? This is difficult to assess as most series have a rather short follow-up, or else the patients with a longer follow-up are not separated from the rest. Schneider et al. (1986), with an average follow-up of 5 years, experienced 34% recurrences and 48% extension. The only work that specifically studied the long-term results (5 years and over) of the McCash procedure is that by Foucher et al. (1992), who concluded that the open wound shares the prognosis of limited fasciectomy with no difference so far as the 'activity' of the disease is concerned (i.e. recurrence plus extension).

Indications

The obvious advantage of this technique is its low rate of complications. Also, it was probably very attractive for both surgeons and patients in the days of McCash when the complications of fasciectomy were so numerous. Nowadays, a closer attention to skin incisions, the miniaturization of instruments and the routine use of magnifying loupes, as well as a more careful hemostasis, have dramatically lowered the rate of complications with closed techniques.

The main drawback of the open palm technique is the duration of functional impairment because of the dressing, splinting and physiotherapy throughout the healing time (up to 8 weeks).

This technique should therefore not be regarded as the standard procedure for Dupuytren's disease. It is certainly not suited for uncooperative patients, who would not be able to cope with this postoperative regimen. McCash (1964) also felt it was not indicated for elderly patients, whereas Allieu (1988) recommends it for the elderly; neither of them justify their position. It is not best indicated in single ray lesions, where closed techniques will lead to a faster result. It is not recommended either when the palmar skin gap is wider than 2 cm as spontaneous healing would take a very long time. When faced with such a gap one may choose to either cover the defect primarily with a full-thickness skin graft or, secondarily after granulation, with a split-thickness graft. The author agrees with Schneider (1991) who, after performing many open palm operations, has restricted its indications to multiple and severe contractures of the MP joints that, when released, would leave a deficit in palmar skin for closure.

Acknowledgment

All clinical figures in this Open Palm section are reproduced courtesy of Professor D. Leviet, Paris, France.

References

Allieu Y, Tessier J (1986) La technique de la 'paume ouverte' dans la traitement de la maladie de Dupuytren. In: Tubiana R, Hueston JT, eds, *La Maladie de Dupuytren. Monographies du GEM.* L'Expansion Scientifique Française, Paris: 160–64.

Allieu Y (1988) La 'paume ouverte' dans le traitement de la maladie de Dupuytren. Technique et indications. *Rev Chir Orthop* **74**: 46–49.

Beltran JE, Jimeno-Urban F, Yunta A (1976) The open palm and digit technique in the treatment of Dupuytren's contracture. *Hand* **3**: 73–77.

Borden J (1974) The open finger treatment of Dupuytren's contracture. *Orthop Rev* **8**: 25–29.

Bourgery JM, Jacob NA (1832) *Traité complet de l'anatomie de l'homme comprenant la médecine opératoire,* 154. CA Delaunay, Paris.

Briedis J (1974) Dupuytren's contracture: lack of complications with the open palm technique. *Br J Plast Surg* **27**: 218–19.

Bruner JM (1974) Technique of selective aponeurectomy for Dupuytren's contracture. In: Hueston JT,

Tubiana R, eds, *Dupuytren's Disease*, 93–94. Churchill Livingstone, Edinburgh.

Conolly WB (1974) Spontaneous healing and wound contraction of soft tissue wounds in the hand. *Hand* **6**: 26–32.

Conway H, Stark RB (1954) Arterial vascularization of the soft tissues of the hand. *J Bone Joint Surg* **36A**: 1238–40.

Dupuytren G (1832) Rétraction permanente des doigts. In: *Leçons orales de clinique chirurgicale faites à l'Hôtel-Dieu de Paris,* 2–24. Germer Baillière, Paris.

Foucher G, Schuind F, Lemarechal P et al. (1985) La technique de la paume ouverte pour le traitement de la maladie de Dupuytren. *Ann Chir Plast Esthet* **30**: 211–15.

Foucher G, Cornil C, Lenoble E (1992) Open palm technique for Dupuytren's disease. *Ann Chir Main (Ann Hand Surg)* **11**: 362–66.

Gelberman RH, Panagis JS, Hergenroeder PT, Zakaib GS (1982) Wound complications in the surgical management of Dupuytren's contracture: a comparison of operative incisions. *Hand* **14**: 248–54.

Lubahn JD (1999) Open palm technique and soft-tissue coverage in Dupuytren's disease. *Hand Clin* **15**: 127–36.

Lubahn JD, Lister GD, Wolfe T (1984) Fasciectomy and Dupuytren's disease: a comparison between the open-palm technique and wound closure. *J Hand Surg* **9A**: 53–58.

McCash CR (1964) The open palm technique in Dupuytren's contracture. *Br J Plast Surg* **17**: 271–80.

McCash CR (1974) The open palm technique in Dupuytren's contracture. In: Hueston JT, Tubiana R, eds, *Dupuytren's Disease*, 129–33. Churchill Livingstone, Edinburgh.

McGregor IA (1967) The Z-plasty in hand surgery. *J Bone Joint Surg* **49B**: 448–57.

Noble J, Harrison DH (1976) Open palm technique for Dupuytren's contracture. *Hand* **8**: 272–78.

Orlando JC, Smith JW, Goulian D (1974) Dupuytren's contracture: a review of 100 patients. *Br J Plast Surg* **27**: 211–17.

Schneider LH (1991) The open palm technique. *Hand Clin* **7**: 723–28.

Schneider LH, Hankin FM, Eisenberg T (1986) Surgery of Dupuytren's disease: a review of the open palm method. *J Hand Surg* **11A**: 23–27.

Tubiana R, Thomine J-M, Brown S (1967) Complications in surgery of Dupuytren's contracture. *Plast Reconstr Surg* **39**: 603–12.

SKIN FLAPS, SKIN GRAFTS, AND DERMOFASCIECTOMY

Raoul Tubiana

The use of skin replacement to relieve Dupuytren's contracture is not new. It was advocated by Rogue de Fursac and by Berger in France in 1892 who made, in cases of long-standing disease, a wide excision of the palmar skin and fascia and replaced it with a pedicle skin flap from the chest. Davis (1919) in England, Blair (1924) in the USA and Lexer (1931) in Germany employed skin grafting. Skinner (1941) used tunnel grafting placed transversely under the area of devitalized skin.

Lexer practiced an extensive excision of the palmar aponeurosis associated with excision of the palmar skin in the ulnar side of the palm (Figures 6.66 and 6.67). A palmar skin flap, based distally, covered the radial aspect of the palm, and the skin over the central and

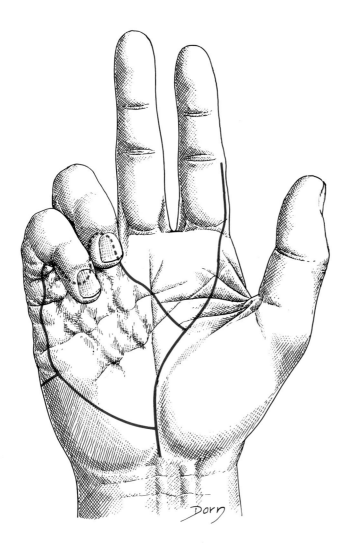

Figure 6.66 Incision for Lexer's extensive fasciectomy.

ulnar aspects of the palm was replaced by a Wolfe–Krause skin graft (full-thickness).

Piulachs and Mir y Mir (1952) from Barcelona used a similar technique. The radial palmar flap was replaced by a hypothenar flap turned over the base of the ring and little fingers. The central palmar zone was covered by a full-thickness skin graft (Figures 6.68 and 6.69). Note that in these early procedures the skin grafts were placed in the palm, whereas at present they are widely used in the fingers.

Skin flaps

Skin flaps now have only rare indications but the technique should be known as it may come in useful.

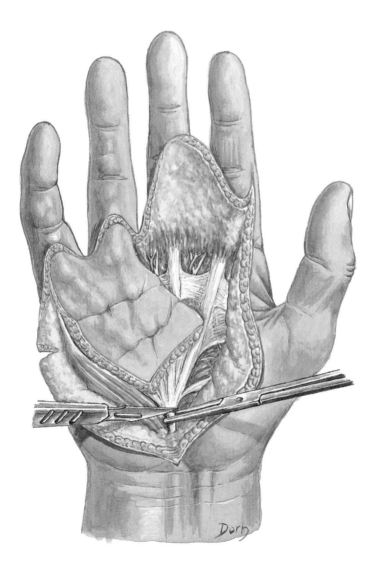

Figure 6.67 The skin in the ulnar side of the palm and the mid-palmar aponeurosis are excised. A palmar skin flap based distally is turned over the radial aspect of the palm. The palmar skin excised is replaced by a full-thickness skin graft.

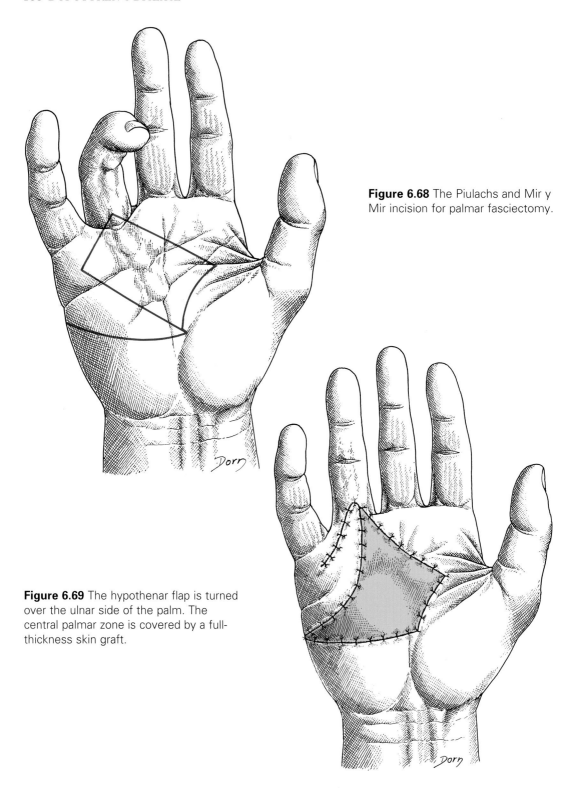

Figure 6.68 The Piulachs and Mir y Mir incision for palmar fasciectomy.

Figure 6.69 The hypothenar flap is turned over the ulnar side of the palm. The central palmar zone is covered by a full-thickness skin graft.

Figure 6.70 (a and b) Ulnar palmar flap.

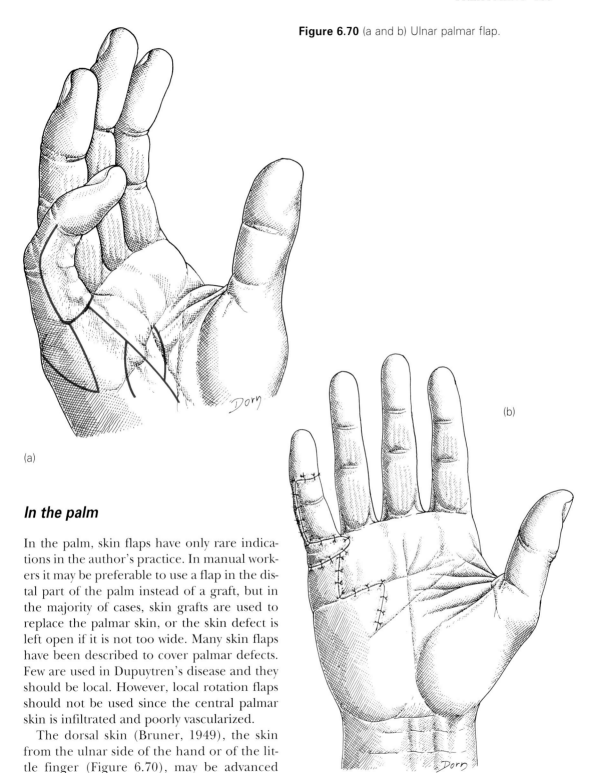

(a)

(b)

In the palm

In the palm, skin flaps have only rare indications in the author's practice. In manual workers it may be preferable to use a flap in the distal part of the palm instead of a graft, but in the majority of cases, skin grafts are used to replace the palmar skin, or the skin defect is left open if it is not too wide. Many skin flaps have been described to cover palmar defects. Few are used in Dupuytren's disease and they should be local. However, local rotation flaps should not be used since the central palmar skin is infiltrated and poorly vascularized.

The dorsal skin (Bruner, 1949), the skin from the ulnar side of the hand or of the little finger (Figure 6.70), may be advanced

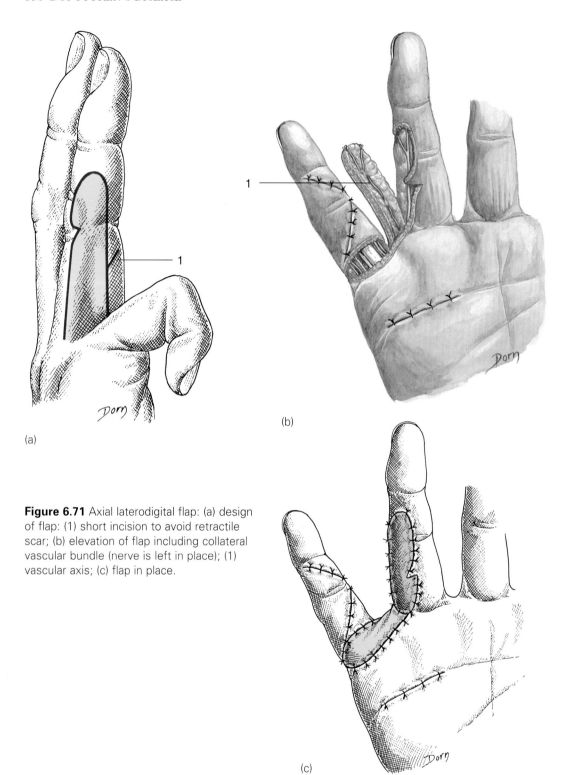

(a)

(b)

(c)

Figure 6.71 Axial laterodigital flap: (a) design of flap: (1) short incision to avoid retractile scar; (b) elevation of flap including collateral vascular bundle (nerve is left in place); (1) vascular axis; (c) flap in place.

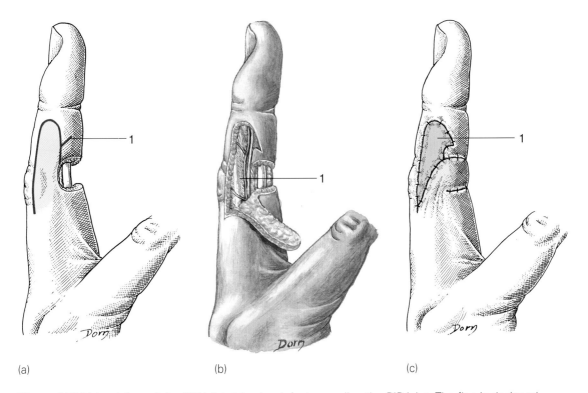

Figure 6.72 Volar defect of the PIP joint: (a) volar defect regarding the PIP joint. The flap is designed on the middle phalanx: (1) skin incision to avoid retractile scar; (b) flap elevated: (1) vascular bundle; (c) graft: (1) skin graft on donor site.

onto the palm after being dissected free. The design of these flaps must be accomplished carefully because they are poorly vascularized at their extremities, and this limits their capacity to provide cover. Laterodigital flaps can be brought to the distal part of the palm (Figure 6.71) or to the volar aspect of the finger (Figures 6.72 and 6.73). The subsequent skin defect is covered by a skin graft. The use of skin from an amputated finger or cheiloplasty produces good-quality skin coverage in the palm but can be used only very occasionally, after a severe recurrence, especially in the little finger (see Figure 7.15, page 234).

In the finger

In the fingers full-thickness skin grafts are more generally used than skin flaps. Advancement flaps [Hueston, 1966 (Figure 6.74); Lane, 1981 (Figure 6.75)] or island flaps such as the Joshi 'creeping flap' (see Figure 6.74) may be used to cover the areas in which flexor tendons have become exposed, when the flexion sheath is opened. The flaps are designed after the tourniquet is deflated; the two collateral arteries of the finger should be preserved. A skin graft can be used to cover an exposed tendon, but there may be subsequent adhesion that will reduce the range of

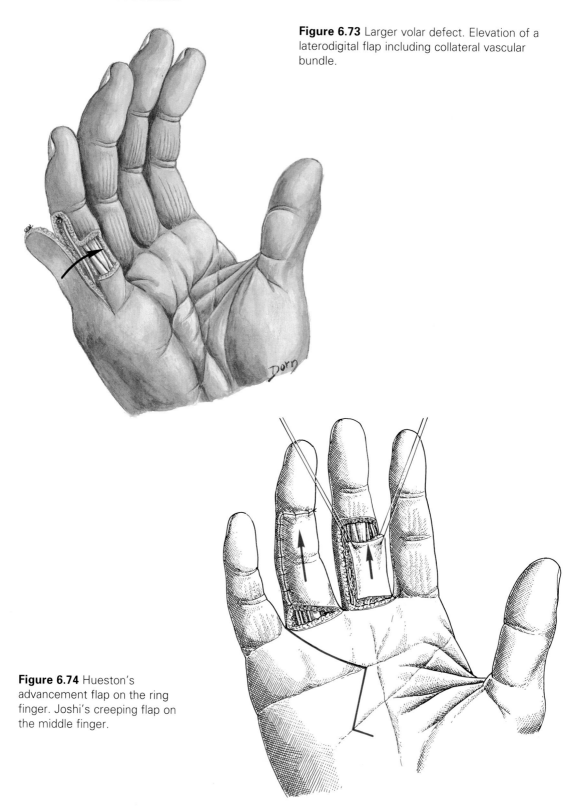

Figure 6.73 Larger volar defect. Elevation of a laterodigital flap including collateral vascular bundle.

Figure 6.74 Hueston's advancement flap on the ring finger. Joshi's creeping flap on the middle finger.

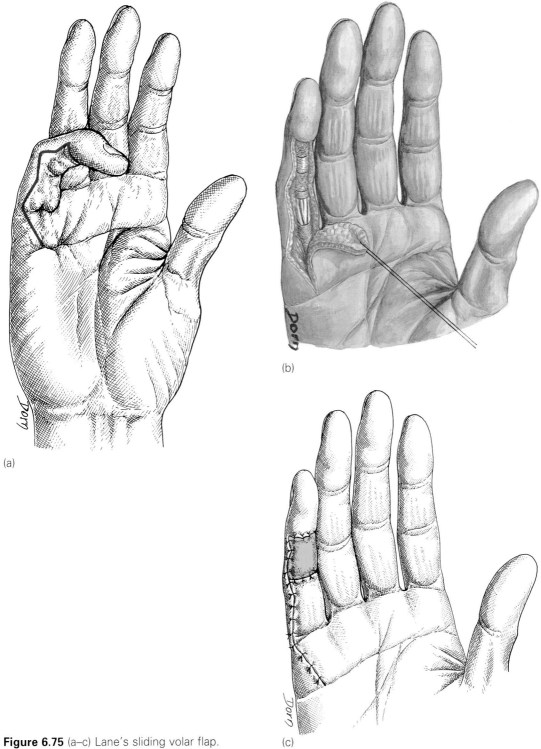

Figure 6.75 (a–c) Lane's sliding volar flap.

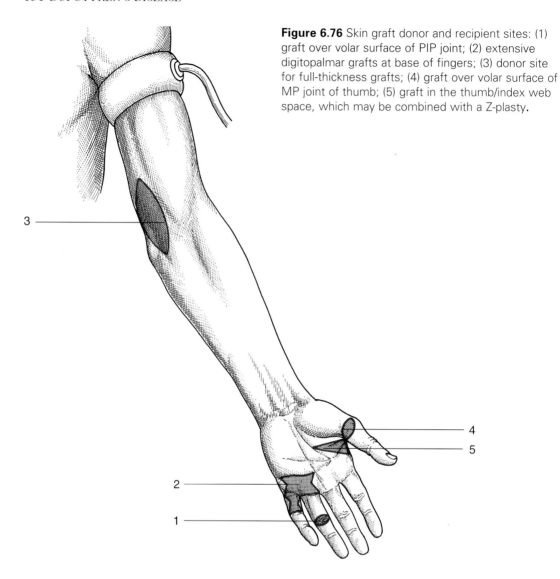

Figure 6.76 Skin graft donor and recipient sites: (1) graft over volar surface of PIP joint; (2) extensive digitopalmar grafts at base of fingers; (3) donor site for full-thickness grafts; (4) graft over volar surface of MP joint of thumb; (5) graft in the thumb/index web space, which may be combined with a Z-plasty.

motion. The author prefers to cover exposed tendons with a flap. Heterodigital flaps are only used when the arterial supply of the finger is insufficient for a homodigital flap (see Figure 7.1, page 224).

Skin grafts

The observation that recurrence did not occur beneath a skin graft, reported by Piulachs and Mir y Mir (1952), Gordon (1957) and Hueston (1962), has popularized the use of skin grafts in the treatment of Dupuytren's disease.

Some surgeons remain sceptical about the prophylactic effect of the graft. McFarlane and co-workers (1990) think that grafting is unnecessary if all diseased fascial cords are excised except in severe recurrent cases. The fact is that despite an increasingly widespread use of grafts, recurrences have only exceptionally been found beneath them. How do these skin grafts work? Some authors think that they have a prophylactic action. Rudolph and co-workers (1977) discovered that there was an absence of myofibroblasts under full-thickness skin grafts, and that this may explain the lack of proliferation of retractile tissue. Other authors think that recurrence is secondary to retained diseased fascia precursor cells in the dermis, and the absence of a recurrence is simply due to the absence of diseased skin and of scarring of the graft to the healthy deeper tissues. Exceptional cases of recurrence under the graft may be caused by a partial necrosis of the graft.

The prophylactic effect of these grafts is limited to the area they cover. The progression of the disease seems to be unchanged in the surrounding tissues.

Thus, skin grafts have several roles in the treatment of Dupuytren's disease:

• The covering of skin defects;
• The replacement of skin of poor viability;
• The treatment of recurrences;
• The prevention of recurrence.

For this purpose the graft can be associated with a fasciectomy (the dermofasciectomy of Hueston) or with an open fasciotomy (Gonzalez, 1974; see 'Fasciotomy', pages 132–38).

Full-thickness skin grafts are preferred both for their biologic effects and for their physical qualities. They give a more esthetic skin coverage while having less tendency to retract than partial-thickness skin grafts. They can be taken from the groin (Gonzalez, 1974). The author prefers to harvest the skin graft from the glabrous skin of the medial aspect of the upper arm, below the tourniquet, which is placed as high as possible. On the medial aspect of the upper arm there is a large area of fine, supple skin that is highly suitable for replacing palmar skin (Figure 6.76). Care is taken to remove fat from the graft. After excis-

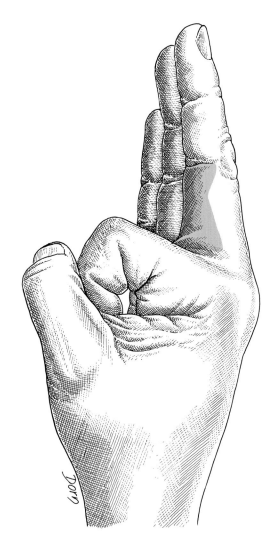

Figure 6.77 Skin graft extending from one lateral edge of the proximal phalanx to the other.

ing a longitudinal ellipse, it is usually possible to close the resulting wound directly. The scar is not very obvious and is not subjected to stretching movements as is true of the flexion crease at the elbow.

Partial thickness skin grafts, taken from the ulnar side of the hand, may be used to cover

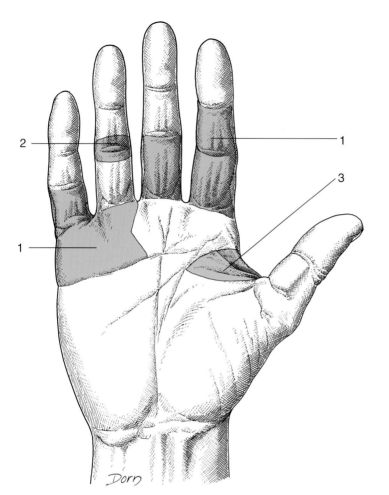

2

1

1

3

Dorn

Figure 6.78 Different sites of skin grafts: (1) dermato-fasciectomy; (2) 'fire-break' graft; (3) skin graft for correction of thumb web space contracture.

small defects. The size, site and shape of a graft must be tailored to each case and certain principles must be adopted.

The site for grafting must be chosen with care. Obviously, it must correspond to the site of a skin defect or skin infiltration or to a usual site of recurrence. This means that the grafts are usually placed on the palmar aspect of the digits and in the first web. The state of the underlying tissues must be suitable, and it is preferable to avoid placing the graft on exposed flexor tendons, however good the take may be. Finally, it is important to place the graft in a strategic area in which one can

predict new joint contractures (Hueston's fire-break grafts). Thus it should be sited at or just proximal to the PIP joint (that is, the most threatened site). It must extend from one lateral edge to the other, and the shape should be such as to avoid a scar retraction (Figures 6.77 and 6.78). Some surgeons place the graft across the entire palm after a wide fasciotomy (McGregor, 1986) in order to break the longitudinal tensile forces and to prevent reunion of divided cords. Most surgeons confine the grafts to the digit and its base because recurrence in the proximal part of the palm is less likely to be produced. The edges of the graft

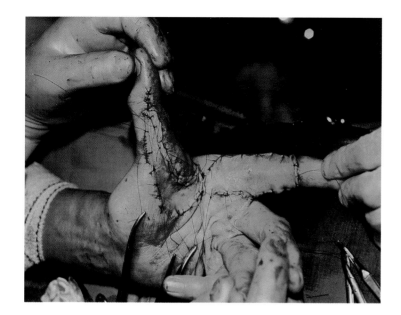

Figure 6.79 Grafted zones on the radial aspect of the hand.

should be placed in the zones in which the skin is little affected by finger movements: the lateral borders of the fingers, diagonally lengthwise on the phalanges and in the transverse skin creases. The size of the graft should be sufficiently large to stop a reproliferation of fibrous tissue, thus preventing new retractions. It is also important to remember that recurrences may arise around the grafted zone. One should not graft those areas involved in prehension or in which sensation must be conserved. This is particularly important on the radial aspect of the hand where sensitive skin must be retained not only on digital pulps but also on the radial side of the index finger and on the medial side of the thenar eminence (Figure 6.79). Arm, forearm, and submalleolar donor sites (Searle and Logan, 1992) give robust enough skin grafts for most patients. In manual workers, it may be preferable to avoid grafts in the distal palm where they will be in close contact with tool handles. If not avoided, the patient should be instructed to use a glove to cover the graft area.

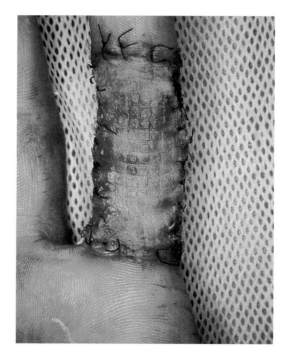

Figure 6.80 The graft is sutured using interrupted sutures.

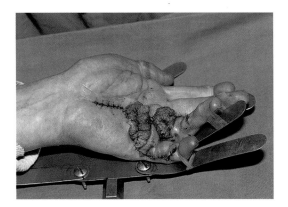

Figure 6.81 Compressive suture over the graft.

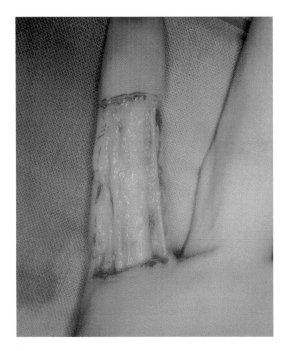

Figure 6.82 Palmar skin excision on the proximal and middle phalanges of the little finger.

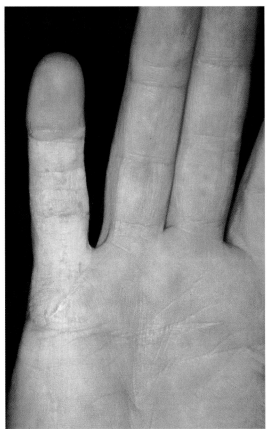

Figure 6.83 Little finger, aspect, 4 years after.

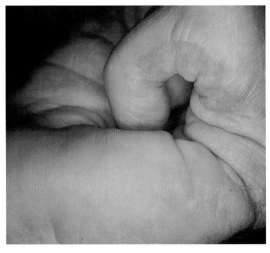

Figure 6.84 Little finger 4 years later.

The outline of the graft is drawn first, taking account of the loss of substance, the devascularized areas at risk for necrosis, and those elements already mentioned concerning the site and shape. It should extend on to one or more fingers and in the palm up to the distal

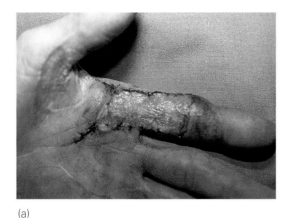

(a)

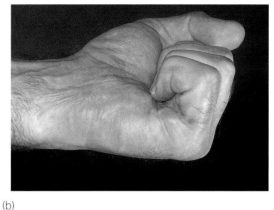

(b)

Figure 6.85 (a and b) Secondary dermofasciectomy after recurrence on the radial aspect of the hand.

transverse skin crease. Occasionally, several grafts are envisaged. The skin is excised, with an accentuation of the angles on the periphery. If there is a severe contracture of the PIP joint, a Kirschner wire may be placed obliquely across the joint, maintaining the joint in the maximal extension obtained.

The tourniquet is deflated. No pin is left in place until capillary refill is examined to ensure that the extended finger is not compromising digital artery function. A rigorous hemostasis is performed while carefully avoiding damage to the digital arteries. The vascularity of the skin is confirmed, and further skin excision is performed as necessary. The shape and size of the graft can be determined by using a sterile transparent paper. If several grafts are required, the pieces of paper are placed side by side, and an ellipse can then be drawn around them.

After being rinsed with saline, the hand is placed in a wet compressive dressing. If there is a persistent oozing of blood, the tourniquet may be inflated as required. The required shape of graft is then drawn on the medial aspect of the upper arm, above the flexion crease of the elbow. The long axis must be longitudinal. The skin graft is lifted using a scalpel with a large blade, keeping deep to the dermis. The donor site is then sutured.

The graft may be applied with the tourniquet inflated, but it is preferable to remove the tourniquet entirely and perform hemostasis once again.

The graft is sutured, using interrupted sutures (Figure 6.80) and leaving the ends long enough to be tied over a stent on a compressive dressing with tulle gras (Figure 6.81). Gaps are left on the transverse margins of the skin graft for the evacuation of liquid. We do not make holes in the graft. Before placing the dressing, one should irrigate again under the graft, using a syringe with a blunt ophthalmologic needle; the dressing is then rapidly applied. Perfect hemostasis takes time. This is not a procedure for hurried surgeons.

A dorsal plaster splint may be used to immobilize the wrist and grafted fingers for 7 days, at which time the dressing and the pin, if it has been used, are removed. There is usually a 100% take of the graft when digital arteries have not been damaged. Grafts mature to become soft and supple and of adequate color (when they are taken from the glabrous skin from the medial aspect of the arm) (Figures 6.82–6.84).

Dermofasciectomy

Hueston (1969) proposed deliberate excision of the skin associated with the involved under-

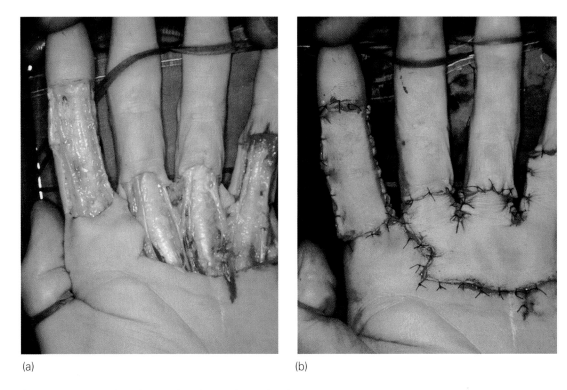

(a)   (b)

Figure 6.86 (a and b) Hueston's primary dermofasciectomy.

lying fascia, with subsequent placement of skin grafts in order to prevent local recurrence under the grafted area. This technique has been called dermofasciectomy. When the skin is excised along with a virgin lesion, after a prognostic estimation that recurrence is very likely, this was termed by Hueston a 'primary graft'. When the skin is excised along with a recurrence, the term 'secondary graft' is used. We have already seen that Lexer, Piulachs and Mir y Mir practiced dermofasciectomies in the first half of this century. It is stressed by Hueston that skin replacement is reserved for those young patients with an active diathesis to the production of Dupuytren's contracture, as evidenced by a short history with rapid progression of deformity and skin fixation, particularly in the little finger, but also elsewhere.

The usual precautions are taken at operation to preserve the digital theca intact. The dissection of the neurovascular bundles and of the digital theca is safer and simpler at the primary operation than after recurrence, and the correction of the PIP joint deformity is more often complete. The digits recover surprisingly well from such a radical procedure (Figure 6.85).

In the years following dermofasciectomy, Hueston and other surgeons have found that extension of the disease has occurred elsewhere but not beneath the graft. Gordon (1964) treated 42 hands by removal of the fascia and involved skin, and its replacement by autogenous skin. Not one has developed recurrence in the grafted area.

The author's experience is similar. Many dermofasciectomies have been carried out, primary grafts (Figure 6.86) mostly in the little finger or in the thumb ray, and secondary grafts for recurrence. Cases have been examined several times. Like Hueston, the author has noticed many extensions, even at the margin of the grafts, but no cord beneath them (Tubiana and Leclercq, 1985). For Hueston, skin replacement was the all-important factor in disease control. Searle and Logan (1992) believe that dermofasciectomy should be thought of as a subtotal preaxial amputation of the digit, removing all tissue that might result in further joint flexion contracture.

Although dermofasciectomy has not been popular for a long time, results reported by Tonkin et al. (1985), Ketchum and Hixson (1987), Makela et al. (1991), Searle and Logan (1992), and Kelly and Varian (1992) have all shown very rare recurrence under the graft.

Kelly and Varian (1992) re-examined 32 (24 cases) of the 41 dermofasciectomies reported by Tonkin et al. in 1985. The follow-up period ranged from 11–17 years, with an average of 13 years. Extension of the disease outside the grafted ray was found in 19 cases (79%). Recurrence of the disease within the same ray as in the skin graft was found in 15 digits (47%). Of these, two were under the graft. Of the 10 found outside the graft, seven were nodules without recurrent contracture. They concluded their retrospective study on dermofasciectomies: '... this procedure must remain the operation of choice in the management of aggressive Dupuytren's disease.'

François Iselin (pers. comm., 1998), who has great experience of this disease, kindly supplied the late results of two homogenous study groups operated on by him between 1975 and 1984: 511 primary forms operated by fasciectomy and 129 actual or potential recurrences operated by dermofasciectomy. After more than 5 years' follow-up, he observed 49 recurrences after the 511 fasciectomies (10%) and only two recurrences after the 129 dermofasciectomies (1.5%). However, of these 129 dermofasciectomies, 41 extensions have been observed in a 2–10-year follow-up. This can be explained by the invasive factor in this type of cutaneous juvenile disease. He adds: 'the bothering extensions have been

proposed a new dermofasciectomy, each time well accepted because of the positive result of the previous one.'

Another recent retrospective study on dermofasciectomy by Logan et al. (1998) reports 135 consecutive patients operated on between 1986 and 1995 for diffuse Dupuytren's disease. One hundred and three patients having had 143 dermofasciectomies were reviewed independently of the senior author (AML), 32 being lost to follow-up and five having died. Follow-up was from 2.1 to 11.5 years (average 5.8 years). Of 103 patients reviewed, 82 were male and 21 were female. Average age at the time of dermofasciectomy was 69.2 years (range 37.3–87.6). Of the 143 dermofasciectomies 110 were carried out as a primary procedure and 33 for recurrent disease. The number of previous fasciectomies carried out on the ray undergoing dermofasciectomy for recurrent disease is recorded in Table 6.1 and the site of dermofasciectomies in Table 6.2. Recurrence under a skin graft is sometimes difficult to ascertain clinically and would require a positive histology in some cases. In

Table 6.1 Secondary dermofasciectomies.

No. of previous operations on the same day	No. of rays
1	26
2	5
4	2
	Total 33

Note: The majority of previous operations were fasciectomies.

Table 6.2 Site of dermofasciectomies.

Ray	No. of dermofasciectomies
Thumb	4
Index	2
Middle	7
Ring	34
Little	96

Logan et al's series (1998) there were nine certain and three less certain recurrences (all doubtful recurrences were included). No patient had more than one recurrence, giving a recurrence rate per ray of 8.4% and per patient of 11.6%. Eight recurrent cords were diagnosed and four recurrent nodules. Only one cord had progressed to recontracture.

Logan et al. concluded: 'While encouraging reports of the use of injected collagenase are beginning to emerge and whilst others are examining growth factor profiles in active Dupuytren's disease as therapeutic targets [Lappi et al. 1992], dermofasciectomy is presently the best surgical technique for controlling the more diffuse Dupuytren's disease with skin involvement.'

The present author's conclusions are the same. The use of skin grafts is increasingly more popular. In his last article (1998) McGrouther writes: 'Retention of the original skin increases the likelihood of recurrence. For this reason I have now almost universally adopted the procedure of insertion of a skin graft after a complete removal of fascia in the proximal segment of the digit.' Without being this radical, the author routinely uses primary skin grafts after fasciectomy on young patients under 45 years who have PIP joint involvement, and secondary grafts for the treatment of recurrence.

References

Berger P (1892) Traitement de la rétraction de l'aponévrose palmaire par une autoplastie. *Bull Acad Med Paris* **56**: 608.

Blair VP (1924) The full thickness skin graft. *Ann Surg* **80**: 298.

Bruner JM (1949) The use of the dorsal skin flap for the coverage of palmar defects after aponeurectomy for Dupuytren's contracture. *Plast Reconstr Surg* **4**: 599.

Davis JS (1919) *Plastic Surgery, its Principles and Practice.* London (cited by Skoog (1948)).

Gonzalez RI (1974) Open fasciotomy and full thickness skin graft in the correction of digital flexion deformity.

In: Hueston JT, Tubiana R, eds, *Dupuytren's Disease,* 123–28. Churchill Livingstone, London.

Gordon SD (1957) Dupuytren's contracture: recurrence and extension following surgical treatment. *Br J Plast Surg* **9**: 286–88.

Gordon SD (1964) Dupuytren's contracture. The use of free skin grafts in treatment. *Transactions of the 3rd Congress of the International Society of Plastic Surgeons, Washington, 1963,* 963–67. Excerpta Medica, Amsterdam.

Hueston JT (1962) Digital Wolfe grafts in recurrent Dupuytren's contracture. *Plast Reconstr Surg* **29**: 342–44.

Hueston JT (1966) Local flap repair of fingertip injury. *Plast Reconstr Surg* **37**: 349–50.

Hueston JT (1969) The control of recurrent Dupuytren's contracture by skin replacement. *Br J Plast Surg* **22**: 152–56.

Hueston JT (1984) 'Firebreak' grafts in Dupuytren's contracture. *Aust N Z J Surg* **54**: 277–81.

Kelly C, Varian J (1992) Dermofasciectomy – a long-term review. *Ann Hand Upper Limb Surg* **11**: 381–82.

Ketchum LD, Hixson FP (1987) Treatment of Dupuytren's contracture with dermofasciectomy and full thickness skin graft. *J Hand Surg* **12A**: 659–63.

Ketchum LD (1992) The use of full thickness skin graft in Dupuytren's contracture. *Hand Clin* **7**: 731–41.

Lane CS (1981) The treatment of Dupuytren's contracture with flexor tendon sheath involvement. The sliding volar flap. *Ann Plast Surg* **6**: 20–23.

Lappi DA, Martineau D, Maher PA et al. (1992) Basic fibroblast growth factor in cells derived from Dupuytren's contracture: synthesis, presence, and implications for treatment of the disease. *J Hand Surg* **17**: 324–32.

Lexer E (1931) *Die gesamte Wiederherstellungschirurgie,* 2nd edn. Leipzig.

Logan AM, Armstrong JR, Huerren J (1998) Dermofasciectomy in the management of Dupuytren's disease. Paper presented at the *7th Congress of the International Federation of Societies for Surgery of the Hand,* Vancouver.

Makela EA, Jaroma H, Harju A et al. (1991) Dupuytren's contracture: the long-term results after day surgery. *J Hand Surg* **16B**: 272–74.

McFarlane R, McGrouther D, Flint M (1990) *Dupuytren's Disease: Biology and Treatment.* Churchill Livingstone, Edinburgh.

McGregor IA (1986) Traitement de la maladie de Dupuytren par aponévrotomie et greffe. In: Tubiana R, Hueston JT, eds, *La Maladie de Dupuytren,* 3rd edn, 165–71. L'Expansion Scientifique Française, Paris.

McGrouther DA (1998) Dupuytren's contracture. In: Green DP, Hotchkiss RN, Pederson WC, eds, *Green's Operative Hand Surgery*, 4th edn, Vol. 1, 563–91. Churchill Livingstone, New York.

Piulachs P, Mir y Mir L (1952) Considerations sobre la enfermedad de Dupuytren. *Fol Clin Int* **II**: 415–16.

Rogue de Fursac (1892) *Correction de la retraction permanente des doigts à l'aide d'un lambeau cutané*. Thèse soutenue le 29 janvier 1892 à la Faculté de Médecine de Paris.

Rudolph R, Guber S, Suzuki M, Woodward M (1977) The life cycle of the myofibroblast. *Surg Gynecol Obstet* **145**: 389–94.

Searle AE, Logan AM (1992) A mid-term review of the results of dermofasciectomy for Dupuytren's disease. *Ann Hand Upper Limb Surg* **11**: 376–80.

Skinner HL (1941) Dupuytren's contraction. Operative correction by use of tunnel skin graft. *Surgery* **10**: 313.

Tonkin MA, Burke FD, Varian JPW (1985) The proximal interphalangeal joint in Dupuytren's disease. *J Hand Surg* **10B**: 358–64.

Tubiana R, Leclercq C (1985) Recurrent Dupuytren's disease. In: Hueston JT, Tubiana R, eds, *Dupuytren's Disease*, 2nd edn. Churchill Livingstone, Edinburgh.

TREATMENT OF ECTOPIC LESIONS

Caroline Leclercq

Knuckle pads

Knuckle pads usually cause more cosmetic than functional problems to the patients, for example they may interfere with wearing rings and may be tender when knocked. Therefore there is a low demand for surgical removal from patients when knuckle pads occur in Dupuytren's disease. Also, there is a general reluctance on the surgeon's part to operate on these nodules because of their high recurrence rate after simple excision, although a few authors do not share these pessimistic views (Iselin et al., 1988).

After introducing the concept of dermofasietomy as a prophylaxis of recurrence in palmar lesions, Hueston applied it to dorsal disease. He performed an *en bloc* excision of an elliptic zone, including the skin and knuckle pad, from the most proximal to the most distal skin fold overlying the dorsum of the PIP joint, and covered the defect with a full-thickness skin graft. With this technique he experienced a reduction in the number of recurrences (Hueston, 1985).

Knuckle pads often adhere to the outer surface of the extensor tendon and their removal leaves a bare, tendinous surface devoid of perimysium. The authors have experienced difficulties in grafts taking over such a bed (Figure 6.87). Therefore, rather than skin grafting the defect the authors prefer to close it by direct suture when possible, or else to cover it by two large dorsal rotation flaps (Hueston's dorsal flap) (Figure 6.88). These flaps heal in 2 weeks and do not interfere with early motion.

Another potential complication after surgical excision of knuckle pads is PIP joint stiffness. This has been reported with all techniques, including simple excision of the nodule; its mechanism remains unclear. Is it due to adhesions of the extensor apparatus, prolonged immobilization, or postoperative edema? It is more likely to occur in patients with pre-existing joint problems, such as degenerative arthritis or diabetic conditions (see 'Associated conditions' in Chapter 5, pages 108–109) but remains unpredictable otherwise.

Therefore, aside from the removal of isolated knuckle pads (without other manifestations of Dupuytren's disease) for diagnostic purposes,

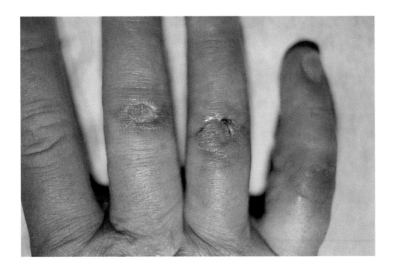

Figure 6.87 Skin grafting after the removal of knuckle pads on the middle and ring fingers: partial graft loss on the middle finger.

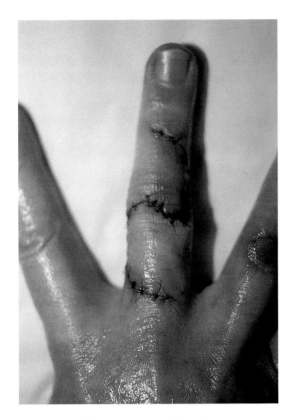

Figure 6.88 Two large dorsal flaps have been used to cover the defect after the removal of a knuckle pad and the overlying skin.

nodules around the excision scar, which are embedded in the scar tissue and usually prove very difficult to remove, putting the plantar nerves at risk if a second excision is attempted. In the past there have been some disastrous confusions of these highly cellular nodules, recurring early after excision, with fibrosarcoma, leading on several occasions to an amputation of the foot, as reported by Pickren et al. (1951).

Recurrence seems less frequent when the plantar nodule is removed together with a wide excision of the surrounding plantar fascia (Gordon, 1964; Aviles et al., 1971; Haedicke, 1989). Again, as with knuckle pads, the incidence of recurrence seems least likely if the overlying skin is removed together with the nodule and the defect covered with a full-thickness skin graft (Hueston, 1985). However, these grafts do not always take well, they are unsightly and may produce hyperkeratosis at the skin–graft junction.

For all the above reasons, the removal of plantar nodules should only be undertaken when they cause a genuine functional impairment.

Plantar lesions

Plantar nodules are usually painless, in fact a number of patients are unaware of them until their feet are examined. As with knuckle pads, these lesions share a high risk of recurrence after excision (Allen et al., 1955; Gordon, 1964; Aviles et al., 1971; Hueston, 1985). Recurrence occurs in the form of peripheral

surgical excision should only be performed when there is a serious impairment, and the patient must be warned of the potential risks of recurrence and joint stiffness.

References

Allen RA, Woolner LB, Ghormly RK (1955) Soft tissue tumors of the sole. *J Bone Joint Surg* **37A**: 14.

Aviles E, Arlen M, Miller T (1971) Plantar fibromatosis. *Surgery* **69**: 117–20.

Gordon SD (1964) Dupuytren's contracture: plantar involvement. *Br J Plast Surg* **17**: 421.

Haedicke GJ, Sturim HS (1989) Plantar fibromatosis: an isolated disease. *Plast Reconstr Surg* **83**: 296–300.

Hueston JT (1985) The management of ectopic lesions in Dupuytren's disease. In: Hueston JT, Tubiana R, eds, *Dupuytren's Disease*, 2nd edn, 204–10. Churchill Livingstone, Edinburgh.

Iselin F, Cardenas-Baron L, Gouget-Audry I, Peze W (1988) La maladie de Dupuytren dorsale. *Ann Chir Main* **7**: 247–50.

Pickren JW, Smith AG, Stevenson TWJ, Stout AP (1951) Fibromatosis of the plantar fascia. *Cancer* **4**, 846.

COMPLICATIONS AFTER SURGERY

Raoul Tubiana

'A complication is something not anticipated by the surgeon. An early complication is due to the surgeon's technique, a late complication is due to the patient's genetic constitution. The only way to prevent a surgical complication is not to operate.' Hueston (1991)

In the past, complications during and after fasciectomies were frequent and diminished or negated the benefits that the patient had gained from surgery. The prevention of complications has been, and is still, a major problem for surgeons.

There is certainly a correlation between surgical complications, the severity of the deformities and extensive operations; but more frequently such complications arise from faulty surgical indications, inadequate operative technique and poor postoperative care.

Operative complications

The avoidance of complications depends largely on surgical skill. The experience of the operator with this type of surgery has a definite influence on the percentage of complications (Tubiana et al., 1967). Nerves, arteries and skin are the structures most at risk.

Injury to the neurovascular bundle

This occurs most frequently at two sites: in the distal part of the palm, near the web and distally, in the finger, at the level of the proximal interphalangeal joint.

At the web space
It should be noted that the neurovascular bundles, which are quite separate from the diseased tissue in their palmar course, become closely associated distal to the distal transverse palmar crease. It is important to remember that the common digital arteries and nerves do not divide at the same level. The artery divides more distally and the digital vessels are exposed to injury, especially when abnormal fascial structures are present between the nerve and artery divisions. These injuries have usually occurred during the relatively blind subcutaneous dissection between separate palmar and digital incisions. It is preferable to use the direct exposure offered by a digito-palmar incision.

At the PIP joint level
It is at this point, also, that the neurovascular bundles are at most risk. They can be displaced superficially and medially by the digital cords that surround them and their sudden emergence under the skin at the level of the PIP joint renders these pedicles particularly vulnerable. It is necessary therefore to locate the arteries and nerves in normal tissue and isolate them with silastic loops and follow them. Nerve injuries must be repaired primarily in order to diminish residual anesthesia and trophic changes and to prevent painful neuromas.

Correction of longstanding PIP joint deformity must be carried out cautiously. Obliteration or rupture of neurovascular pedicles may occur at the PIP joint level during vigorous correction of a markedly contracted finger. It would be wise to attempt a gentle correction of the PIP joint only after taking the precaution of flexing the metacarpophalangeal joint.

The vascular status of the finger can be assessed when the tourniquet is deflated. If the finger is pink and warm in complete extension there is an adequate vascular supply. However, if the digit remains white, this may be caused by a spasm or by excessive tension on the vessels. The finger should be flexed immediately and warm saline-soaked gauze applied to the digit. If these measures are not successful the vessel is explored. Smooth-muscle relaxant agents (20% lignocaine and papaverine) are applied directly to the vessel. An adventitial stripping may be useful. Compression of the vessel may be caused by a fascial band or by transposition of a skin flap, especially a Z-plasty, which should be released. Insufficient blood supply may be caused by an injury to the two collateral arteries; and since there is a real risk of necrosis of the finger, an arterial repair or a vein graft is then required.

Trauma to the arterial wall without transection may lead to development of a pseudo-aneurysm (Hueston, 1973).

Skin integrity

Skin integrity may be altered by extensive or too superficial dissection. Skin viability should be checked with the tourniquet deflated; dead skin should be debrided and grafted when necessary, or left to heal by secondary intention when the areas of skin deficit are small.

Postoperative complications

These are numerous and often interdependent. Once initiated, a sequence of edema, delayed healing and delayed mobilization may occur and ultimately result in a loss of joint mobility (Tubiana et al., 1967).

Hematomas

This is the most frequent complication and the cause of many other complications: infection, wound dehiscence, skin necrosis and joint stiffness. Hematomas were most commonly seen after marked undermining for extensive fasciectomies and transverse palmar skin incisions that had been sutured. A hematoma creates a dead space, is a source of fibrosis and a nidus for infection. If a hematoma has developed, it should be removed in the operating room. The wound is washed and hemostasis is secured. The incision may be left partly open or closed without tension over a drain. A voluminous fluff dressing is applied (Tubiana et al., 1981).

Wound dehiscence and skin necrosis

The infiltration of the skin by the sclerotic lesions is a factor predisposing to poor healing. Wound disruption is probably a result of insufficient vascularity of the skin after undermining and may be classified as the lowest grade of skin necrosis.

The danger of skin necrosis can be reduced by a dissection of the skin flaps with conservation of as much of the subcutaneous tissue as possible and by manipulation of the skin by means of traction threads to avoid excessive trauma to the skin by instruments. Undermining of tissue should be kept to a minimum. Extensive undermining of the palmar skin, which is already poorly vascularized in its central zone, certainly enhances the possibility of cutaneous complications. Closure with undue tension should be avoided. Digital skin complications are generally less severe than those of palmar origin, since they tend to limit themselves to the involved finger. When they arise on the palm, all fingers are at risk. Utmost care must be paid to the design of skin flaps in order to avoid partial necrosis, frequent on the tips of the flaps after a Z-plasty on patients with thick skin. Of course, no flap should be designed where a cord crosses its base or a nodule in the center of the base of the flap. It is preferable not to wait passively for the eschar to separate spontaneously but to excise it expeditiously. Generally, wounds in the palm are left open and allowed to heal by secondary intention. Digital wounds with exposed flexor tendons are better covered by a skin flap taking account of the digital vascular supply (see 'Skin flaps, skin grafts, and dermofasciectomy', pages 186–203).

Infection

Primary postoperative infection is rare. However, the risk of postoperative infection is increased if pre-existing conditions exist such as skin maceration or diabetes mellitus. Infection is generally seen following dehiscence on skin necrosis. Wound cultures and antibiotic treatment are immediately required.

Deep pyogenic infection is treated in a similar manner to that following other hand surgical procedures: in the operating room, the wound is opened and a saline irrigation is administered. If there is suspicion of infection of the flexor tendon sheath, the sheath is opened proximally and distally for irrigation.

Edema

Edema is associated with extensive fasciectomies and lengthy tourniquet times. It is also frequently associated with hematoma and infection and constitutes a source of joint stiffness. Persistent edema may be an early sign of reflex sympathetic dystrophy (RSD) (see pages 212–14). There are several measures that will help to reduce postoperative edema. Hand elevation and active exercises are mandatory.

Stiffness

Loss of finger joint mobility may be the result of the preceding complications. Digital nerve and artery injury contributes to postoperative joint stiffness and cold intolerance. Joint stiffness may also be a sign of RSD, even in the absence of pain.

Postoperative painful complications

Normally, there should be little pain after a fasciectomy. If severe pain should develop, an immediate wound inspection is mandatory. Pain may be due to excessive constriction of

the dressing or to a hematoma. Appearance of a painful neuroma after section of a digital nerve is characterized by an electric pain at the point of pressure. Diffuse hand pain in the weeks following a fasciectomy may be a sign of RSD. All painful physiotherapy must be stopped immediately.

Reflex sympathetic dystrophy (RSD)

Howard (1959) popularized the term 'flare reaction' for this condition. RSD is feared after fasciectomies because of its unpredictable nature, the length of its course and the possibility of permanent disability. It is especially feared in those who are emotional and anxious, often women. This syndrome usually appears 3–6 weeks after surgery and includes diffuse hand pain, edema, diminished hand function, joint stiffness, skin trophic changes and, later, bone decalcification (Lankford, 1999). This symptomatology is not complete at the beginning and it is of the utmost importance that treatment be instituted as early as possible. Scanning helps for early diagnosis (Constantinesco et al., 1986; Foucher, 1995; Mackinnon and Holder, 1984) even if it is not specific to this syndrome (see pages 212–17).

In practice, any abnormal postoperative evolution after any surgical procedure for Dupuytren's disease (edema, diffuse pain, joint stiffness) must be carefully observed for RSD and early treatment instituted. It consists of calcitonin, sympathetic blocks and sedation, in combination with gentle, non-painful hand therapy. The efficacy of the treatment in the individual patient is variable, but the earlier treatment is instituted, the more efficacious it will be.

Prevention of RSD is difficult since it remains a syndrome of unknown cause. However, in patients at risk, especially in anxious patients, in women (Zemel, 1991), or in patients demanding long extensive procedures for advanced widespread disease or recurrences, preventive measures should be set up: a long-acting regional anesthetic technique should preferably be used and the operation should be performed with great care to avoid all hematoma and any other complications that might become a source of undue pain or restriction of movement.

Zemel et al. (1987) have shown clearly the higher incidence of flare reaction in women following surgery for Dupuytren's disease: 'during a 15-year interval, the same authors operated on 163 hands in women and 24.5% of these hands exhibited a flare reaction. During the same time period, 383 hands of men with Dupuytren's disease were operated upon and only 12.5% had a flare reaction.'

The literature demonstrates a wide disparity in the reported incidence of RSD after fasciectomy. McFarlane et al. (1990) note that in a series of 1339 patients, 4.2% developed RSD. They attribute these disparities to a lack of uniform diagnostic criteria of RSD.

Recurrence

Recurrence is not considered to be a surgical complication as it depends mostly on the patient's genetic constitution. However, any operation for Dupuytren's disease is an injury to the hand and can initiate a series of biologic changes that may lead to uncontrolled fibrous reaction.

Conversely, most surgeons believe that recurrence does not depend on the extent of the fasciectomy, unlike Millesi (1974) who believes that 'prophylactic removal of originally healthy parts of the palmar aponeurosis contributes to an improvement in the long-term result, by reducing the amount of tissue that is potentially liable to pathological changes.' Even Hueston, in his limited fasciectomies, tried to prevent early reunion of divided cords by using 'fire-break grafts'. Recurrence rates differ greatly according to the diathesis from low-risk Japanese to high-risk young Scottish and Irish.

Prevention of complications

The prevention of complications has been, and still is, a major preoccupation for surgeons. In fact, not only has the incidence of complications associated with fasciectomies in Dupuytren's disease considerably decreased in the last few decades but the treatment of these complications has improved in such a way that most complications, with the exception of RSD and neurovascular injuries, simply prolong the period of morbidity for 2–3 weeks (McFarlane et al., 1990). Thomine, in 1964, reviewed the complications of 195 fasciectomies carried out at the orthopedic clinic of the Hôpital Cochin in Paris by a group of surgeons with varying degrees of experience. Fasciectomies were carried out according to McIndoe's technique (McIndoe and Beare, 1958). There were 103 complications including 31 hematomas, 26 wound dehiscences, 24 cases of skin slough, and 15 nerve injuries. In 29 cases, there was joint stiffness causing a permanent disability. Two secondary amputations were required. Such was the state of surgery for Dupuytren's disease in a general orthopedic service at that time. Things have changed with the development of hand surgery. The Dupuytren's Disease Committee of the International Federation of Societies for Surgery of the Hand evaluated the percentage of complications in a multicenter study at 19% (McFarlane, 1986). McFarlane et al. (1990) summarized the complications reported in a series of 1339 cases: infection 1.3%, hematoma 2.2%, skin slough 4.7%, nerve injury 1.5%, arterial injury 0.8%, gangrene of the finger 0.1%, loss of flexion 4.6%, sympathetic dystrophy 4.2%, and other 2.7%.

In a personal series of fasciectomies performed between 1970 and 1976, reviewed by Leclercq (Tubiana and Leclercq, 1985), there were 10% complications and all the patients regained complete flexion, in spite of the severity of many cases (the average preoperative scoring was 4.7) (See page 250 for more details).

The improvement of the incidence of complications and the diminution of sequelae are the result of a variety of factors:

- Primarily, the spread of hand surgery and better surgical technique, using magnification;
- A better understanding of the position of the contracted cords;
- The abandoning of extensive aponeurectomies that required considerable undermining and an increase in more limited aponeurectomies;
- The use of longitudinal digitopalmar incisions, which allow the dissection of both the cords and the neurovascular bundles along their entire length. 'The ability to expose contracted tissue through open incisions rather than by tunneling beneath intact skin is one of the major advances in Dupuytren's surgery.' (Jabaley, 1999);
- The absence of skin sutures placed under tension; it is better to leave the skin edges slightly separated or to use a skin graft;
- A thorough knowledge of reported complications and a comprehensive approach to the management of these complications.

Some surgeons, hoping to reduce the risk of complications, routinely use a McCash open palm technique (1964) and thus avoid hematomata and wound dehiscence. The delay caused by waiting for wound healing would seem to favor joint stiffness (Schneider et al., 1986). The open-palm technique has certainly reduced the incidence of complications and has specific indications, especially when a transverse palmar incision is used. McCash's procedure had merit at a time when hematoma and skin necrosis were frequent. It should not be used routinely when advanced surgical techniques and appropriate surgical indications can prevent complications in a less onerous way, since the gain in operative time, in the McCash procedure, is balanced by the lengthening of the postoperative period. The

favorable influence sometimes claimed (Fietti and Mackin, 1995), of the open-palm technique on the incidence of RSD has not yet been proved by any statistical data.

A problem occasionally arises in a patient who has had RSD after a previous procedure and requires surgery because of severe and progressive contractures on the contralateral hand. The history of dystrophy is not an absolute contraindication to another operation, but certain precautions should be taken. It is necessary to wait until the pain has settled, which may take several months. It does not seem that preoperative treatment by drugs or blocks has any preventive effect. Surgery should be limited, postoperative evolution should be carefully observed, and early treatment against RSD instituted if any abnormal symptoms appear.

References

Boyer MI, Gelberman RH (1999) Complications of the operative treatment of Dupuytren's disease. *Hand Clin* **15**: 161–46.

Costantinesco A, Brunot B, Demangeot JL et al. (1986) Apport de la scintigraphie osseuse en trois phases au diagnostic précoce de l'algoneurodystrophie de la main. *Ann Chir Main* **5**: 93–104.

Fietti VG Jr, Mackin EJ (1995) Open-Palm technique in Dupuytren's disease. In: Hunter JM, Mackin EJ, Callahan AD, eds, *Rehabilitation of the Hand – Surgery and Therapy* 4th edn, 981–94. CV Mosby, St Louis.

Foucher G (1995) *L'Algodystrophie de la main.* Springer, Paris.

Howard LD Jr (1959) Dupuytren's contracture. A guide for management. *Clin Orthop* **15**: 118.

Hueston JT (1973) Traumatic aneurysm of the digital artery: a complication of fasciectomy. *Hand* **5**: 232–34.

Hueston JT (1991) Unsatisfactory results in Dupuytren's contracture. *Hand Clin* **7**: 759–63.

Jabaley ME (1999) Surgical treatment of Dupuytren's disease. *Hand Clin* **15**: 109–26.

Lankford LL (1999) Reflex sympathetic dystrophy. In: Tubiana R, ed., *The Hand*, Vol. 5. WB Saunders, Philadelphia.

Mackinnon S, Holder LE (1984) The use of three-phase radionuclide bone scanning in the diagnosis of reflex sympathetic dystrophy. *J Hand Surg* **9A**: 556–63.

McCash CR (1964) The open palm technique in Dupuytren's contracture. *Br J Plast Surg* **17**: 271.

McFarlane RM (1986) Epidemiologie de la maladie de Dupuytren. In: Tubiana R, Hueston, JT, eds, *La Maladie de Dupuytren*, 3rd edn, 106–10. L'Expansion Scientifique Française, Paris.

McFarlane RM, McGrouther DA, Flint MH (1990) *Dupuytren's Disease, Biology and Treatment*. Churchill Livingstone, Edinburgh.

McIndoe AH, Beare RLB (1958) The surgical management of Dupuytren's contracture. *Am J Surg* **95**: 197.

Millesi H (1974) The clinical and morphological course of Dupuytren's disease. In: Hueston J, Tubiana R, eds, *Dupuytren's Disease*, 49–60. Churchill Livingstone, Edinburgh.

Schneider LH, Hankin FM, Eisenberg T (1986) Surgery of Dupuytren's disease: a review of the open palm method. *J Hand Surg* **11A**: 23.

Thomine M (1964) Contribution à l'étude de la maladie de Dupuytren et son traitement chirurgical. Thèse, Paris.

Tubiana R (1963) Les temps cutanés dans le traitement chirurgical de la maladie de Dupuytren. *Ann Chirurg Plast* **8**: 157–68.

Tubiana R, Leclercq C (1985) Recurrent Dupuytren's disease. In: Hueston JT, Tubiana R, eds, *Dupuytren's Disease*, 2nd edn, 200–203. Churchill Livingstone, Edinburgh.

Tubiana R, Thomine JM, Brown S (1967) Complications in surgery of Dupuytren's contracture. *Plast Reconstr Surg* **89**: 603–12.

Tubiana R, Fahrer M, McCullough CJ (1981) Recurrence and other complications in surgery of Dupuytren's contracture. *Clin Plast Surg* **8**: 45.

Zemel NP (1991) Dupuytren's contracture in women. *Hand Clin* **7**: 707.

Zemel NP, Balcomb TV, Stark HH et al. (1987) Dupuytren's disease in women: evaluation of long-term results after operation. *J Hand Surg* **12A**: 1012–16.

A STUDY OF REFLEX SYMPATHETIC DYSTROPHY AFTER SURGERY FOR DUPUYTREN'S DISEASE

Jean-Jacques Comtet

'There is no surgical act which does not produce a significant or minor repercussion in the organism' (Leriche, 1945)

Reflex sympathetic dystrophy (RSD), after an operation for Dupuytren's disease is the great fear of the hand surgeon. It transforms a lack of extension with variable disability to a lack of flexion that is functionally more serious. To a lesser degree, one may observe isolated loss of flexion without any other sign of RSD (Schneider et al., 1986).

The definition and criteria for RSD are still debatable (Lankford, 1988; Attal, 1997; Cooney, 1997; Doury, 1997; Wong and Wilson, 1997). Postoperative complications of Dupuytren's disease are often difficult to classify. Are isolated symptoms such as pain, edema and stiffness, vasomotor changes or are they part of RSD, and if so which type of RSD?

Since pain is not consistent and difficult to quantify, we have chosen to analyze and compare some symptoms that constitute a part of the general syndrome of RSD. However, these are not always sufficient in quality or quantity to confirm the diagnosis of RSD. The features that we have chosen to analyze are:

- Joint stiffness, because it is a constant symptom, it is measurable and it constitutes the most obvious sequela of RSD;
- Edema, because it is frequent, unpleasant and because it plays a role in the development of joint stiffness;
- Increased uptake on bone scan because it gives precise documentation. The value of the bonescan has been documented in several publications (Constantinesco et al., 1986; Foucher, 1995; Kline et al., 1993). However, the sensitivity and specificity of this investigation have been debated (Lee and Weeks, 1995).

Method

In a continuous series of 47 patients, operated upon by the same surgeon between March 1989 and June 1992, we have selected 37 cases in which edema has been measured before the surgical procedure and then each week for 3 weeks following the surgery. Among these 37 patients, 28 patients consented to have a technetium scan before the surgical procedure, and in 26 patients, two more scans were performed (on the 8th postoperative day and before the 45th day), and in two cases one scan was performed within 6 weeks of the operation.

The patients were placed into three categories according to the severity of joint stiffness:

Group 1: (stiff) Lack of active flexion persisting 6 months after the operation. The extremity of one or more fingers was at least 20 mm from the distal palmar crease.

Group 2: (intermediate) Lack of active flexion persisting for 3 months, but at 6 months' distance to the distal palmar crease was 0–20 mm.

Group 3: (lack of stiffness) Active flexion normal after 3 months.

The edema was measured as the percentage of the volume of the hand prior to the operation (Brand, 1985). A curve documenting the variation of edema as a function of time was established for each patient. The average curve for the group was also noted in terms of stiffness and gender. Curves were also established for different surgical interventions: palmar, digital and digitopalmar. We attempted to define the critical threshold for edema for which the risk of stiffness was significant. We

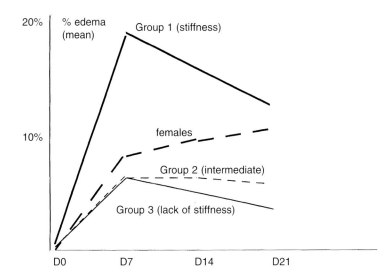

Figure 6.89 Evaluation of edema (mean; as a percentage of the volume of the hand). This is shown during the first 3 weeks (from Day 0 to Day 21), in the three groups: (1): stiffness; (2): intermediate; and (3): lack of stiffness, and in women.

have documented both the absolute and average values for this threshold. We have studied these thresholds using contingency tables (2×2) in which these thresholds were related to stiffness.

The analysis of the scans was performed by the same specialist in nuclear medicine (Prof. Espinasse). Three-phase scintigraphy was used: immediate phase (vascular), early (tissue) and delayed (bone). The increased uptakes were divided into local, segmental and regional (Kline et al., 1993). Local increased uptakes in only one joint were not included. Segmental increased uptake affected part of the hand (e.g. one or two digital rays). Regional increased uptake affected the whole hand and digits in a diffuse fashion. Increased uptake of more than 10% compared with the contralateral side was considered pathologic. Results of the scans were compared, using tables, to the edema and stiffness. Results were determined in relation to the type of increased uptake, early or late and segmental or diffuse.

Results

Results of the edema measurements

In this series of 37 cases where it was possible to measure edema, the average age was 56 years. There were 32 males and 5 females. The edema was less than 2% in five cases of the 37 (16%) and varied between 0 and 25% of the normal volume of the hand. In most of the cases, edema occurred during the first week and the average is represented by the descending line of the first week (Figure 6.89).

Group 1:
Stiffness was characterized by significant edema from the first week. The average volume of edema at the end of the third week remained more significant than the other two groups ($P = 0.002$, T-test).

The edema average in groups 2 and 3 was not significantly different. In these two groups, edema at the end of the third week did not exceed 13%.

Table 6.3 Relationship of edema at the 3rd week and stiffness. Group 1 versus Groups 2 + 3. Threshold in absolute value at 13%.			
	Group 1 (stiffness)	Groups 2+3 (intermediate stiffness or no stiffness at 90 days)	Total
Edema > 13% (absolute value)	2	0	2
Edema < 13% (absolute value)	1	34	35
TOTAL	3	34	37

Group 1: lack of active flexion persisting 6 months after the operation.
Group 2: intermediate.
Group 3: lack of stiffness after 3 months.
Sensitivity 66%, specificity 100%, positive predictive value 97%.

Table 6.4 Relationship of edema at the 3rd week and stiffness. Group 1 versus Groups 2 + 3. Threshold average at 4%.			
	Group 1 (stiffness)	Groups 2+3 (intermediate stiffness or no stiffness at 90 days)	Total
Edema > 4% (average)	3	12	15
Edema ≤ 4% (average)	0	22	22
TOTAL	3	34	37

Group 1: lack of active flexion persisting 6 months after the operation.
Group 2: intermediate.
Group 3: lack of stiffness after 3 months.
Sensitivity 100%, specificity 64%, positive predictive value 67%.

We tried to define the threshold of the severity of edema between the two groups. The establishment of this threshold of edema in absolute values at 13% at the end of the third week has allowed the prediction of severe stiffness with a specificity of 100%, a sensitivity of 66% and a positive predictive value of 97% (Table 6.3). The establishment of an average threshold of edema at 4% provides a sensitivity of 100% and a specificity of 64% (Tables 6.3 and 6.4).

Group 2:
Intermediate stiffness was characterized in 8 out of 12 cases by a secondary aggravation of edema after the first week. Therefore the curve for average edema decreases only very slightly.

The existence of the secondary increase in the curve for edema following the first week results in a risk of severe or intermediate stiffness of 38%.

The five women in this series all had this type of curve, increasing between the end of the first week and the third. At the third week, the average edema curve for women was higher than the average for Group 2. At the end of the third week, the average of edema was 5.5% ± 4.9 for digito-palmar surgery, 4.4% ± 6 for palmar surgery and 2% ± 1.8 for digital surgery.

Results of technetium bone scan

Among the 28 cases who underwent a bone scan, the average age was 56 years. There were 24 males and four females. 21 patients (15%) demonstrated increased uptake postoperatively, segmentally and/or regionally and either early or delayed. The number and percentage of regional increased uptake, either early or delayed as a function of stiffness is presented in Table 6.5.

The number and percentage of regional increased uptake, either early or delayed, is

Table 6.5 Regional increased uptake on bone scan. Number of cases of regional increased uptake, early or delayed as a function of stiffness.*		
	Early increased uptake	Late increased uptake
Group 1 (severe stiffness) n=3	2 (66%)	3 (100%)
Group 2 (intermediate) n=5	1 (20%)	2 (40%)
Group 3 (no stiffness at 90 days) n=20	4 (20%)	5 (25%)

*Local and segmental increased uptake are not included.

Table 6.6 Delayed increased uptake on bone scan. Number of cases and percentage of delayed increased uptake, both segmental and regional as a function of stiffness.

	No increased uptake	Segmental increased uptake	Regional increased uptake
Group 1 (severe stiffness) n=3	0 (0%)	0 (0%)	3 (100%)
Group 2 (intermediate) n=5	1 (20%)	2 (40%)	2 (40%)
Group 3 (no stiffness at 90 days) n=20	6 (30%)	8 (40%)	6 (30%)
Total bone scans n=28	7 (25%)	10 (36%)	11 (39%)

*Purely local increased uptake was not included.

Table 6.7 Edema persisting for the first 3 weeks versus the results of the bone scan.

	Maximum observed	Minimum observed	Average
Normal bone scan (n=7)	11%	1%	4.7% (SD 3.4)
Delayed regional increased uptake (n=11)	25%	0%	12.7% (SD 7.6)

Significance 0.019 (T test).

Table 6.8 The relationship of delayed regional increased uptake on bone scan and stiffness. Group 1 versus Groups 2 + 3.

	Group 1 Severe stiffness n=3	Groups 2 + 3 Intermediate or no stiffness n=25	TOTAL n=28
Increased uptake	3	7	10
No increased uptake	0	18	18

Sensitivity 100%, specificity 72%, positive predictive value 75%.

shown in Table 6.6. Of the 26 cases where there were two postoperative scans, the appearance of secondary increase in uptake was observed in three cases. The relationship between maximum, minimum and average quantity of edema as a function of late regional increased uptake on bone scan is shown in Table 6.7. The relationship of delayed regional increased uptake and stiffness are shown in Table 6.8.

Conclusion and discussion

After surgery for Dupuytren's disease, changes may appear locally in the territory of the surgery or beyond (Kline et al., 1993). In our series, these changes were demonstrated by edema greater than 2% in over 89% of cases, segmental and/or regional increased uptake in 75% of our series, severe stiffness in 8% and transitory stiffness in one third of cases.

Correlations exist between these three type of changes. They confirm the concept that RSD is a disorder of which edema, stiffness and hyperfixation on bone scan are the usual symptoms. We must add pain to these objective symptoms, which is a major symptom but difficult to quantify. For this reason we did not include it in this study.

The percentage of severe stiffness in this series (8%) allows us to consider these cases as real RSD. Indeed, this percentage is similar to the percentage of RSD observed in the literature after surgery for Dupuytren's disease of approximately 5–12% (MacFarlane, 1983; Michon and Merle, 1986; Schneider et al., 1986).

These postoperative changes are more frequently present in a minor degree without constituting the complete and typical syndrome of RSD. A limited transitory stiffness has been observed in our intermediate group and this represents approximately one-third of the cases. In a series of women who underwent surgery for Dupuytren's disease, moderate or severe stiffness was found in one third of the cases (Zemel et al., 1987).

Hence a spectrum exists, from a postoperative course without even minor changes, which is infrequent, to the full-blown syndrome of RSD. 'Postoperative disease' is found after surgery for Dupuytren's disease as in other surgical fields (Leriche, 1940, 1945; Schuind and Burny, 1997). Schuind et al. have observed a postoperative increase in blood flow in 80% of cases on patients who have had surgery for various indications and have not developed RSD.

One may consider that postoperative edema in Dupuytren's disease is a normal phenomenon when it remains within certain limits. Beyond those limits, edema has pathological significance and one must fear that there will be persistent stiffness. These limits are difficult to define because of the great variations observed. One may consider edema at risk of becoming pathologic if it is either marked from the onset, persistent after 3 weeks, increasing secondarily in the first week, or greater than 4% at any point in time.

Edema is more marked in women or in certain individuals (Barclay, 1958). Edema is also more significant when the surgery is more extensive. This may be similar to Zemel's findings (Zemel et al., 1987) of a 'flare reaction' in women who had had surgery for Dupuytren's disease. He observed a 'flare reaction' more frequently if an extensive fasciectomy had been performed or if carpal tunnel surgery was associated with the intervention.

The bone scan results confirm the great frequency (75%) of segmental and/or regional changes after Dupuytren's disease surgery. In the literature, the value of segmental increased uptake on bone scan in the early diagnosis of RSD has been emphasized (Kline et al., 1993). However, our results suggest that scan results are better correlated with edema and stiffness when one considers regional rather than segmental increased uptake.

Our results are in favor of delayed increased uptake being of greater diagnostic value than the early (tissue) phase. The diagnostic value of the delayed phase of the bone scan has already been highlighted (Kline et al., 1993).

The appearance of a secondary increase in bone scan uptake can be observed after the 8th day. These late changes are more rare for increased uptake on bone scan than for edema. The second scan examination was performed after the 3rd week but edema was not measured after the 3rd week. One must conclude that secondary changes appear during the first 3 weeks.

These different manners of appearance of edema and increased bone scan uptake evoke a cumulative stimulus at the origin of the postoperative changes. The quantity of stimulus required to trigger these changes may be reached either immediately owing to the aggressiveness of the stimulus (for example due to the extent of the surgery) or the susceptibility of the patient, or later owing to the persistence of local irritation such as delayed wound healing. The mediators of this stimulus are yet to be clarified. It would be interesting, in the future, to see if the changes we have observed after surgery for Dupuytren's disease have the same frequency after other types of hand surgery. The particular frequency of RSD after Dupuytren's surgery and the vascular manifestations often seen in this syndrome (Comtet and Bourne-Branchu, 1986), suggest that there is some relationship between Dupuytren's disease and RSD that is yet to be determined precisely.

References

Attal N (1997) Algodystrophies. Aspects cliniques, physiopathogéniques et thérapeutiques. In: Evaluation et traitement de la douleur. Proceedings of the *39th Congrès National d'Anesthésie et de Réanimation*. Société Française d'anesthésie et de réanimation (SFAR), 73–92, Elsevier, Paris.

Barclay TL (1958) Edema following operation for Dupuytren contracture. *Plast Reconstr Surg* **23**: 348–60.

Brand PW (1985) *Clinical Mechanics of the Hand*, 180. Mosby, St Louis.

Comtet JJ, Bourne-Branchu B (1986) La maladie de Dupuytren est-elle d'origine vasculaire? In: Tubiana R, Hueston JT, eds, *Monographies du groupe d'Etude de la Main*, 79–83. L'Expansion Scientifique Française, Paris.

Constantinesco A, Brunot B, Demangeat JL et al. (1986) Apport de la scintigraphie osseuse en trois phases au diagnostic précoce de l'algoneurodystrophie de la main. *Ann Chir Main* **5**: 93–104.

Cooney WP (1997) Somatic versus sympathetic mediated chronic limb pain. *Hand Clinics* **13**: 355–61.

Doury PCC (1997) Algodystrophy. *Hand Clinics* **13**: 327–37.

Foucher G (1995) L'algodystrophie de la main. Springer, Paris.

Kline SC, Beach V, Holder LE (1993) Segmental reflex sympathetic dystrophy: clinical and scintigraphic criteria. *J Hand Surg* **18A**: 853–59.

Lankford LL (1988) Reflex sympathetic dystrophy. In: Green DP, ed., *Operative Hand Surgery*, 2nd edn, Vol. 1, 633–933. Churchill Livingstone, New York.

Lee GW, Weeks PM (1995) The role of bone scintigraphy in diagnosing reflex sympathetic dystrophy. *J Hand Surg* **20A**: 458–63.

Leriche R (1940) Les algies diffusantes post-traumatiques. In: Leriche R, ed., *La chirurgie de la douleur*, 129–50. Masson, Paris.

Leriche R (1945) La chirurgie à l'ordre de la vie, 153. Zeluck, Paris.

McFarlane RM (1983) The current status of Dupuytren's disease. *J Hand Surg* **8A**: 703–8.

Michon J, Merle M (1986) Difficultés et complications dans la chirurgie de la maladie de Dupuytren. In: Tubiana R, Hueston JT, eds, *La Maladie de Dupuytren*, 3rd edn, 186. L'Expansion Scientifique Française, Paris.

Schneider LH, Hankin FM, Eisenberg T (1986) Surgery of Dupuytren's disease: a review of the open palm method. *J Hand Surg* **11A**: 23–27.

Schuind F, Burny F (1997) Can algodystrophy be prevented after hand surgery? *Hand Clinics* **13**: 455–76.

Wong GY, Wilson PR (1997) Classification of complex regional pain syndromes. *Hand Clinics* **13**: 319–25.

Zemel NP, Balcomb TV, Stark HH et al. (1987) Dupuytren disease in women: evaluation of long-term results after operation. *J Hand Surg* **12A**: 1012–16.

SURGICAL INDICATIONS

Raoul Tubiana

'The goal in treatment of Dupuytren's disease is painless full correction of deformity with full recovery of flexion allowing resumption of normal hand activities in one month with sustained correction thereafter' (Hueston, 1991)

Timing

The decision to operate is based on functional problems. The general rule is that one should not operate in the absence of a contracture.

The discovery of a palmar nodule that does not move with movement of the fingers does not constitute an indication for surgery. The progression of Dupuytren's disease is extremely irregular. There might be a nodule present for many years, without causing a contracture, or the nodule may even regress spontaneously. Sometimes the nodule, when it first appears, causes discomfort; such discomfort is not an indication for surgery. However, the surgeon should consider the extremely rare possibility of fibrosarcoma in the young patient with severe pain, particularly night pain (Hurst, 1996). Hueston (1963) believed that surgery should be considered when the patient is unable to put the palm of the hand and the fingers simultaneously flat on a table. A positive 'tabletop' test (see Figure 5.9) should distinguish between MP contractures and PIP joint contractures; the former can be corrected fully after being present for a considerable period of time because the collateral ligaments *cannot* retract in flexion. Whereas, in the PIP joint, collateral ligaments retract in flexion and can rapidly produce a joint stiffness that is more difficult to treat.

For Hurst (1996) an MP flexion contracture of 30° or any PIP contracture (perhaps it should be greater than 20–25°) that interferes with function is an indication for surgery.

It is also important to take account of the age, general state of the patient, and his or her motivation.

Choosing an operation

There is no universal operation for Dupuytren's disease and the aim of surgery is not simply to release joint contracture or to excise diseased fascia. There are several factors involved in the choice and the extent of surgery. Some relate to the experience of the surgeon in certain procedures and on the desire to prevent complications, but the main factors in the selection of the best operation for each individual are based on the evaluation of the prognosis. The surgeon must take into account when choosing an operation the risk of complications and of recurrence, and the nature of the postoperative period.

General prognostic factors

The most important factors to be considered when assessing the prognosis are:

1) General factors: family history, age of onset, gender of patient, associated pathologies, rate of progression of the contracture.
2) Local factors: distribution of lesions, severity of deformity and the effect of previous surgery.

General factors

There is now considerable evidence that surgery controls the contracture but has no effect on the disease progression. The rate of progress of the disease is individual and seems to depend on the following factors:

Family history
This indicates by its severity the likelihood of rapid progress, but few patients have an accurate knowledge of the hands of elderly relatives.

The age of onset
The younger the age of onset, the worse the prognosis, because, not only is there a correspondingly longer lifespan for continued progress of lesions, but the pathological process is usually more active and more diffuse in younger patients. The decision to operate is generally made earlier in a patient who is younger than 45 years of age and has a rapidly progressive disease. One becomes less interventionist with elderly patients, or uses simple procedures such as limited excision or fasciotomy to minimize deformity and avoid severe handicap deformities.

The gender of the patient
This influences the prognosis because, in women, the onset is usually later and the progress slower: 'The most significant difference between men and women in Dupuytren's disease is the higher incidence of flare reaction in women following the operation.' (Zemel, 1991) (see 'Complications after surgery', pages 206–11). Most authors fear postoperative PIP joint stiffness in women (Hueston, 1974).

Progression of the disease
The natural progress of the disease is the best indication for the prognosis, since it seems that the rate of recurrence is higher in those patients with a rapidly progressive disease. Young patients seem to be more inclined to present with a rapidly progressing recurrence than older patients. A limited procedure is usually sufficient in older patients.

Hueston (1963) grouped together predisposing factors for rapid progression under the term 'diathesis' that is, an inherited tendency to the disease: positive family history, early onset of the disease, bilateral diffuse lesions, and ectopic deposits such as knuckle pads or plantar nodules, which are evidence of a stronger diathesis. Thus, when a patient presents with several of these factors, a rapid progression of the disease must be considered and the treatment altered accordingly. These factors also influence the rapidity and severity of the development of a recurrence. Both true recurrences and extension of the disease are often seen together and seem to reflect the 'rate of activity' of the disease (Millesi, 1974). This rate seems to depend on a process that is unique for each patient.

Geographic distribution
Dupuytren's disease is now disseminated all over the world although it is admitted that cases in non-Caucasian populations are less severe. Even in Europe or in the USA, the evolution rate of the disease may be different from one country or state to another. 'It may well be that the form of disease seen in the Mississippi is less virulent than that observed in continental Europe, the British Isles, Australia or even the coastal areas of the US' (Jabaley, 1999). This is certainly true. However, surgical indications are not based on the geographic distribution of the disease, but on individual factors, already mentioned.

Associated pathologies
In addition to these factors, there are certain frequently associated pathologies such as epilepsy, alcoholism, smoking or diabetes, which worsen the prognosis of Dupuytren's disease. The association of Dupuytren's disease with vasomotor phenomenon and sweating is rightly considered a potential source of postoperative edema and stiffness (Desplas, 1951). Only limited surgery is indicated.

Local factors

Site of the lesions
Distribution of lesions in the hands is infinitely variable. Unilateral lesions have, for

McFarlane, a better prognosis than bilateral lesions, but there may be a long interval before involvement of the second hand.

Lesions on the ulnar side of the hand are by far the most frequent, with production of MP and IP deformities, perhaps, as was suggested by Hueston, because of the lesser stretching influence on these digits solely reserved for power gripping.

Contracture of the little finger often has a more severe prognosis than contractures on the other digits (James and Tubiana, 1952). A hyperextension of the distal phalanx coexists always with a marked flexion of the PIP joint (boutonnière-type deformity) and a central cord often coexists with an abductor digiti minimi cord. These deformities may be difficult to correct completely.

Recurrence seems to be particularly frequent when the Dupuytren's disease is located on the fifth ray without involvement of the other rays. Sometimes, only the little finger is contracted and the palm has no lesion. Early local recurrences are the rule in such cases, and should be treated by dermofasciectomy.

Radial-sided Dupuytren's disease can often be left unoperated in elderly patients because of the slow progress of first web space contraction and the rare production of MP and IP deformity of the thumb. Conversely, we have seen that in young adults, radial-side lesions may cause a contracture of the thumb web, which is a serious functional upset that requires surgical treatment. Mild radial-side Dupuytren's disease is often seen in diabetes.

Severity of the deformity

Contracture of a single MP joint may be corrected by a limited palmar fasciectomy or even by a simple fasciotomy if the cord is well defined. A contracture of the PIP joint requires a digital incision to excise or divide all the cords. The importance of a deformity also depends on its site. A contracture of more than 70° of the MP joint is still corrected by simple excision or division of the fibrous cord. However, a PIP joint contracture of 70° may be difficult to correct.

This contracture may entail, in addition to the fibrous cords, a retraction of the flexor sheath and perhaps stiffness of the volar plate and collateral ligaments. For this reason, when the contracture of the PIP joint reaches or passes 70°, it is indicated in the authors' scoring system by the sign D+. In a similar way, the 'severe forms' (S) are indicated when the total score for all the deformities added in several digits reaches or passes 8, or in cases with a score of less than 8 but with a single ray scoring 4 D+ (PIP joint contracture of 70° or more).

Results of previous surgery

Results of previous surgery are a good indication of the reactive state of the patient. Residual joint stiffness should be a warning against another operation. Early recurrence will indicate an aggressive disease and the need for a local skin replacement, if further surgery has to be performed.

Prevention of operative complications

The prevention of the many and serious possible operative and postoperative complications takes precedence over the prevention of recurrences and even over the complete correction of the deformity. McCash's open-palm technique is a procedure designed to prevent the complications resulting from skin closure (McCash, 1964). This procedure is particularly useful for surgeons who do not have much experience in Dupuytren's surgery. However, an experienced rehabilitation team and co-operative patients are needed.

Nature of the postoperative period

The surgeon should take into consideration the duration and quality of the postoperative period.

The average time needed for skin-healing after a limited digitopalmar aponeurectomy, when the skin is sutured, is 2–3 weeks; that for the open palm procedure is an average of 5–8 weeks. However, the recurrence rate is the same (Schneider et al., 1986; Foucher et al., 1985).

Prevention of recurrence

A radical fasciectomy, including the excision of apparently healthy tissue, is not the answer for prevention of recurrence. In the proximal part of the palm, in which the aponeurotic structures are well defined and can accordingly be thoroughly excised, recurrences are rare (Millesi found fewer than 10%). The recurrences, like initial lesions, often arise in the distal part of the palm, an area in which the normal aponeurotic tissue is relatively less important. The natatory cord is the site of frequent recurrences. Recurrences are mostly seen in those areas in which the aponeurosis adheres intimately to the skin.

Prevention and treatment of recurrences are discussed in Chapter 8.

Respective indications for the different surgical procedures

Bearing these different factors in mind, the advice to any particular patient may be:

1) No surgery at present because of the absence of deformity and likelihood of very slow progress. A non-surgical treatment may be indicated.

    Before any surgery for Dupuytren's disease, the surgeon should explain to the patient what to expect from the chosen operation and the risk of recurrence from a strong diathesis.

2) Fasciotomy is indicated for the treatment of well-defined palmar cords with MP joint deformity, particularly in the elderly.

3) Limited regional fasciectomy is the most frequently performed procedure in the authors' practice. In this procedure, the macroscopic Dupuytren's tissue infiltrating the palm and the fingers is removed through zig-zag longitudinal digitopalmar incisions. The skin is sutured, using local advancement techniques and all tension is avoided. If there is a need, the wound can be left open a few millimeters.

4) McCash's open palm technique is not used routinely in the authors' practice. However, an open palm procedure associated with digitopalmar incisions (see Figure 6.60, page 177) has several indications:
    a) diffuse palmar lesions with severe skin adhesion;
    b) the presence of multiple ray involvement;
    c) to avoid skin grafts in patients with intercurrent pathology.

    In these patients, it is justified to minimize the risk of complications and to reduce the operating time. These same considerations are also relevant in the treatment of recurrences.

5) Primary dermofasciectomy is reserved for those patients with a high risk of recurrence, especially the young, with a rapidly progressive disease. Its use is particularly indicated on the little finger.

6) Secondary dermofasciectomy is advised for the treatment of recurrences.

References

Desplas B (1951) A propos de la maladie de Dupuytren. *Mem Acad Chir* **77**: 425–28.

Foucher G, Schuind F, Lemarechal P et al. (1985) La technique de la paume ouverte pour le traitement de la Maladie de Dupuytren. *Ann Chir Plast Esthet* **30**: 211–15.

Hueston JT (1963) *Dupuytren's Contracture.* E & S Livingstone, Edinburgh.

Hueston JT (1974) Prognosis as a guide to the timing and extent of surgery in Dupuytren's contracture. In: Hueston JT, Tubiana R, eds, *Dupuytren's Disease*, 1st edn, 61–62. Churchill Livingstone, Edinburgh.

Hueston JT (1991) Unsatisfactory results in Dupuytren's contracture. *Hand Clin* **7**: 759–63.

Hurst LC (1996) Dupuytren's fasciectomy: zig-zag plasty technique. *Techn Hand Surg* **64**: 519–29.

Jabaley ME (1999) Surgical treatment of Dupuytren's disease. *Hand Clin* **15**: 109–26.

James JIP, Tubiana R (1952) La maladie de Dupuytren. *Rev Chir Orthop* **38**: 352–406.

McCash CR (1964) The open palm technique in Dupuytren's contracture. *Br J Plast Surg* **17**: 271.

McFarlane RM, McGrouther D, Flint M (1990) *Dupuytren's Disease. Biology and treatment.* Churchill Livingstone, Edinburgh.

Millesi H (1974) The clinical and morphological course of Dupuytren's disease. In: Hueston JT, Tubiana R, eds, *Dupuytren's Disease*, 49. Churchill Livingstone, Edinburgh.

Millesi H (1985) The clinical and morphological course of Dupuytren's disease. In: Hueston JT, Tubiana R, eds, *Dupuytren's Disease*, 2nd edn, 114–21. Churchill Livingstone, Edinburgh.

Schneider LH, Hankin FM, Eisenberg T (1986) Surgery of Dupuytren's disease: a review of the open palm method. *J Hand Surg* **11A**: 23–27.

Zemel NP (1991) Dupuytren's contracture in women. *Hand Clin* **7**: 707–11.

Zemel NP, Balcomb TV, Stark HH et al. (1987) Dupuytren's disease in women: evaluation of long-term results after operation. *J Hand Surg* **12A**: 1012–16.

7

Salvage procedures

Raoul Tubiana

INTRODUCTION

Eicher and Moberg in 1970 described three salvage procedures used in patients with very severe Dupuytren's contracture, as an alternative to amputation of the finger. These were the cross-finger skin flap, PIP joint arthrodesis and wedge osteotomy proximal to the PIP joint.

Moberg (1973) had a large experience of cross-finger flaps (not only in Dupuytren's disease) (Figure 7.1), which in his view did not prevent an early return to work. He recommended delaying separation of the syndactylism for several months. In spite of Moberg's recommendations, cross-finger flaps are now rarely used for Dupuytren's disease. In case of skin loss on the volar surface of the finger, full-thickness skin grafts are the first choice. If a skin flap seems preferable over bare flexor tendons, several other flaps may be used (see Chapter 6, pages 186–203).

Moberg's osteotomy removes a dorsal wedge from the proximal phalanx (Figure 7.2) The PIP joint arc of motion is moved to a better functional position, but there is a risk of joint stiffness.

SEVERE PIP JOINT CONTRACTURES

Severe PIP joint contractures are difficult to treat especially if they are long standing or if

there is a recurrence on a finger already operated upon. We have already described our attitude towards PIP joint contracture in a first-time Dupuytren operation (see 'Fasciectomy', Chapter 6, pages 161–62). Resection of the volar plate check reins (see Figure 6.44, page 161) (Watson et al., 1979) is efficient as a primary procedure, when the volar plate and the collateral ligaments are not contracted. However, if there is scar tissue or if the PIP joint flexion is severe and long standing, possibly of several years' duration, it is not possible to straighten the finger despite the resection.

Andrew (1991) studied seven PIP joints in amputated digits severely affected by Dupuytren's disease and he attempted a release of various structures that might have been responsible for the joint contracture. No improvement was noted with excision of the skin, neurovascular bundles, Dupuytren's cords, oblique retinacular ligaments or with transverse division of the flexor sheath at the level of the PIP joint. Division of the check rein ligaments produced, at maximum, a 5° improvement. The most effective procedure was the release of the accessory collateral ligaments, producing full extension on five fingers. Release of the proximal attachment of the central part of the volar plate produced full extension in the two remaining digits.

This interesting study on amputated digits does not reflect operative findings when

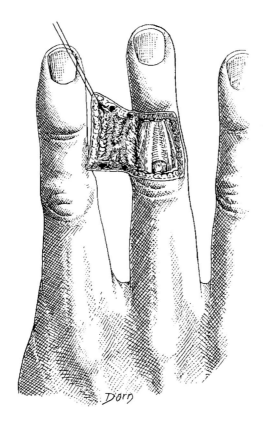

Figure 7.1 (a) Elevation of the flap on the dorsal aspect of P2, sparing the areolar tissue of the extensor tendon. (b) Palmar view (left) and dorsal view (right): (1) Flap in place; (2) skin graft on donor site.

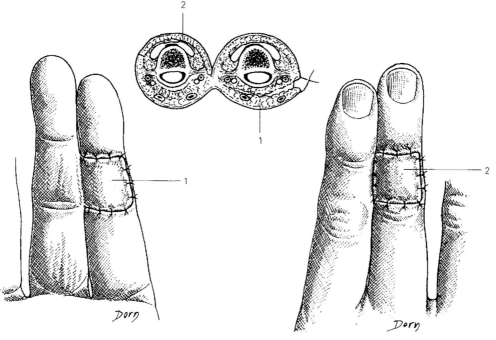

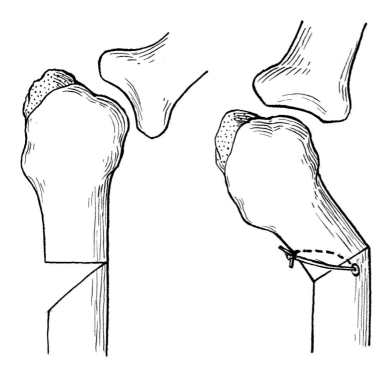

Figure 7.2 Wedge osteotomy on the proximal phalanx. (Reproduced with permission from Eicher and Moberg, 1970.)

fasciectomy is performed for the first time. It is obvious that resection of Dupuytren's cords improves PIP joint contracture and that division of the volar plate check reins produces more than 5° improvement. However, the situation is different after severe recurrence. Some surgeons have applied the technique of volar capsulectomy on PIP joint contracture in Dupuytren's disease, as described by Curtis (1974), mainly for post-traumatic joint stiffness. This procedure consists of a partial excision of the volar plate on either side of the flexor tendon together with the accessory volar ligaments; a small ribbon of volar plate is left over the central portion of the joint (Figure 7.3).

We have already mentioned our reluctance to perform capsuloligamentous release in Dupuytren's contracture, and in spite of the correction of PIP joint contracture obtained at the time of operation. Relapse of PIP joint extension deficit is frequent after long-standing flexion contracture because of the flexor muscles' loss of elasticity and secondary changes in the extensor mechanism (see 'Proximal interphalangeal joint contracture', Chapter 6, pages 161–63).

Other procedures have been used for the treatment of severe PIP joint contractures.

SKELETAL TRACTION

Skeletal traction as an adjunct to surgery has been used before and after fasciectomy in severe Dupuytren's contracture.

Postoperative traction

Postoperative traction using an external fixation device, as reported by Beard and Trail (1996), improved the initial correction in 17 of 18 fingers treated by limited fasciectomy.

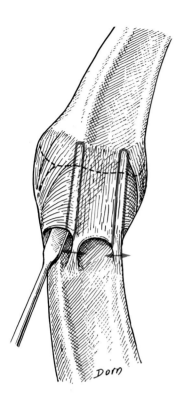

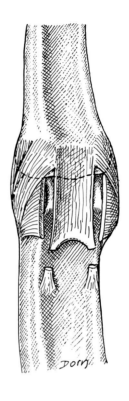

Figure 7.3 Curtis's volar capsulectomy.

Unfortunately only five maintained improved function after one year due to complications included infection, loosening, recurrence, etc. Citron and Messina (1998) also had poor results using postoperative traction, with a high incidence of reflex sympathetic dystrophy (RSD). For them 'fasciectomy followed by traction provides too great an insult to the hand, with resultant stiffness'.

Preoperative continuous elongation technique

Described by Messina in 1989, the continuous elongation technique (referred to as TEC: Tecnica di extensiona continua) consists of applying an external fixator to the contracted ray, then exerting a progressive continuous passive extension. Two self-drilling pins are

inserted in the metacarpals of the involved ray and the adjacent one. The external fixator is then attached to these pins, and to a K wire inserted through the distal metaphysis of the middle phalanx and bent to form a traction loop. The loop is connected to a threaded screw, and distraction initiated on the second day, allowing a 1–2 mm/day lengthening (Figure 7.4). According to the authors, full extension is usually achieved after 2–3 weeks of distraction (Figure 7.5).

Initially used in isolation, this method is now advocated as a preoperative procedure in severely retracted fingers (Messina and Messina, 1991, 1993). The fasciectomy is performed at the time of wire removal, otherwise the deformity would recur very rapidly.

Biochemical studies of the elongated fascia did not reveal signs of collagen fiber rupture or bleeding (Brandes et al., 1994). There

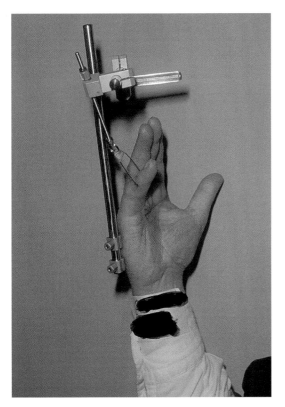

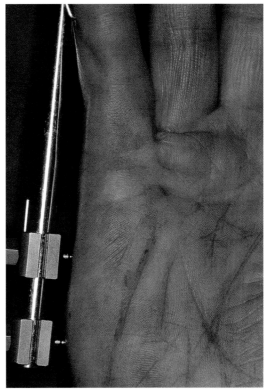

Figure 7.4 Patient treated by TEC device elongation of three retracted fingers in Dupuytren's disease. (Reproduced with permission from Messina, 1989.)

Figure 7.5 In the same patient as in Figure 7.4, the middle, ring and little fingers are extended at the end of continuous elongation (at 3 weeks). The elongation was carried out at home by the patient himself and is controlled every week on an ambulatory basis. The fasciectomy is performed at the same time as the TEC device is removed. (Reproduced with permission from Messina, 1989.)

seems to be an increase of the enzymatic activity of fibroblasts, which increases degradation and synthesis of collagen fibers, thus providing an explanation for the extension of the tissue without trauma (Bailey et al., 1994). Brandes et al. have also noticed in the elongated fascia the appearance of 'stress' fibers in the endothelial cells of both arterioles and veinules. 'There is remodeling of the internal organization of the tissue, but when distrac-tion is removed the diseased process resumes. Traction alone is not enough' (Citron and Messina, 1998).

This technique was applied by its promoter to 85 severely retracted fingers in 56 hands (Stages III and IV), including 37 recurrences. Full extension was achieved in all cases. Complications included one PIP joint subluxa-tion, and three swan-neck deformities probably related to disruption of the palmar plate.

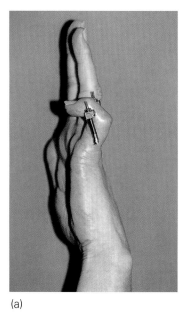
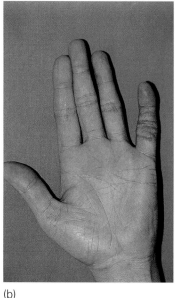
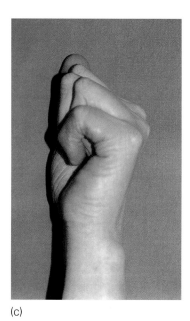

(a)   (b)   (c)

Figure 7.6 (a) Severe PIP joint contracture of the little finger. A DAP device is in place; (b) 3 weeks later a fasciectomy of the little finger, associated with a skin graft, is performed. Postoperative result in extension; (c) and in flexion. (Reproduced with permission from Djermag, 1999.)

Others have also experienced PIP joint stiffness and RSD. At 6 years' follow-up, Messina (unpublished data, 1998) observed a recurrence in eight patients.

Preoperative TEC is certainly useful in extremely retracted fingers that would otherwise require an amputation. In severe retractions, it creates better conditions for the surgical approach and reduces the complexity of the procedure.

Other fixators for preoperative traction

Several series on skeletal traction in the treatment of the flexed PIP joint in Dupuytren's disease have been published recently, using different types of external fixator (von Borchardt and Lanz, 1995).

In addition to the TEC fixator described by Messina and Messina (1991), which can apply longitudinal traction to several fingers simultaneously and to various joints in that finger independently, less bulky fixators may be used on the PIP joint alone. They must be small enough to be used on the central fingers.

Hodgkinson (1994) uses the Pipster device (i.e. the Proximal InterPhalangeal Skeletal Traction Extendor). The 'S' Quattro, devised by Fahmy (1990) has been used by Beard and Trail (1996), and the Verona fixator is used by Citron and Messina (1998) as well as the DAP (i.e. the Distracteur Articulaire Progressif) as devised by Djermag (1999) (Figures 7.6–7.8).

This technique, of the continuous extension of Dupuytren's contracture prior to fasciectomy, demonstrates the possibility of reversing contractures which were 'thought for 160 years

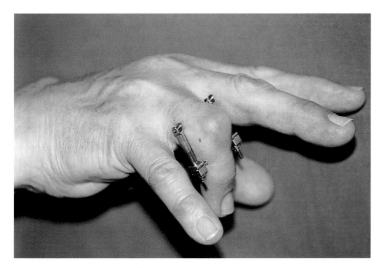

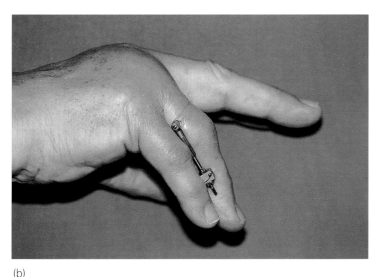

Figure 7.7 (a) Contracture of the PIP joint of the ring finger treated by continuous preoperative elongation (DAP device); (b) the finger is extended and will be operated on. (Reproduced with permission from Djermag, 1999.)

(a)

(b)

to be progressive, degenerative and irreversible' (Messina and Messina, 1993). Preoperative continuous traction may be indicated for severe Dupuytren's disease but only in suitably co-operative patients. However, as stated by Citron and Messina (1998), it must be only one component of a carefully planned program.

A. Messina, who now has several years of follow-up of his technique, has noted the absence of recurrence and extension after preoperative continuous elongation followed by fasciectomy. He therefore thinks that preventive skin grafting is no longer necessary (unpublished presentation, 2000). If this report is confirmed by other long-term follow-up studies, it will have important consequences for the treatment of Dupuytren's contracture.

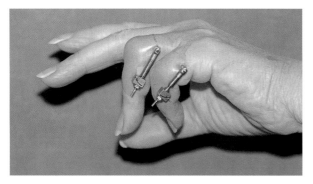

(a)

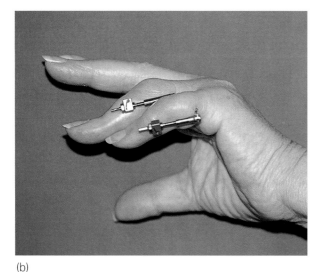

(b)

Figure 7.8 (a) Preoperative continuous elongation (DAP device) on two fingers; (b) extension obtained after 3 weeks. (Reproduced with permission from Djermag, 1999.)

TOTAL ANTERIOR TENOARTHROLYSIS

Another approach to severe PIP joint contractures is the 'total anterior tenoarthrolysis'. This procedure has been described by Saffar and Rengeval (1978) for the treatment of severe contracture of the finger after flexor tendon surgery. It consists of detaching *en bloc* the flexor apparatus and the volar plate from the underlying skeleton. This procedure, after sliding of the soft tissue, allows straightening of the finger, and is mainly a change of the active range of motion into a more functional arc. It can only be used if there is good vascularization and innervation of the finger, with articular cartilages in good condition and tendons that are still working (Pittet-Cuenod et al., 1991). A midlateral approach on one side of the finger is performed, extending from the digitopalmar skin crease to the end of the distal phalanx. At the base of the finger, the incision extends obliquely in the palm or follows the digitopalmar skin crease (Figure 7.9). The neurovascular bundles are protected and

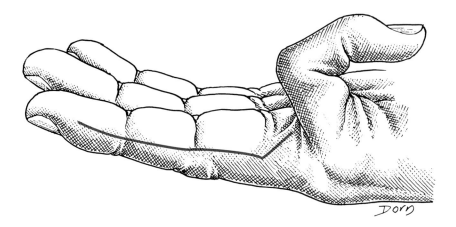

Figure 7.9 Total anterior tenoarthrolysis. Incision.

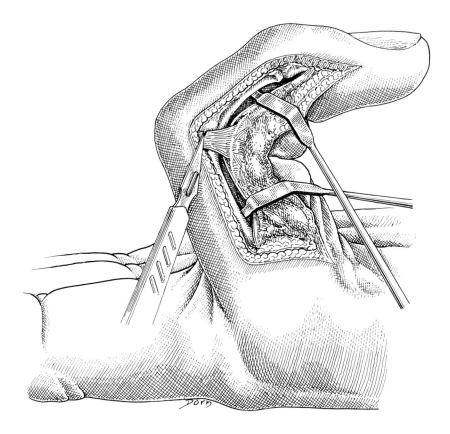

Figure 7.10 Periosteal incision on the lateral sides of the proximal and middle phalanx. Accessory ligaments of the PIP joint are cut under vision.

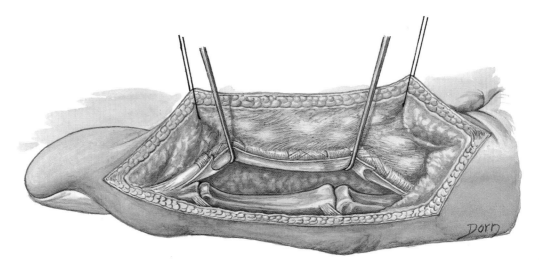

Figure 7.11 The volar tissues slide along the skeleton. It is not always necessary to free the DIP joint.

the subcutaneous fibrous tissue is cut transversally up to the periosteum of the lateral aspect of the phalanx. Direct contact is made and a periosteal incision is made on the lateral sides of the proximal and middle phalanx, which allows a volar subperiosteal elevation. Two retractors are used to raise the periosteum, forming a bridge at the PIP joint (Figure 7.10). The volar plate, which is in continuity with the periosteum, is freed: the accessory ligaments of the PIP joint are cut under direct vision, progressively, while trying to extend the finger after each partial section. The DIP joint volar plate, if necessary, may be freed in a similar way (Figure 7.11), but is best covered by DIP arthrodesis combined with shortening (Foucher and Legaillard, 1996). The volar tissues slide along the skeleton. The flexor profundus tendon must not be divided. The skin defect at the base of the finger is covered with a skin graft.

This salvage operation has been used with satisfactory results in Dupuytren's contracture by Saffar (1983), Michon (quoted by Saffar), Foucher (1996) and Leclercq (pers. comm.).

PIP JOINT ARTHROPLASTY

On occasion, in severe recurrent disease, especially involving the little finger, PIP joint arthroplasty may be considered (Haimovici, 1978). A volar or a lateral approach is used so that the extensor apparatus is not disturbed. The authors are reluctant to use procedures that may lead to an instability or occasionally a limitation of flexion. It is important to remember that a lack of extension causes less functional impairment than a loss of flexion. There are, however, patients in whom the contracture is so severe that no satisfactory surgical correction can be expected using these procedures.

PIP JOINT ARTHRODESIS

A PIP joint arthrodesis in a functional position, as proposed by Moberg, can still be a salvage procedure on a stiff contracted joint (Figures 7.12–7.14). After surgery, a PIP joint contracture, incompletely corrected but still capable of full flexion to the palm, contributes more to

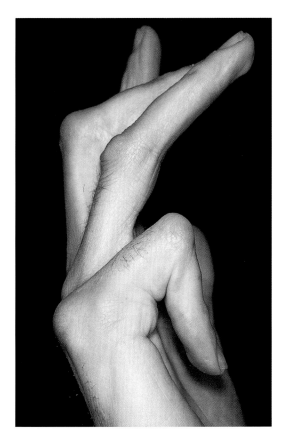

Figure 7.12 Very severe contracture of the little finger.

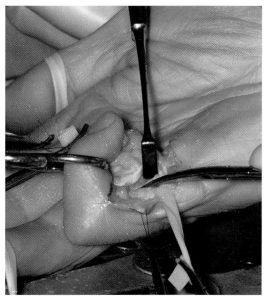

(b)

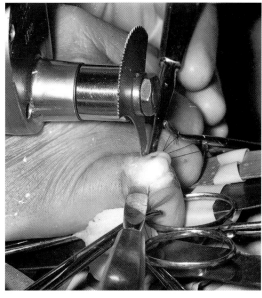

(c)

Figure 7.13 Same patient as in Figure 7.12. (a) Installation of the patient's hand on the malleable operative splint; (b) palmar fasciectomy and fasciectomy at the level of the proximal phalanx allow extension of the MP joint but only partial correction at the PIP joint; (c) a dorsal approach allows a PIP joint resection arthrodesis.

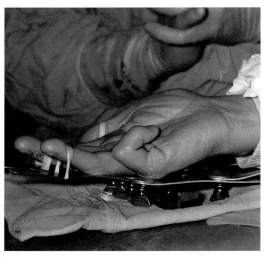

(a)

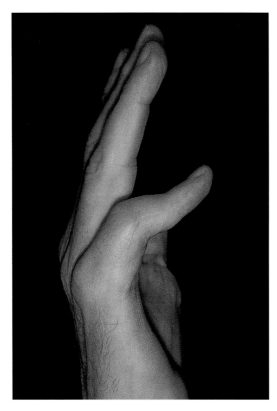

Figure 7.14 Result. The MP joint has a full range of mobility.

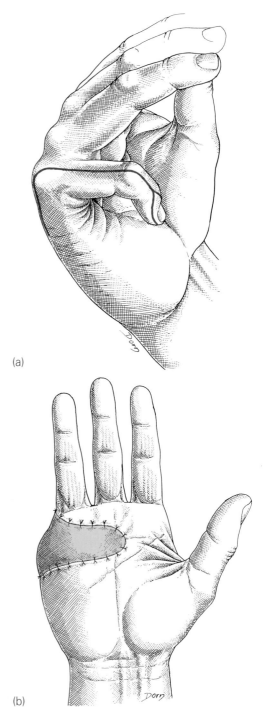

(a)

(b)

Figure 7.15 (a and b) Amputation of the little finger with cheiloplasty.

prehension than a stiff PIP from arthrodesis. PIP joint arthrodesis is only indicated when the joint is stiff and has lost full flexion, or when flexion contracture of the interphalangeal joints, not compensated by MP joint hyperextension, prevents grasping of normal objects.

Moberg systematically added a bone graft to secure the consolidation of the fusion. The present author has used compression arthrodesis with shortening of the phalanges (Lister intraosseous wiring combined with a Kirschner wire).

AMPUTATION

There is virtually never an indication for a primary amputation of a finger in

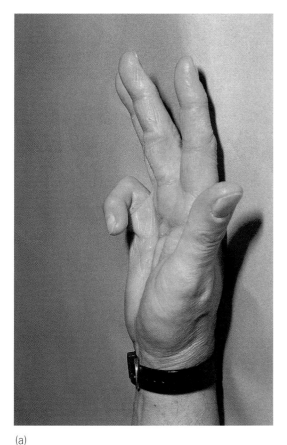

(a)

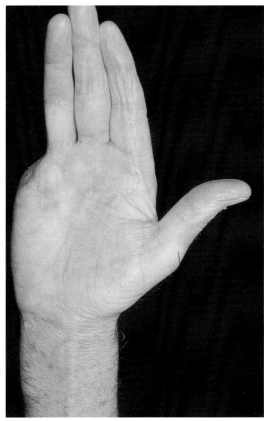

(b)

Figure 7.16 (a) The little finger had already been operated on three times; (b) the patient and the surgeon agreed on an amputation.

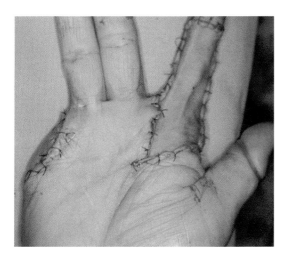

Figure 7.17 Severe recurrence on the little finger that has been amputated. In the same operation a dermofasciectomy is carried out on the index finger.

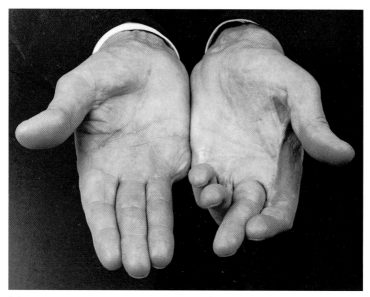

(a)

Figure 7.18 (a) Aggressive bilateral Dupuytren's contracture operated on eight times; (b) after an amputation of the right little finger and large dermofasciectomies on the radial aspect of the left hand, a useful functional result is obtained.

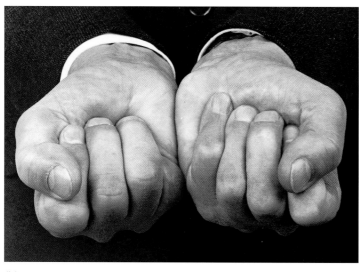

(b)

Dupuytren's disease. Amputation is reserved for recurrence of the disease on a finger with uncorrectable interphalangeal deformity and vascular and nerve lesions, especially of the little finger. The skin of the amputated finger may be used as a skin flap (cheiloplasty) (Figure 7.15a and b.) Figures 7.16–7.20 show some examples of severe Dupuytren's disease treated by salvage procedures.

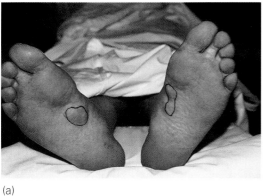

(a)

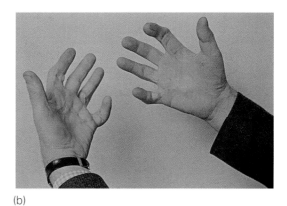

(b)

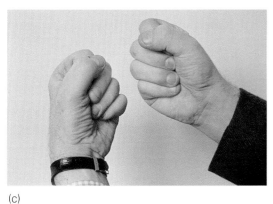

(c)

Figure 7.19 (a) Another aggressive bilateral form of Dupuytren's disease with plantar nodules; (b and c) this patient had six operations before dermofasciectomies were performed on the radial and ulnar sides of both hands resulting in a good functional result.

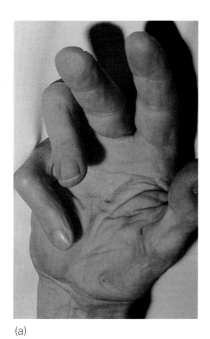

(a)

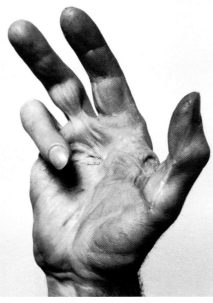

(b)

Figure 7.20 (a) All the fingers present Dupuytren's contracture; (b) dermo-fasciectomies on the thumb and first web. Amputation of the little finger with cheiloplasty. The patient later had a PIP joint arthrodesis on the ring finger.

REFERENCES

Andrew JG (1991) Contracture of the proximal interphalangeal joint in Dupuytren's disease. *J Hand Surg* **16B**: 446–48.

Bailey AJ, Tarlton JF, van der Stappen J et al. (1994) The continuous elongation technique for severe Dupuytren's disease: a biochemical mechanism. *J Hand Surg* **19B**: 522–27.

Beard AJ, Trail IA (1996) The 'S' Quattro in severe Dupuytren's contracture. *J Hand Surg* **21B**: 795–96.

Brandes G, Messina A, Reale E (1994) The palmar fascia after treatment by the continuous extension technique for Dupuytren's contracture. *J Hand Surg* **19B**: 528–33.

Citron N, Messina JC (1998) The use of skeletal traction in the treatment of severe primary Dupuytren's disease. *J Bone Joint Surg* **80B**: 126–29.

Curtis RM (1974) Volar capsulectomy in the proximal interphalangeal joint in Dupuytren's contracture. In: Hueston JT, Tubiana R, eds, *Dupuytren's Disease*. Churchill Livingstone, Edinburgh.

Djermag Y (1999) *Traitement des formes sévères de la maladie de Dupuytren par distracteur articulaire progressif.* Communication à l'Académie Nationale de Chirurgie le 5 mai 1999.

Eicher E, Moberg G (1970) Möglichkeiten zur Vermeidung von Amputationen bei schwerer Dupuytren'scher Kontraktur. *Handchirurgie* **2**: 56–60.

Fahmy NR (1990) The Stockport serpentine spring system for the treatment of displaced comminuted intra-articular phalangeal fractures. *J Hand Surg* **15A**: 303–11.

Foucher G, Legaillard P (1996) Anterior tenoarthrolysis in flexion contracture of the fingers. A propos of 41 cases. *Rev Chir Orthop Rep App Mot* **82**: 529–34.

Haimovici N (1978) Die Alloarthroplastik. Therapicalternative bei der arthrogenen Beugekontracture der Finger bei Dupuytren'scher Krankheit. *Handchirurgie* **10**: 135–48.

Hodgkinson PD (1994) The use of skeletal traction to correct the flexed PIP joint in Dupuytren's disease: a pilot study to assess the use of the Pipster. *J Hand Surg* **19A**: 534–37.

Lister G (1978) Intraosseous wiring of the digital skeleton. *J Hand Surg* **3**: 427–35.

Messina A (1989) La TEC (Tecnica di estensione continua) nel morbo di Dupuytren grave. Dall'amputazione alla ricostruzione. *Riv Chir Mano* **26**: 253–56.

Messina A, Messina J (1991) The TEC treatment (continuous extension technique) for severe Dupuytren's contracture fingers. *Ann Chir Main Memb Super* **10**: 247–50.

Messina A, Messina J (1993) The continuous elongation treatment by the TEC device for severe Dupuytren's contracture of the fingers. *Plast Reconstr Surg* **7**: 84–90.

Moberg E (1973) Three useful ways to avoid amputation in advanced Dupuytren's contracture. *Orthop Clin North Am* **4**: 1001.

Pittet-Cuenod B, Della Santa D, Chamay A (1991) Total anterior tenoarthrolysis to treat inveterate flexion contraction of the fingers: a series of 16 patients. *Ann Plast Surg* **26**: 358–64.

Saffar Ph (1983) Total anterior teno-arthrolysis. Report of 72 cases. *Ann Chir Main* **2**: 345–50.

Saffar Ph (1988) Total anterior tenoarthrolysis. In: Tubiana R, ed., *The Hand*, Vol. III, 297–303. WB Saunders, Philadelphia.

Saffar Ph, Rengeval JP (1978) La ténoarthrolyse totale antérieure. Technique de traitement des doigts en crochet. *Ann Chir* **32**: 579–82.

Von Borchardt B, Lanz U (1995) Die präoperative kontinuierliche Extensionsbehandlung hochgradiger Dupuytrenscher Kontrakturen. *Handchir Mikrochir Plast Chir* **27**: 269–71.

Watson HK, Lovallo JL (1987) Salvage of severe recurrent Dupuytren's contracture of the ring and small fingers. *J Hand Surg* **12A**: 287.

Watson HK, Light TR, Johnston TR (1979) Checkrein resection for flexion contracture of the middle joint. *J Hand Surg* **4**: 67–71.

8

Results of surgical treatment

Caroline Leclercq

RECURRENCE

The term 'recurrence' has various meanings in the Dupuytren's disease literature. Some authors restrict its use to secondary flexion contractures of the fingers (Dickie and Hughes, 1967). Others gather local recurrence of the disease and extension, and evaluate their results in terms of 'global activity' (Millesi, 1974). Yet other authors publish their results in terms of range of motion, without separating local recurrence from joint stiffness or scar contracture (Orlando et al., 1974; Noble and Harrison, 1976). These varied interpretations may explain why the recurrence rate varies so greatly from one series to the other, from 22% (Dickie and Hughes, 1967) to 77% (Mantero et al., 1986). It thus seems important to start out with a clear definition of recurrence as related to Dupuytren's disease.

Definition

'Recurrence' means the reappearance of Dupuytren's tissue in a zone previously operated on (and thus cleared of abnormal fascia at the time of surgery). This definition includes the reappearance of isolated nodules, without contracture, but excludes the appearance of new lesions in a zone previously unaffected, which forms on *extension* of Dupuytren's disease (Figure 8.1). The overall

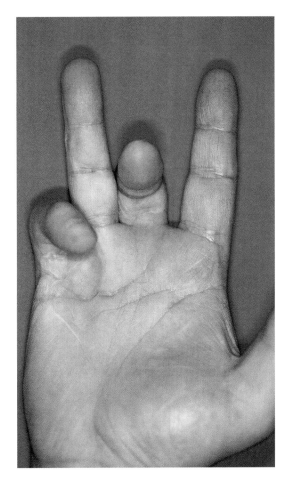

Figure 8.1 Recurrence of Dupuytren's disease on the little finger (previously operated on), and extension on the middle finger (previously unaffected).

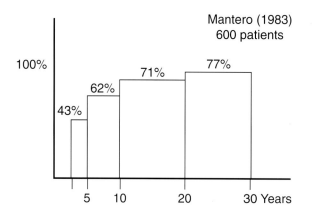

Figure 8.2 Recurrence in Mantero's series (*n* = 600 patients): evolution with time.

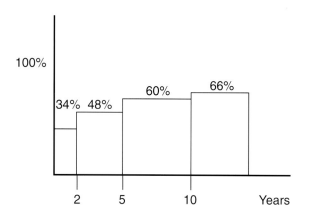

Figure 8.3 Recurrence in Tubiana's series (*n* = 38 patients): evolution with time.

activity of the disease, as defined by Millesi (1974), includes recurrence and extension.

It is equally important to distinguish recurrence from skin contracture at the operation site, which is not always easy and requires careful clinical examination. Scar contractures are generally mobile and are less prominent when the fingers are flexed. The recurrence is deeper, not mobile, and does not lessen with finger flexion.

Frequency of recurrence

The incidence of true recurrence reported in the relevant literature is wide-ranging. This variability depends on two factors: partly in various interpretations of the term 'recurrence' as above, and partly, and most importantly, the duration of postoperative follow-up.

Initially recurrence was thought to occur early after surgery (Hueston, 1963), within the first two postoperative years; and analysis of the early series, which had a short follow-up, shows a fairly low rate of recurrence: Gonzalez (1971), 10% recurrence; Dickie and Hughes (1967), 22%; Hueston (1963), 30%; Rank and Wakefield, reviewed by Hueston (1978), 40%; Honner et al. (1971), 54%. Only McIndoe's series has a long-term follow-up. It was reviewed by Hakstian (1974) who followed

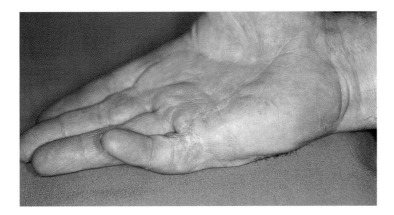

Figure 8.4 Stage I recurrence after two operations.

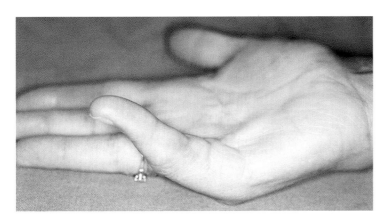

Figure 8.5 Stage II recurrence 10 years after operation.

patients for 10 years and observed a recurrence rate of 34%. However, the term defining recurrence was restrictive.

In 1974, Millesi questioned this early occurrence of recurrence, having noticed that 48% of his recurrences appeared after the third postoperative year. Then Dickie and Hughes (1967), who analyzed their results each year, noticed an annual increase of 5.5% in the disease's activity (recurrences and extensions) of their series up to the fourth postoperative year. In 1986, Mantero et al., who had followed up 600 patients for up to 30 years, produced a logarithmic progression of the numbers of recurrence. They noticed that a 43% recurrence rate occured between the third and fifth postoperative years, and they found a

77% recurrence rate among those who could be followed up between 20 and 30 years (Figure 8.2).

In 1985, the author reviewed Tubiana's series of 89 patients who had been operated on more than 8 years previously (Tubiana and Leclercq, 1986; Leclercq and Tubiana, 1999). Of these 89, the author was able to examine 38 after 8–14 years (average 10 years). Surgery was performed bilaterally in 12 patients, amounting to 50 hands reviewed. The author found a 66% rate of recurrence, which followed the same type of progression with time as in Mantero et al.'s series (1986) (Figure 8.3). Of these recurrences, 18% were limited to a mere palmar nodule (27% of all recurrences), 12% were Stage I (Figure 8.4), and 36% were Stages

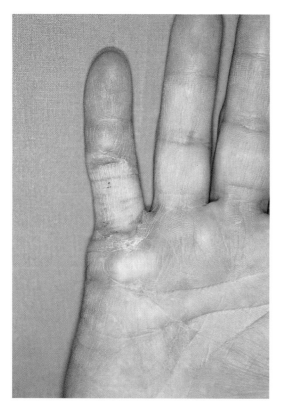

Figure 8.6 Nodular recurrence immediately proximal to a skin graft covering the volar aspect of the proximal phalanx.

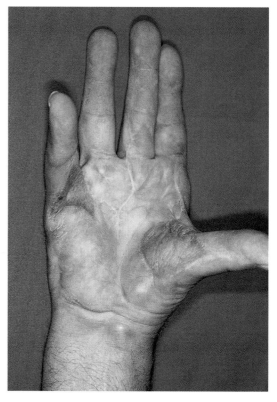

Figure 8.7 Early recurrence and extension in a young man with severe involvement. There is no recurrence under the skin grafts.

II or III (Figure 8.5). An extension of the disease was present in 62% of patients, isolated in 16%, and associated with a recurrence in 46%. The global activity rate as defined by Millesi (addition of recurrences and extension) was therefore 82%. A skin graft was performed in 11 cases and recurrence occured in 9. It was never located under the graft but rather along the edge of the graft (Figures 8.6 and 8.7). This corroborates Hueston's etiological hypothesis of a dermal origin of the disease, and confirms the result of series of dermofasciectomy (Hueston, 1985; Tonkin et al., 1984); see 'Dermofasciectomy', pages 199–203.

Functional impairment linked to Dupuytren's disease is difficult to assess. It varies greatly with the patients' ages and activities. We have attempted an objective scoring of this impairment (Tubiana and Leclercq, 1985). According to this score 62% presented with a potential impairment preoperatively, versus 24% at 10-year follow-up. Thus even if recurrence is rather frequent, it is not often incapacitating. Although surgery is not able to cure the disease, it is useful. (Details of the whole Tubiana series form the end section of this chapter, see page 250.)

More recent series agree with these figures, with recurrence rates similar to that in Tubiana's series. All of them have a much longer follow-up than earlier series:

- Mantero et al. (1986) followed their patients for up to 30 years and reported a global rate of 63% recurrence;
- Norotte et al. (1988) followed 58 patients for more than 10 years. Of 69 hands operated on, 71% had a recurrence after 10 years;
- Foucher et al.'s series (1992) showed a lower incidence of recurrences (46%) but his 54 patients were reviewed at 5.6 years on average.

These figures suggest that recurrence occurs very frequently in Dupuytren's disease, as demonstrated when the patients are followed for long enough and when all signs of recurrence, including nodules, are taken into account. In Tubiana's series, 27% of recurrences were merely nodular. If these nodules had not been included, the global recurrence rate of the series would have been 48% and not 66%.

Progression of the number of recurrences with time is similar in all long-term series as in Mantero's (Tubiana and Leclercq, 1985; Norotte et al., 1988). An average of 30% of patients experience a recurrence during the first and second postoperative years, then another 15% during the third to fifth years,

10% between 5 and 10 years, and less than 10% after 10 years. Thus, even though patients are free of recurrence at 5 years, there is still a 10–15% chance that they develop one later on. From Norotte et al.'s series, it appears that the most severe recurrences (Stages II and above in Tubiana's grading) occurred early, whereas recurrences appearing later usually remained discrete (Stages 0 or I).

Factors influencing recurrence

Certain factors, grouped under the term 'Dupuytren's diathesis' by Hueston (1963b), are well known as pejorative prognostic factors. These include a young age of occurrence, a family history of Dupuytren's disease and the presence of ectopic lesions (see Chapter 5). Other factors have since been regarded as possible risk factors, such as gender (women), race, associated diseases, and some local factors.

When reviewing Tubiana's series (Tubiana and Leclercq, 1985), the author has studied all these factors in order to determine their precise influence on recurrence (Table 8.1).

Table 8.1 Factors influencing recurrence in Tubiana's series.

	Factors	No. of patients	No. of recurrences	%
Age	< 45 years old	16	16	100
	45–65 years old	18	12	66
	> 65 years old	4		44
Gender	F	3	3	
	M	35	22	64
Family history	Yes	14	11	78
	No	24	14	58
Ectopic lesions	Knuckle pads	15	8	53
	Feet	2	2	
Associated conditions	Epilepsy	1	1	
	Diabetes	1	1	
Localization	Thumb	4	3	75
	Fifth finger	7	6	85

Age

Among the 38 patients reviewed, 6 were younger than 45 years old at the time of surgery. All 6 of these developed a recurrence (nodular in 3, with a contracture in 3). Among the 23 patients aged 45–65 at the time of surgery 15 (66%) developed a recurrence, and among the 9 patients aged over 65, 4 (44%) developed a recurrence, thus suggesting a strong positive correlation of early age of onset with recurrence.

Family history

Of the 15 cases with knuckle pads, 53% developed a recurrence, and the 2 cases with plantar lesions developed a recurrent nodule. None of the reviewed patients was affected with Peyronie's disease. Although these figures are too small for statistical analysis, they tend to show that knuckle pads did not have a detrimental effect on recurrence in our patients [in contradiction to Hueston (1963b) and other series such as Norotte et al., where all the patients with ectopic lesions developed a recurrence].

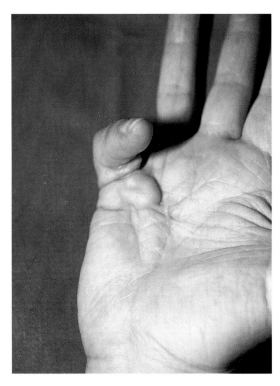

Figure 8.8 Early and severe recurrence localized to the little finger in a woman.

Gender

All 3 female patients had a recurrence (Figure 8.8). This is in contradiction to studies by Tonkin et al. (1984) and by Zemel et al. (1987) who found a lower recurrence rate in women than in men.

Associated diseases

Our only patient with epilepsy developed a severe recurrence, and our only patient with diabetes developed a minor recurrence limited to a palmar nodule. Norotte et al.'s series shows the same high recurrence rate in their diabetic patients (82%), epileptic patients (75%), and alcoholic patients (83%) as compared to the whole series (71%). None of the large studies of these associated diseases in the literature report any specific rate of recurrence after surgery.

Local factors

The author has also tried to determine if some specific localizations or the initial severity were detrimental prognostic factors:

• Involvement of the thumb was present in 20 of the 50 hands. It was always associated with involvement of other digits, and the thumb itself was operated on in 4 cases only, with 3 recurrences. Among the 16 other cases where the thumb was involved but not operated on, a recurrence occured in the operated finger in 14 cases (87%); it is possible that the thumb involvement in itself is not a 'risk' factor but more the extent of the disease, involving several rays;

- Little finger involvement was isolated in 7 patients (including 2 of the 3 women). Six of the 7 developed a recurrence, which was rapid and severe in 3;
- Local severity of the disease was calculated for each hand using Tubiana's scoring system (see 'Assessment of lesions', pages 97–107). Extension was included in the calculation so as to determine the global involvement of each hand, both initially and at follow-up. Table 8.2 indicates that the greater the initial score the greater the global involvement at the latest follow-up. This was also reported in other series (Vigroux and Valentin, 1992);
- A severe contracture of the PIP joint has been recognized as a detrimental factor (Foucher et al., 1992). In Tubiana's series, correction of the PIP contracture obtained at surgery was incomplete in 3 cases and in all 3 cases there was an early and severe recurrence. This correlates with Vigroux and Valentin (1992) who

found a statistically significant correlation between failure to achieve full PIP extension at surgery and unsatisfactory results. But PIP involvement is often present in more severe cases, and it may well be the initial severity of the disease rather than PIP involvement *per se* that has a pejorative prognostic value.

Type of operation

It is extremely difficult, from the literature, to get a precise idea of incidence of the type of procedure on the recurrence rate. To try to clarify this point, the author gathered three Dupuytren's disease surgeons, who used three different techniques, at a Round Table meeting and asked them to assess their results after more than 5 years using the same criteria and the same grading system as in Tubiana's series:

- Regional fasciectomy was performed by Valentin. Review of his 56 patients by Vigroux and Valentin (1992) showed a 45% recurrence rate at 10 years;
- Open palm was performed by Foucher. Of his 54 patients reviewed at an average of 5.6 years, 46% had developed a recurrence (Foucher et al., 1992);
- Dermofasciectomy and skin grafting was performed by Varian. Of his 32 patients, 47% developed a recurrence (Kelly and Varian, 1992).

Table 8.2 Preoperative and late postoperative assessment 10 years later.				
Scoring	No. of cases	Mean preoperative	Mean postoperative	%
<5	31	3.3	1.6	48
5–10	16	6.2	3.8	61
>10	3	12.8	9.6	75
Total	**50**	**4.7**	**2.8**	**60**

In light of these results, there does not seem to be a significant relationship between the type of procedures and the rate of recurrence. However, all three authors stated that there is a significant relationship between the initial degree of PIP contracture and the rate of recurrence.

In Tubiana's series a skin graft was performed in 11 cases, 9 of which later presented with a recurrence outside the grafted area. But skin grafting was not a routine procedure in the series and was used only in severe cases (e.g. severe local involvement or strong diathesis).

Postoperative complications

Early postoperative complications included one hematoma, one nerve division, one delayed healing, one limited skin necrosis, and one superficial infection. The last 3 of these 5 cases developed a recurrence. In Norotte et al.'s series, postoperative complications occured in 15 cases, with 86% recurrence, which is higher than average in their series (71%) but those 15 cases were all among the initially severe ones, which were also shown to have a higher rate of recurrence.

From this series and the author's experience, there seem to be two different types of recurrence in two different population groups:

- Late and minimal recurrence, affecting older patients with initially localized and slowly evolving disease. The recurrence manifests as the progressive reappearance of a cord or nodule, which develops slowly;
- Massive and early recurrence, which mainly manifests in young patients, generally involves the whole area operated on, with extension to zones previously unaffected. It tends to occur in the first two postoperative years and may develop into a more severe contracture than initially present (3 cases in our series).

The isolated form affecting the little finger is often severe but localized and it is more common in women. Recurrence tends to be early and severe but often remains limited to the fifth digital ray and may not be accompanied by extension to other rays (7 cases in Tubiana's series, with 3 early and severe recurrences).

Treatment of recurrence

Reoperation is not always necessary when contracture is limited, particularly in the elderly. We are more likely to intervene when the patient is younger, especially when there is a contracture of the PIP joint. It is not necessary to undertake a complete fasciectomy as classically described but rather to excise only the tissues responsible for the contraction. This intervention should be carried out under magnification because the dissection is particularly difficult and not without risk to vessels and nerves. The patient must be warned of the possibility that amputation of the finger may result.

The dissection begins by identifying the neurovascular bundles proximal to the area of recurrence. These are then followed through the length of the digit. The fibrous tissues limiting extension are progressively excised. If there is a contracture affecting the flexor sheath, transverse incisions are made. It may also be necessary to incise the check rein ligaments of the volar plate to free a contracture of the PIP joint. When contracture is severe, it is sometimes preferable to undertake an arthrodesis and shortening at the PIP joint.

There then remains the problem of skin cover. Some surgeons close primarily with a local flap when necessary. This technique may be justified when the progression of disease is very slow. After a lengthy dissection, some prefer to leave the wound open, especially when several rays are affected. This helps to shorten the length of the intervention and to avoid some early complications. Our preference tends towards the use of a graft to fill the

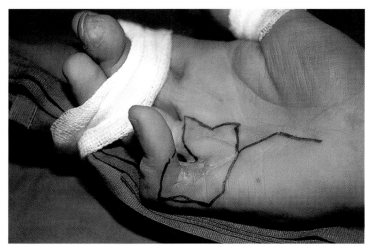

(a)

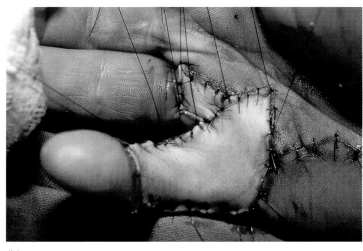

(b)

Figure 8.9 (a) Severe recurrence on the ring and little fingers in a 25-year-old man: planned skin excision. Note the lateral extent of excision, up to the junction of palmar and dorsal skin; (b) immediate postoperative view.

defect, as grafts discourage recurrence locally. We use full-thickness skin as this contracts less than split skin.

Full-thickness skin grafts

In 1952, Piulachs and Mir y Mir demonstrated that there are no recurrences under skin grafts. Hueston popularized the use of these grafts while noting that the prophylactic effect of full-thickness grafts is not completely explained (Hueston, 1962, 1974). Long-term series of dermofasciectomies have shown that recurrence is extremely infrequent under skin grafts (Kelly and Varian 1992; Searle and Logan, 1992).

The graft is harvested from the medial aspect of the same arm, which allows surgery to be undertaken under regional anesthesia with a tourniquet on the proximal arm. The size and shape of the graft are tailored according to the size of the defect. The area to be grafted must be chosen carefully, taking account of the following factors (Figure 8.9):

- Excision should include all areas where skin is affected;
- Exposed flexor tendons must be covered with well-vascularized tissue, e.g. skin flaps;
- The graft should be positioned proximal to the most affected joint (usually the PIP);
- The edges of the graft should be planned to avoid formation of scar contractures; at the level of the fingers, the skin is excised up to the junction of the palmar and dorsal skin;
- The graft should be sufficiently large to avoid formation of a new contracture; make sure that the continuity of the diseased tissue is interrupted;
- Grafts should not be placed in areas important for prehension.

The use of full-thickness grafts must follow the normal rules of the technique, namely deflation of the tourniquet to obtain perfect hemostasis, subsequent reinflation of the tourniquet before positioning the graft, irrigation of the site with saline, and the application of a pad covering the entire graft surface. The dressing is left in place for 6–8 days and is then replaced with a lighter dressing to allow gentle mobilization of the digit. Physiotherapy and dynamic splinting are delayed until the graft has completely taken (see 'Skin grafts', pages 194–99).

Digital amputation

In the presence of a severe or longstanding contracture with severe infiltration of the finger by recurrence, especially if there is a neurovascular deficit, amputation of a digit can be decided on after discussion with the patient. It is often the little finger that is involved. Amputation is at the level of the MP joint, and the skin over the ulnar border of the digit can be used to cover the palmar surface. If the central rays are involved, amputation can be transmetacarpal or transcarpal as proposed by Leviet (1978).

Occasionally, amputation is decided on intraoperatively, in the face of acute ischemia of the finger once the tourniquet is released. Attempts at revascularization are of uncertain value when the vascular pedicles may have been damaged by previous interventions. Placing the finger in flexion may re-establish blood flow but the ischemia may be irreversible. It is preferable to acquire the patient's consent prior to amputation. In all cases the patient should be warned of this possibility when operating on a recurrence.

Prevention of recurrence

Owing to the many preceding studies, it is now possible to predict the likelihood of recurrence in a number of cases and adapt the operative procedure accordingly. The only surgical technique capable of controlling the disease locally is dermofasciectomy and skin grafting (although it does not prevent recurrence outside the grafted area). Our current attitude in patients with several risk factors is to perform primary dermofasciectomy and skin grafting in all areas where the skin is adherent to the fascial lesions.

References

Dickie WR, Hughes NC (1967) Dupuytren's contracture: a review of the late results of radical fasciectomy. *Br J Plast Surg* **20**: 311–14.

Foucher G, Cornil C, Lenoble E (1992) Open palm technique for Dupuytren's disease: a five year follow-up. *Ann Chir Main* **11**: 362–66.

Gonzalez RI (1971) Dupuytren's contracture of the fingers: a simplified approach to the surgical treatment. *Calif Med* **115**: 25–31.

Hakstian RW (1974) Late results of extensive fasciectomy. In: Hueston JT, Tubiana R, eds, *Dupuytren's Disease*, 79–84. Churchill Livingstone, Edinburgh.

Honner R, Lamb DW, James JIP (1971) Dupuytren's contracture: long term results after fasciectomy. *J Bone Joint Surg* **53**: 240–46.

Hueston JT (1962) Digital Wolfe grafts in recurrent Dupuytren's contracture. *Plast Reconstr Surg* **29**: 342–44.

Hueston JT (1963a) The Dupuytren's diathesis. In: Hueston JT, ed., *Dupuytren's Contracture*, 51–63. Churchill Livingstone, Edinburgh.

Hueston JT (1963b) Recurrent Dupuytren's contracture. *Plast Reconstr Surg* **31**: 66–69.

Hueston JT (1974) Skin replacement in Dupuytren's contracture. In: Hueston JT, Tubiana R, eds, *Dupuytren's Disease*, 119–22. Churchill Livingstone, Edinburgh.

Hueston JT (1978) Review of Rank and Wakefield's series.

Hueston JT (1985) Dermofasciectomy and skin replacement in Dupuytren's disease. In: Hueston JT, Tubiana R, eds, *Dupuytren's Disease*, 2nd edn, 149–53. Churchill Livingstone, Edinburgh.

Kelly C, Varian J (1992) Dermofasciectomy: a long-term review. *Ann Chir Main* **11**: 381–82.

Leclercq C, Tubiana R (1999) Recurrence in Dupuytren's contracture. In: Tubiana R, ed., *The Hand*, Vol. V, 484–92. Saunders, Philadelphia.

Leviet D (1978) La translocation de l'auriculaire par ostéotomie intracarpienne (in French with English summary). *Ann Chir* **32**: 609–12.

Mantero R, Ghigliazza GB, Bertolloti P et al. (1986) Les formes récidivantes de al maladie de Dupuytren (analyse d'une casuitique). In: Tubiana R, Hueston JT, eds, *La Maladie de Dupuytren*, 3rd edn, 208–209. Expansion Scientifique Française, Paris.

Millesi H (1974) The clinical and morphological course of Dupuytren's disease. In: Hueston JT,

Tubiana R, eds, *Dupuytren's Disease*, 49–60. Churchill Livingstone, Edinburgh.

Noble J, Harrison DH (1976) Open palm technique for Dupuytren's contracture. *Hand* **8**: 272–78.

Norotte G, Apoil A, Travers V (1988) A ten year follow-up of the results of surgery for Dupuytren's disease. A study of 58 cases (in French and English). *Ann Chir Main* **7**: 277–81.

Orlando JC, Smith JW, Goulian D (1974) Dupuytren's contracture: a review of one hundred patients. *Br J Plast Surg* **27**: 211–17.

Piulachs P, Mir y Mir L (1952) Considerations sobre la enfermedad de Dupuytren. *Fol Clin Int* **II**: 415–16.

Searle AE, Logan AM (1992) A mid-term review of the results of dermofasciectomy for Dupuytren's disease. *Ann Chir Main* **11**: 375–80.

Tonkin MA, Burke FD, Varian JP (1984) Dupuytren's contracture: a comparative study of fasciectomy in one hundred patients. *J Hand Surg* **9B**: 156–62.

Tubiana R, Leclercq C (1985) Recurrent Dupuytren's disease. In: Hueston JT, Tubiana R, eds, *Dupuytren's Disease*, 2nd edn, 200–203. Churchill Livingstone, Edinburgh.

Vigroux JP, Valentin LP (1992) Natural history of Dupuytren's contracture treated by surgical fasciectomy: the influence of diathesis (76 hands reviewed at more than 10 years). *Ann Chir Main* **11**: 367–74.

Zemel NP, Balcomb TV, Skark HH et al. (1987) Dupuytren's disease in women: evaluation of long-term results after operation. *J Hand Surg* **12A**: 1012–16.

PERSONAL SERIES

Caroline Leclercq and Raoul Tubiana

This series includes all of Professor Tubiana's personal cases treated between 1970 and 1976. This forms a group of 183 patients, 89 of whom were treated in his private practice and 94 in his public practice. All patients were operated on with the same technique, i.e. limited fasciectomy with primary skin closure (or full-thickness skin graft):

- Number of patients: 183;
- Gender: male 160 (87%), female 23 (13%);
- Age at onset: <25 years (3%), 25–35 years (17%), 35–45 years (16%), 45–55 years (20%), 55–65 years (13%), >65 years (4%);
- Bilaterality: 83%;
- Number of rays involved: 1 (11%), 2 (14%), 3 (28%), 4 (27%), 5 (17%); (These high figures attest to the severity of many of the cases who were referred to Professor Tubiana.)
- Family history: 22%;
- Associated diseases: diabetes (1%), epilepsy (3%);
- Ectopic lesions: knuckle pads (17%), Ledderhose (5%), Peyronie's disease (1%);
- Postoperative complications: RSD (3%), hematoma (1%), nerve division (2%), skin dehiscence (0%), skin necrosis (0%), finger ischemia (1%), infection (0.5%);
- Postoperative range of motion: *complete joint flexion in all patients.*
- Recurrence: only the patients from the private practice (*n* = 89) were reviewed at long term (8–14 years). The recurrence rate was 66%. Details of recurrence are in the previous section in this chapter.

9

Hand therapy

Evelyn J Mackin and Terri M Skirven

INTRODUCTION

The successful removal of the affected fascia in Dupuytren's disease requires a delicate surgical technique and excellent knowledge of anatomy in order to prevent damage to the digital nerves and vessels. Equally important is a skilled and experienced hand therapist to monitor a carefully orchestrated postoperative mobilization program. Postoperative complications need to be recognized and dealt with early.

Some of these complications are persistent edema, infection, stiffness of the entire hand, hematoma, and early recurrence of flexion contractures. Patients must understand that approximately 6–8 weeks' of postoperative therapy and splinting may be required if the good results attained at surgery are to be maintained, and that night extension splinting may be necessary for 6 months or longer in some cases.

POSTOPERATIVE THERAPY

Undue postoperative swelling and pain are ominous signs that a reflex sympathetic dystrophy (RSD) may be occurring. If it develops, RSD can prolong morbidity and result in permanent disability with loss of digital flexion. Since patients almost always have full flexion even with long-standing and severe contractures, the loss of full flexion is often more disabling than the lack of full extension. If RSD develops, treatment must be given immediately (Walsh, 1984a).

Some degree of hematoma or blood clot is inevitable after extensive dissection and closure of transverse incisions over the concavity of the palm. If the therapist suspects a hematoma, the surgeon should be notified even though the hematoma may be small and not require any surgical attention. The area may heal satisfactorily with splinting, wound and scar care. However, the hematoma may be treated successfully by removing the sutures over the area of tension and allowing the hematoma to drain. If the hematoma is large and not recognized and properly drained, some degree of necrosis at the suture line is likely, and this will be followed by infection (McFarlane, 1986). The result is frequently swelling and stiffness of the hand.

Since postoperative splinting must be initiated immediately to hold the patient's fingers in extension during the period of wound healing, careful attention must be given to splint fabrication, and the patient must be seen by the therapist on a regular schedule. Should a hematoma begin to develop, causing additional swelling, the splint may no longer fit properly. If, in addition, the patient fails to attend his scheduled therapy appointments, a constricting wrist strap can increase the edema, resulting in further problems, for example more fibrosis, thicker scar (Mackin and Byron, 1990).

Evolution

Since the postoperative Dupuytren's hand can change dramatically in as little as a few days because of the dynamics of the healing process, careful evaluation must be performed and documented from the first visit. The evaluation battery should include wound and edema assessment, active range-of-motion (ROM), passive range-of-motion (ROM), and sensibility evaluation (Fietti and Mackin, 1995).

Edema is initially recorded using circumferential measurements taken with a flexible tape measure. Tapes for measuring the circumference are available commercially (North Coast Medical, Inc., Campbell, CA). These measurements should be taken at specific landmarks on the hands and fingers to improve reproducibility. When the wounds are healed, volumetric measurements replace circumferential measures. The volumeter, based on Archimedes' principle of water displacement, measures hand volume and is commercially available. Brand and Wood (1977) introduced the volumeter to measure hand volume more objectively. Measurements should be taken before and after treatment. A marked increase in swelling accompanied by pain may indicate an inflammatory reaction, which can occur if exercises are too vigorous or if the patient is using the hand for more than light activities of daily living.

Active and passive range-of-motion measurements are taken with a goniometer.

Finger flexion is frequently limited, especially when the incision extends into the digit. This limitation is due to swelling and volar scar formation combined with the prolonged positioning of the digit(s) in extension, which is necessary to maintain the degree of extension obtained at surgery. Measurement is made of the distance from the finger pulp(s) to the distal palmar crease (DPC) during active flexion, because this measurement relates to the function of grasp (Tonkin et al., 1984). Extension must also be closely monitored. Maintaining the degree of extension obtained at surgery may be difficult due to weakness or attenuation of the extensor tendon. This is often compounded by the resistance to finger extension that results from the volar incision scar. As the scar matures and becomes stiffer, resistance to extension increases and the patient is at risk of losing range of motion in extension and may develop a flexion contracture. Measurements at each joint in both flexion and extension are taken initially and repeated at appropriate intervals (Mackin and Byron, 1990) to ensure that progress is being made and that treatment methods are effective.

Sensibility may be affected as a result of Dupuytren's surgery. The diminished sensation often recovers spontaneously but should be monitored because it may influence functional recovery (Mackin and Byron, 1990). Semmes Weinstein monofilaments may be used to evaluate light touch sensibility with the periodic re-evaluation every 4–6 weeks.

The wounds may be closed with the appropriate Z-plasties or skin graft, or the wound may be left open as described by McCash (1964). Therapy usually begins on the third to fifth postoperative day. It includes custom splint fabrication, wound care, edema control, and active and passive ROM exercises. As healing progresses, flexion splinting and scar management also may be indicated (Fietti and Mackin, 1995).

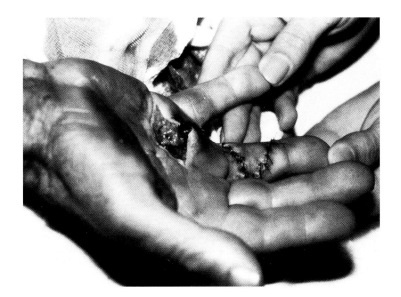

Figure 9.1 McCash (1964) found that transverse incisions in the palm could be left unsutured to heal secondarily, resulting in a cosmetically acceptable scar with little or no morbidity.

Open palm technique

The open palm technique of McCash prevents hematoma and may contribute to the overall reduction of complications (Tubiana, 1985). Since the wounds drain freely, hematomas do not occur and skin sloughs are uncommon (Gelberman et al., 1982). Diminished postoperative pain is an advantage of leaving the surgical incision open. This becomes even more noticeable when the patient begins active motion of the hand. Early motion reduces edema and stiffness.

Patients are often apprehensive about the appearance of the open wound unless well prepared by their surgeon. The therapist must explain the wound healing process to the patient or they may not comply with treatment requirements (Figure 9.1).

Since the open palm technique allows free drainage of the wound, whirlpool treatment assists in wound management by cleansing and debriding the wound. A whirlpool bath clear-rinse procedure is used. Chlorazene™, an antibacterial agent, is added to the agitating water. Whirlpool bath temperature should be close to 36.7°C (98°F) or at body temperature (37°C; 98.6°F). The patient's extremity is positioned with the elbow in flexion so that the mildly agitating water just covers the hand, thus avoiding as much as possible a dependent position. Active flexion/extension exercises are carried out in the bath (Fietti and Mackin, 1995; Mackin and Byron, 1990). When the whirlpool bath treatment is completed, the patient's hand is rinsed with clear water (Bohannon, 1982; Niederhuber et al., 1975). A contraindication to a whirlpool bath is the presence of edema, which may increase with the heat of warm water. Walsh (1984b) evaluated the swelling response in normal subjects receiving whirlpool therapy at 37.6°C (99.7°F) and 40°C (104°F). He found an increase in edema at 40°C (104°F). The risk of increasing edema is decreased by maintaining the water temperature closer to 37°C (98.6°F) and by having the patient remove the hand from the whirlpool and elevate it overhead and perform active fisting for 1 minute (Figure 9.2).

This is repeated every 3–5 minutes (Byron and Muntzer, 1986; Walsh, 1984b).

Between sessions with the therapist, the patient will perform warm saline soaks at home, prepared with one tablespoon of table salt added to a quart (1.136 l) of boiling water. The hypertonic solution is bactericidal. The patient lets the boiling water cool to lukewarm temperature and then soaks the hand for 10–15 minutes, three times a day. As with the whirlpool bath treatment, the hand is rinsed with clear water. Active motion is performed during the soaks. The patient is instructed in redressing the wounds at home in the manner preferred by the surgeon. Generally, a non-adhering sterile dressing is applied directly on to the granulating wound, followed by a sterile dry gauze pad for protection (Figure 9.3). Pads are changed after each whirlpool bath or home saline treatment. The critical factor is to keep the wound clean. A few patients will develop superficial infection with increased exudate. This can be treated with a light application of an antibiotic ointment. This must be applied sparingly in the very center of the wound since it might promote the formation of hypertrophic granulations. The ointment is applied after the whirlpool or saline soak. If granulations become exuberant, they respond to silver nitrate application (Figure 9.4) (Fietti and Mackin, 1995; Mackin and Byron, 1990).

An alternative method for managing an infected wound is with the use of a wet-to-dry dressing, which is helpful in mechanically debriding exudate and eschar from the wound. A sterile pad is saturated with a bacteriocidal agent such as Dakin's solution and applied directly to the wound. The dressing is allowed to dry and is then removed, pulling devitalized tissue with it. The dressing is changed two or three times a day.

Closed palm technique

The postoperative management for the closed palm technique is essentially the same as for

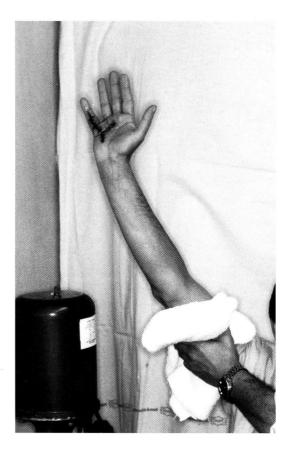

Figure 9.2 If the physiologic effects of whirlpool treatment are desired, attention to the position of the hand in the whirlpool, 'overhead fisting' during the treatment, and the recommended water temperature may help to minimize an increase in edema. (Reproduced with permission from Walsh, 1984b.)

the open palm technique except that whirlpool therapy is not used so long as the sutures remain in the hand and digits. The wounds are kept dry. When the sutures are removed, generally at 7–10 days, whirlpool therapy may be initiated.

If resection into the digit or digits is necessary, the closed digital incision is also bandaged; however, the dressing to the digits must not restrict the patient's exercise pro-

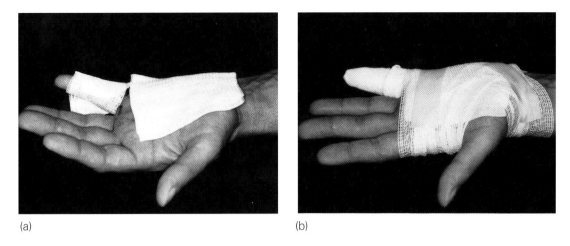

(a)   (b)

Figure 9.3 (a and b) Generally, dry sterile dressings are applied to the wound. They are changed after each whirlpool bath or home saline treatment.

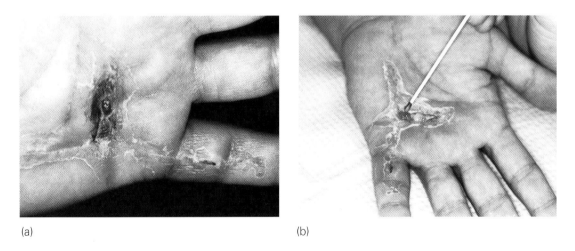

(a)   (b)

Figure 9.4 (a and b) Silver nitrate application.

gram; full active flexion/extension exercises must be possible within the confines of the dressing. A thin piece of gauze cut from a 4 × 4 inches (approx. 10 × 10 cm) sterile gauze pad, placed over the incision and covered with a piece of tube bandage, is effective when the digital incision is bandaged (Fietti and Mackin, 1995) (Figure 9.5).

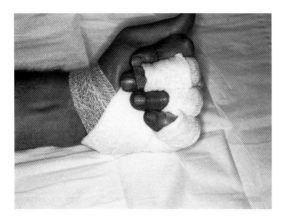

Figure 9.5 Dressings to the digits must not restrict the patients' active flexion/extension exercises.

Closure with skin grafts

The postoperative management after the open palm technique differs from that after closure with skin grafts when early hydrotherapy would be inappropriate due to the shearing forces created by the whirlpool therapy. Skin grafts at this time are not adherent to granular bed and do not have good enough

capillary ingrowth. Whirlpool treatment in the presence of skin grafts should be delayed until the graft has taken. This requires a minimum of 5 days and may take up to 2 weeks.

If a skin graft was necessary at surgery, it must be closely monitored for vascularity during the early phase of healing. Generally, the volar plaster splint applied at surgery is removed and a lighter dressing is applied at the first postoperative visit. Care must be taken to apply the dressing so that it does not abrade or cause pressure to the graft during early mobilization. A palmar pan extension splint is fabricated to maintain extension (Figure 9.6) (Mackin and Byron, 1990).

CONTROL OF EDEMA

Edema is a common reaction in the hand disturbed by the complex surgical dissection required in many Dupuytren procedures. The importance of controlling postoperative edema and thereby avoiding complications must be emphasized. Until good muscular activity is restored, we depend on gravity and external measures to assist the return of blood flow through the lymphatic and venous systems (Fietti and Mackin, 1995).

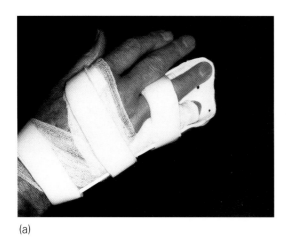

(a)

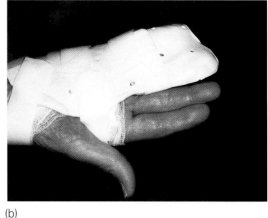

(b)

Figure 9.6 (a and b) Palmar pan extension splint.

The patient's hand is elevated after surgery to minimize limb dependency and thus assist in edema control. The elbow should not be flexed acutely because this will increase venous stasis. During sleep the hand should be elevated on pillows.

In cases of severe pitting edema, external compression using an intermittent compression unit is helpful to reduce swelling. The hand is placed in the sleeve with the fingers in extension. The extremity is elevated on a table or pillows to an angle of 30°–45° to take advantage of gravity while the intermittent pressure is applied. Use of external compression is not contraindicated in the presence of open wounds so long as sterile dressings are used. Felt pads can be positioned around pins to prevent pressure on them. The amount of pressure is adjusted to the condition. Initial treatment might be as low as 30–40 mmHg for 30–60 minutes. [To be effective, unit pressure must exceed capillary pressure (25 mmHg) and be kept below the patient's diastolic pressure.] After mechanical massage by the intermittent compression unit, retrograde massage, a form of intermittent compression, with lanolin, may be applied by the therapist in a further attempt to push the extracellular fluid out of the hand. Care must be taken to avoid contaminating the wound with lanolin (Fietti and Mackin, 1995; Mackin and Byron, 1990).

An inexpensive, effective and easy method to remove edema fluid is by string wrapping (Figure 9.7). A soft cord is wrapped closely and firmly circumferentially around the finger(s). The wrapping begins at the level of the nail bed and proceeds proximally until the cord reaches the web space. Each wrap of the cord is placed snugly up against the previous one so that, upon completion, the entire finger is covered by the series of wraps. The cord is not pulled so tight as to create a tourniquet effect. The hand is then placed in elevation. The cord remains on the hand for 5 minutes. When the cord is removed, the patient is instructed to make a firm fist 10 times. Measurements taken before and after string-

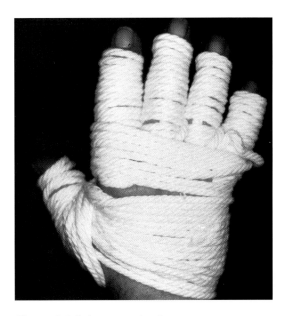

Figure 9.7 String wrapping is an easy, inexpensive and effective intermittent compression technique to reduce edema.

wrapping will show a decrease in edema and an increase in active ROM.

The beneficial effects induced by string wrapping may only be short-term at first. The treatment should be repeated three times a day until return flow circulation is restored adequately.

Flowers (1985) reported that massage and string wrapping are equally effective in the reduction of edema, but a combination of the two, that is retrograde massage to the hand while the string is in place, is more effective than either technique used alone.

Coban wraps (Minnesota Mining and Manufacturing Co., 3M, St Paul, MN) applied to the digits and hand also assist in reduction of edema. Coban tape is applied distally to proximally and must be wrapped without tension. Tightly applied Coban will interfere with circulation of the fingers. An Isotoner glove (an elasticized glove; Aris Isotoner Glove, New York, NY) may also be helpful in controlling edema while allowing the patient to use the hand with minimal restriction. The tips of the glove may be cut off to allow sensory input (Fietti and Mackin, 1995; Mackin and Byron, 1990).

We have found that an effective exercise that incorporates elevation and active motion is to have the patient elevate both arms over the head and make as firm a fist as possible 10 times each hour. This exercise can also be used to maintain good shoulder and elbow motion (Moberg, personal communication).

Macramé and the Valpar Whole Body Work Samples (Valpar Work Samples, Valpar Corp., Tucson, AZ) are examples of activities that may be performed in elevation to decrease edema while increasing active motion and co-ordination.

SPLINTING

Splinting is an important part of postoperative care. In a few patients with minimal disease and pliable skin, and in whom good finger extension has been obtained, postoperative splinting may not be necessary. However, in all other patients a splint to maintain the gains in extension of the digits(s) achieved by the surgical procedure is fabricated at the initial therapy session. The aim of surgery is to regain full extension of the involved digit(s) thus restoring maximal hand function. Usually full extension can be achieved but, in certain cases, the surgeon may have to accept some residual flexion contracture. In some instances the surgeon cannot release a PIP joint contracture to full extension. Since it is unlikely that postoperative therapy will increase the correction obtained at surgery, it is important for the therapist to know the intraoperative ROM and the result the surgeon expects postoperatively so that realistic goals can be set. Awareness of neurovascular status is important in splint application (Fietti and Mackin, 1995).

Splints must be fitted carefully to gently hold the digit(s) in extension during wound healing. Evans (1997) advises against splinting all digital joints in maximal extension during the first 2 weeks after surgery. She prefers instead to position the MCP joints in 30°–40° of flexion and the PIP joints in full extension. This is also Tubiana's opinion, who never splints the MP and IPP joints together in complete extension (see 'Postoperative care' and 'Postoperative rehabilitation', pages 175–77). Evans' rationale is based on the fact that excessive stress to the healing tissue may provoke a negative cellular response and lead to increased fibrosis with or without recurrence. Each time the patient is seen for therapy, the splint should be evaluated so that necessary adjustments can be made. Two weeks after surgery the splint can be adjusted to allow for greater MCP extension if needed. Initially it is removed only for exercise and wound care. As healing progresses, day splinting is gradually reduced but night extension splinting may be necessary for 6 months or longer. The surgeon and therapist may elect to change initial day splinting in specific cases (Fietti and Mackin, 1995; Mackin and Byron, 1990).

In cases of long-standing severe flexion contracture, the surgeon may have been able to obtain full extension at surgery but unable to maintain the position due to compromised circulation. In these cases, the postoperative splint is made so as to position the digit in the degree of extension that does not compromise circulation to the finger. At each subsequent therapy visit, the splint is adjusted gradually to increase extension of the digit in the splint until the degree of extension obtained at surgery is achieved.

In severe cases where a digit shows early signs of recurring contraction (this is most often seen in the little finger PIP joint), a different splint design may be needed. In these cases a splint designed in the authors' clinic by Callahan specifically addresses this problem. The splint (Figure 9.8) employs a length of Velcro loop over the outrigger to provide the extension force instead of a finger loop and rubber band. The Velcro provides a static pull. It may be adjusted to provide increased tension as tolerated by the patient between treatments.

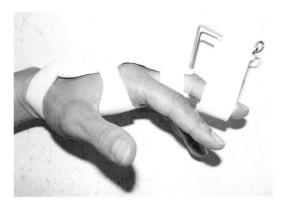

Figure 9.8 Step-up splint.

MODALITIES

Physical agent modalities of heat and cold are helpful in the postoperative program for the Dupuytren's patient. Heat in the form of hot packs, Fluidotherapy, continuous mode ultrasound or paraffin wax is helpful in increasing scar and soft tissue extensibility and can decrease stiffness and pain. Used prior to exercise, heat can greatly enhance the patient's efforts. Following exercise, cold packs may be used to manage any swelling or pain. Contrast baths have also been found to be helpful in controlling swelling and pain. The procedure for contrast baths involves immersing the hand in a container of cold water, 12.8°–18.3°C (55°–65°F), for 1 minute and then removing and placing it in a container of warm water, 35.6°–37.8°C (96°–100°F), for 3 minutes. While in the water, the patient squeezes a sponge and then extends the fingers. This sequence is repeated for 10 minutes. The alternation between heat and cold stimulates circulation and facilitates the resolution of edema.

THERAPEUTIC EXERCISE
Active range of motion

Gentle, basic active finger exercises are begun during the first postoperative visit. The active exercise program includes the following:

1) Finger-blocking:
   a) Active flexion of the PIP joint while holding the MP joint in extension;
   b) Active DIP joint flexion while holding the MP and PIP joints in extension.
2) Active flexion of each finger to the thenar eminence.
3) Active flexion of each PIP joint into the palm as all the other digits are held in extension.
4) Fist-making.
5) Finger abduction and adduction.
6) Finger extension:
   a) Active MP extension;
   b) Active PIP extension while holding the MP joint in a hyperflexed position with the uninvolved hand.
7) Full wrist motion and thumb active ROM.

Ten repetitions of each exercise are performed three to four times daily; however, some patients may require a modified program of a decreased number of repetitions.

Severe PIP joint flexion contractures of the little finger frequently result in hyperextension of the distal joint, an attitude assumed by the digit to compensate for the PIP joint flexion. When these contractures are released at surgery, the surgeons' approach may be to hold the PIP joint in extension by Kirschner wire fixation. Early active DIP joint flexion must be emphasized to encourage tendon gliding and restore system alignment (Fietti and Mackin, 1995).

As motion improves, the exercise program is modified to make the exercises more precise. Usually by the second postoperative week, tendon-gliding exercises can be initiated (Figure 9.9). These exercises optimize flexor tendon motion and as a result joint motion (Wehbe and Hunter, 1985a, 1985b).

As exercises become 'easy', they are discontinued and more difficult exercises and resistance are gradually added. For example, when finger extension is performed easily, the patient may be asked to cross his fingers, such as index over long, long over index, and long

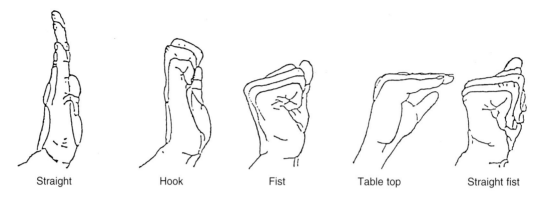

| Straight | Hook | Fist | Table top | Straight fist |

1 Start with fingers and wrist straight every time.
2 Make each type of fist ____ times, hold ____ seconds.
3 Do these exercises ____ times every day.

Figure 9.9 Tendon-gliding exercises, hook, fist and straight fist positions are used to optimize tendon excursion.

over ring. This exercise can be made even more difficult by asking the patient to pass a coin from finger to finger (Fietti and Mackin, 1995; Mackin and Byron, 1990).

Active hand use is encouraged in therapy via functional activities. While the wound is still open (open palm method), light pick-ups and pinch activities may be initiated.

When the wound closes, generally by 4 weeks for the open palm method and 2–3 weeks for the closed palm, gradual, progressive, sustained grip-strengthening exercises are added to the program. When healing permits, strengthening may be added to the program for the patient with skin grafts.

Putty squeezing is an effective method for grip strengthening. Making a 'hot dog' from putty, that is, repetitive squeezing of the putty using only the fingers, strengthens the grip and improves flexion. Exercises should never be overdone. Squeezing the putty 10 times intermittently during the day is a far better regimen than doing it for 10–20 minutes continuously, which might result in pain and edema. Patients must be cautioned

against this. Putty may also be used for extension exercises (Fietti and Mackin, 1995).

Sustained grip activities, such as woodworking and working with leather, help regain full function of the hand. Resistance is increased as tolerated.

Passive range of motion

Gentle PROM is incorporated into the exercise program when joint stiffness is present or when active tendon function is limited and passive motion is performed to maintain joint mobility.

When passive flexion of one or more PIP joints is limited, splinting may be necessary. A web strap may be used to improve passive range of motion. The strap is worn over the involved PIP joints and behind the MP joints. The strap is fabricated from a 2.5 cm-wide webbing with a 2.5 cm-wide buckle. The patient may begin wearing the strap for 30 minutes, three times a day. The patient

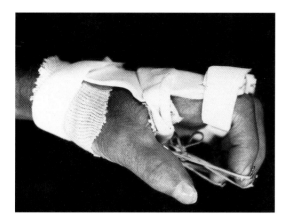

Figure 9.10 Intrinsic stretcher splint.

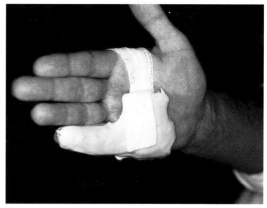

Figure 9.11 Elastomer is mixed with a catalyst and spread on the scar. The mixture is allowed to set, forming an exact mold of the scar and held in place by a closely fitting splint or Coban tape. As the scar compresses, new molds are made to accommodate the changes.

adjusts the tension of the strap until he feels a slight pull on the affected joints. The time the strap is worn may be increased gradually for as long as 2 hours, three times a day (Fietti and Mackin, 1995).

When passive flexion of both the PIP and DIP joints is limited an elastic loop can be used that maintains the PIP and DIP joints in a flexed position with light tension. In general, a low-intensity application of stress at the end ranges of motion is more effective than brief-duration, high-intensity stress.

Owing to prolonged preoperative positioning in MP joint or combined MP/PIP joint flexion, intrinsic tightness may be a problem. The splinting alternatives mentioned here may not be specific enough to resolve this problem because addressing it requires MP joint extension with IP joint flexion. An intrinsic stretcher splint may be required in these cases (Fietti and Mackin, 1995) (Figure 9.10).

Specific instructions should be written clearly for the patient, describing the application of the splint and desired time each splint is to be worn. The patient must be instructed to look for changes in color of the fingertips and increases in tingling, numbness, or swelling of the digit or hand as signs to decrease splint tension. Although passive flexion devices may be necessary during the day to increase flexion, night splinting is reserved for extension (Fietti and Mackin, 1995).

SCAR MANAGEMENT

When the wound has healed, lanolin massage is helpful to soften surgical scar and maintain issue mobility. The palm and digits should be massaged before each exercise session for approximately 10 minutes. A small, deep, circular stroke is used for massage over the scar. After massage, the excess lanolin should be removed to prevent skin maceration (Fietti and Mackin, 1995; Mackin and Byron, 1990).

Silastic 382 medical grade elastomer (Dow Corning Corp., Midland, MI) is an effective adjunct in managing digital and palmar scars (Figure 9.11). A catalyst is added to the material and it is spread over the scar area providing compression to the scar. Its advantage is its ability to conform to the entire scar area, thus producing a reusable mold with pressure over all areas of the scar. It can be applied before complete wound closure by placing a piece of non-adhering gauze over the wound and applying the elastomer over it. Additional pressure is achieved with the palmar pan splint. Elastomer is discontinued when the scar is flat and no longer reactive (Fietti and Mackin, 1995; Mackin and Byron, 1990).

Occasionally a patient may experience hypersensitivity over the healed area. This should be addressed through a program of desensitization. Desensitization involves the stimulation of a hypersensitive area with textures that are normally not noxious. The stimulation is applied for about 10 minutes each waking hour and proceeds through a predefined hierarchy (Mackin and Byron, 1990).

Another means of desensitization is through the use of fluidotherapy, which can be described as a dry whirlpool. The involved hand is immersed in a medium of cellulose particles and warm air is forced through these resulting in a whirlpool effect. Both the temperature of the air and the amount of agitation of the particles can be controlled. The continuous stimulation of the involved hand by the particles has a desensitizing effect and the increased temperature helps to decrease pain and increase tissue extensibility.

Occupation has not been proven to influence the severity or course of Dupuytren's disease but it is a factor in the postoperative management. Sedentary workers often return to work within a few days after surgery whereas a manual worker could be out of work for 3–4 months (McFarlane, 1990).

CONCLUSION

The importance of a carefully supervised, early postoperative active-motion exercise and splinting program cannot be overemphasized.

References

Bohannon RW (1982) Whirlpool versus whirlpool and rinse for removal of bacteria from a venous stasis ulcer. *Phys Ther* **62**: 304–308.

Brand PW, Wood H (1977) Hand Volumeter Instruction Sheet. US Public Health Service Hospital, Carville, LA.

Byron PM, Muntzer EM (1986) *Therapist's Management of the Mutilated Hand. Hand Clinics, Hand Rehabilitation.* WB Saunders, Philadelphia.

Evans RB (1997) The source of our strength. *J Hand Ther* **10**: 18–19.

Fietti VG Jr, Mackin EJ (1995) Open-palm technique in Dupuytren's disease. In: Hunter JM, Mackin EJ, Callahan AD, eds, *Rehabilitation of the Hand: Surgery and Therapy*, 4th edn, 981–94. CV Mosby, St Louis.

Flowers KR (1985) String wrapping versus massage for reducing digital volume. *J Hand Surg* **10**: 583.

Gelberman RH, Panagis JS, Hergenroeder PT, Zakaib GS (1982) Wound complications in the surgical management of Dupuytren's contracture: a comparison of operative incisions. *Hand* **14**: 248–54.

Hueston JT (1974) *Dupuytren's Disease.* Grune and Stratton, New York.

Mackin EJ, Byron PM (1990) Postoperative management. In: McFarlane RM, McGrouther DA, Flint MH, eds, *Dupuytren's Disease*, 368–76. Churchill Livingstone, Edinburgh.

McCash CR (1964) The open palm technique in Dupuytren's contracture. *Br J Plast Surg* **17**: 271.

McFarlane RM (1986) Complications in Dupuytren's disease. In: Boswick JA, ed., *Complications in Hand Surgery*, 294–99. WB Saunders, Philadelphia.

McFarlane RM (1990) In: McFarlane RM, McGrouther DA, Flint MH, eds, *Dupuytren's Disease*, 293. Churchill Livingstone, Edinburgh.

Niederhuber SS, Stribley RF, Koepke GH (1975) Reduction of skin bacterial load with use of therapeutic whirlpool. *Phys Ther* **55**: 482.

Tonkin MA, Burke FD, Vavian JPW (1984) Dupuytren's contracture: a comparative study of fasciectomy and dermofasciectomy in 100 patients. *J Hand Surg* **9**: 156–62.

Tubiana R (1985) Overview on surgical treatment of Dupuytren's disease. In: Hueston JT, Tubiana R, eds, *Dupuytren's Disease*, 2nd edn, 129–30. Churchill Livingstone, Edinburgh.

Walsh MT (1984a) Therapist's management of reflex sympathetic dystrophy. In: Hunter JM, Mackin EJ,

Callahan AD, eds, *Rehabilitation of the Hand: Surgery and Therapy*, 4th edn, CV Mosby, St Louis.

Walsh M (1984b) Relationship of hand edema to upper extremity position and water temperature during whirlpool. *J Hand Surg* **9A**: 609.

Wehbe MA, Hunter JM (1985a) Flexor tendon gliding in the hand. I: in vivo excursions. *J Hand Surg* **10A**: 575–74.

Wehbe MA, Hunter JM (1985b) Flexor tendon gliding in the hand. II: differential gliding. *J Hand Surg* **10A**: 575–79.

10

Conclusions

Raoul Tubiana

We would like to end this book by summarizing those views that appear to be shared by the authors.

1) Numerous and important scientific studies during the last decades, especially on the contractile abilities of myofibroblasts and the nature of the collagen in Dupuytren's disease, have helped us to advance our understanding of the process of contracture in this disease and in its treatment.

A non-operative medical injection therapy for Dupuytren's disease, using Clostridial collagenase injection, is currently in clinical trials to establish its safety and efficacy. The injection of collagenase induces a wide area of lysis in the collagen cord, allowing rupture and thus extension of the injected finger. Early results of this clinical trial are very promising.

While awaiting long-term results of non-surgical treatment, the current treatment for this systemic disease remains essentially surgical.

2) At present, the aim of surgery is not simply to perform a symptomatic correction of joint contracture; the accent tends to be also on the prevention of surgical complications and recurrences.

Many surgical procedures can be used as there is no routine operation for Dupuytren's disease. Treatment must be selective and when making the choice of operation one must take into account the evaluation of the prognosis of the disease, and the risk of complications and recurrences. The evaluation of the prognosis for each individual is based on the assessment of general and local factors which have been described in 'Surgical indications' in Chapter 6, pages 218–22.

3) Under certain conditions, a simple fasciotomy may produce regression of the fibrous tissue, probably owing to suppression of longitudinal tension. A partial fasciectomy may have the same effect. However, continuous longitudinal traction (Messina) may also have the same effect but when this traction is removed the diseased process resumes. In some cases surgical trauma appears to accelerate the evolution of the disease.

4) For a long time the accent has been mainly on the treatment of palmar aponeurotic lesions. This concept should be revised:

a) Palmar fasciectomies, extensive as they can be, cannot release interphalangeal joint contractures;

b) In fact, fibrotic lesions in the fingers are responsible for most contractures at the level of the interphalangeal joints. They have a worse prognosis than palmar lesions, which result in MP contracture and are easily corrected by a limited palmar procedure;

c) Just as the lesions are not restricted to the palm, nor are they restricted to the aponeurosis. It is now accepted that fibrous pathologic formations spread beyond the palmar aponeurosis, and that the dermis and subcutaneous tissues are often contracted. Also, when the lesions are advanced there is secondary contraction of the capsule and ligaments of the digital joints.

5) The skin must be treated with the same thorough care as the fibrous 'aponeurosis' lesions. Poorly planned incisions and faulty closure are responsible for the majority of complications. It is certainly better not to suture the teguments and allow secondary healing than to close the wound under tension or entrap a hematoma. This is not a reason to use McCash's procedure routinely in order to minimize the risk of complications and to reduce the operating time. The open palm technique has, in the authors' practice, only specific indications: diffuse palmar lesions in the presence of multiple ray involvement.

6) It is well known that complications are more common after extended palmar fasciectomies than after limited procedures.

    a) The commonest complications, hematomas, and skin necroses are usually due to extensive undermining of the palmar skin, incomplete hemostasis, and unsuitable incisions and flaps. Most of these can be avoided;

    b) Reflex sympathetic dystrophy (RSD) is still the surgeon's obsessive fear after surgery for Dupuytren's disease. The study by Comtet on the intensity of postoperative edema, digital joint stiffness, and bone scan hyperfixation clearly shows the influence of the extent of surgery on postoperative changes. This is in favor of limited surgical procedures. However, the evolution in favor of these more limited procedures for the correction of deformities must respect an essential principle of surgical safety, namely

that *one must not hesitate to enlarge the approach before performing any fasciotomy or fasciectomy when the exact location of the neurovascular bundles is not definite.* This is also true for needle fasciotomies;

    c) Prevention of RSD is difficult since it remains a syndrome triggered by multiple causes, some of which remain obscure. In practice, any abnormal postoperative evolution after any surgical procedure for Dupuytren's disease, for example edema, diffuse pain or joint stiffness, must be carefully observed for RSD and an early treatment instituted. The earlier the treatment, the more effective it will be;

    d) As recurrence is much more frequent in the distal part of the palm and in the fingers, it is logical that surgical excision should be extended into the affected fingers and their bases, rather than into the proximal and the unaffected part of the palm.

7) Recurrence and postoperative extension of the disease seem to depend essentially on individual factors, the 'Dupuytren's diathesis' well described by Hueston, much more so than on the extent of fasciectomy.

Skin grafting has proved to have a preventive action on the development of local recurrences, but not on extension of the disease. Skin grafts are now much more widely used:

    a) Primary grafting is reserved for those patients with a high risk of recurrence, especially the relatively young (under 50) with a rapidly progressive form of disease;

    b) Secondary dermofasciectomy is advised for the treatment of recurrences.

The possible preventative action of preoperative continuous elongation (Messina's technique, see pp. 228–9) on recurrence has to be confirmed by long-term follow-up studies.

8) Hand therapy is an essential part of postoperative care. Its first aim is to restore *full*

flexion to the fingers. Postoperative splintage should not hold the MP and IPP joints in extension in case of severe pre-operative joint contracture. The authors prefer to splint the MP joints in flexion and the IPP joints in extension so as to relax the neurovascular structures while protecting surgical gains at the PIP joints.

Full extension is difficult to achieve when there is severe PIP joint contracture. Extension splinting in association with exercise may be necessary for 4–6 months.

General bibliography

REFERENCES AND FURTHER READING PRIOR TO 1942

This list includes references from Ferrarini M (1941) *La malattia del Dupuytren*, 409–38. Nistri–Lischi Editori, Pisa, and from Elliot D (1999) Pre-1900 literature on Dupuytren's disease. *Hand Clin* **15**: 175–81.

Abbe R (1884) On Dupuytren's finger contraction; its nervous origin. *New York Med J* **39**: 436.

Abbe R (1888) On Dupuytren's finger contraction; further remarks on the theory of its nervous origin. *Med Record*, **33**: 236.

Abbe R (1894) The surgery of the hand. *New York Med J* **1**: 36.

Abbott AC (1929) Dupuytren's contraction. Review of the literature and a report of a new technique in surgical treatment. *Canadian Med Assoc J* **20**: 250.

Accornero A (1908) Retrazione dell'aponevrosi palmare e degenerazione neuropsichica. *Gazzette Ospedali e Cliniche* **29**: 10.

Adams W (1877) On contraction of the fingers (Dupuytren's contraction) and its treatment by subcutaneous division of the palmar fascia and immediate extension. *Lancet* **i**: 838.

Adams W (1878) Contraction of the fingers (Dupuytren's contraction) and its successful treatment by subcutaneous divisions of the palmar fascia and immediate extension. *BMJ* **1**: 928.

Adams W (1882) Dupuytren's contraction of the fingers in women. *BMJ* **1**: 84.

Adams W (1883) Dupuytren's contraction in a female. *Lancet* **i**: 412.

Adams W (1883) Dupuytren's contraction of the fingers. *Lancet* **i**: 15.

Adams W (1884) Dupuytren's contraction. *Lancet* **i**: 565.

Adams W (1890) Congenital contraction of the fingers. *Lancet* **ii**: 1272.

Adams W (1890) Further observations on the treatment of Dupuytren's finger contraction. *Lancet* **i**: 705.

Adams W (1891) On congenital contraction of the fingers and its association with hammer-toe: its pathology and treatment. *Lancet*, **ii**: 165.

Adams W (1892) *On Contraction of the Fingers and on Hammer-toe*, 2nd edn. J.A. Churchill, London.

Agosti F (1910) Contributo clinico al morbo di Dupuytren. *Annali di Freniatria e Scienze affini* **20**: 175.

Aiello DA (1933) La maladie de Dupuytren et ses rapports avec la glande parathyroïde. Thèse, Genève.

Aievoli E (1897) Aponeurositis palmaris. *Sommario di Patologia chirurgica generale e speciale*, 273. Priore, Napoli.

Aievoli E (1907) Sul concetto della patogenesi della contrattura palmare di Dupuytren. *Archivio di Ortopedia* **24**: 337.

Aievoli E (1911) La contrattura di Dupuytren in rapporto agli infortuni ed alle malattie del lavoro. *Giornale Internazionale delle Scienze Mediche* **33**: 874.

Alajouanine T, Maire R, Guillaume I (1930) Maladie de Dupuytren localisée aux deux derniers doigts de la main gauche et accompagnée d'un syndrome sympathique oculaire de Cl. Bernard-Horner du même côté, survenue 15 ans après une blessure du nerf cubital du côté opposé, avec griffe des deux derniers doigts. *Revue Neurologique* **II**: 679.

Albert E Retrazione dell'aponevrosi palmare. *Trattato di Chirurgia e di Medicina Operatoria* Vol. 2, 542. Vallardi, Milano.

Albinius BS (1734) *Historia Musculorum Hominis. Leidae batavorum.* Bibliothèque de Chirurgie, Paris.

Alderson WE (1886) Dupuytren's contraction. *Lancet* **i**: 388.

Amath CH (1886) De la maladie de Dupuytren. *Gazette Méd Paris* **3**: 25.

Anderson W (1891) Lectures on contractions of the fingers and toes; their varieties, pathology and treatment. *Lancet* **ii**: 1–57.

Anderson W (1891) Ueber die Pathologie und Therapie der Finger-und Zehenkontraktur. *Wiener Mediz Blätter* 445.

Anderson W (1897) *The Deformities of the Fingers and Toes*, 4–43. Churchill, London.

Anger (1875) Des flexions permanents des doigts et de leur traitement. *France Médicale* (cited by Kölliker (1905–7)).

Angus HB (1900) Dupuytren's contractions. *Lancet* **i**: 388.

Annandale T (1865) *The Malformations, Diseases and Injuries of the Fingers and Toes*, 234–44. Edmonston & Douglas, Edinburgh.

Anonimo (1934) La malattia di Dupuytren. *Gazzetta Ospedali e Cliniche* **55**: 9.

Antonioli GM (1927) Sulla malattia di Dupuytren. Contributo clinico ed istologico. *Annali Ital di Chirurgia* **6**: 1011.

Anzilotti A (1935) Tentativi di röntgenterapia del morbo di Dupuytren. *Boll Soc Med Chir di Pisa* **3**: 109.

Apert E (1925) Rétraction de l'aponévrose palmaire. Influence de l'hérédité. Effet heureux de l'émanation de radium. *Gazette Hop* **98**: 1550.

Arcangeli (1892) Sulla malattia di Dupuytren. *Boll Soc Lancisiana Ospedali di Roma* **12**: 173.

Arndt (1888) Aetiologie der Dupuytren'schen Fingerkontraktur. *Deutsche med Wochenschr* **14**: 761.

Audan (1925) Traitement röntgenthérapique de la maladie de Dupuytren. *J Radiol et d'Eléctrol* **9**: 476–77.

Auvray (1929) Double rétraction de l'aponévrose palmaire et de l'aponévrose plantaire chez le même sujet. *Bull Soc Nat Chirurg, Paris* **55**: 1026.

Avignon de Morlac JA (1832) Proposition du débridement de l'aponévrose-palmaire dans certains cas de rétraction permanente des doigts. no. 1832/26, Thèse, Paris.

Baader (1933) Dupuytren'sche Kontraktur und Beruf. *Zentralbl Chir* **40**: 987.

Bäärnhielm G (1905) Beiträge zur operativen Behandlung der Dupuytren'schen Finger-kontraktur. *Hygiea, Iahr* **67**: 719.

Baetzner (1922) Praktische Erfahrungen mit der Pepsin-Pregl-Lösung zur Narbenerweichung u. s. w. *Arch klinisch Chirurgie* **121**: 106.

Bähr F (1895) Aponeuritis palmaris als Unfallsfolge. *Aerztliche Sachverständigen Zeitung* **1**: 124.

Bähr F (1895) Kurze Bemerkung zu den Artikel Bieganski's ueber die Dupuytren'sche Kontraktur. *Deutsche med Wochenschr* **21**: 540.

Bailey S (1892) Dupuytren's finger contraction. *American Practitioner and News*, Louisville, **14**: 133–35.

Baillod IP (1877) Étude sur la rétraction de l'aponévrose palmaire. Thèse, Paris.

Balban (1916) Fall von Dupuytren'scher Kontraktur. *Wiener Klinische Woch* **29**: 1415.

Ballif L, Zoè Caraman (1936) Maladie de Dupuytren bilatérale et double rétraction plantaire dans un cas de polynévrite. *Jahresbericht Chirurg* **42**: 456.

Baptista R (1934) Sobre a mão em garra de Dupuytren. *O Hospital* **6**

Bardeleben A (1872) *Lehrbuch der Chirurgie und Operationslehre*, Vol. 4, 722–28. Reimer, Berlin.

Bardeleben A (1881) *Flessione Permanente Delle Dita* Vol. 4, 600. Instituzioni di Patologia chirurgica e di Medicina operatoria, Jovene, Napoli.

Bardenheuer B (1888) Contractur der Fascia palmaris. In: Billroth, Luecke, *Deutsche Chirurgie*, part 63, 480. Enke, Stuttgart.

Barette Rétraction de l'aponévrose palmaire (maladie de Dupuytren). *Encyclopédie internationale de Chirurgie*, Vol. 6, 693. Baillière, Paris.

Barison F (1932) Morbo di Dupuytren e diabete guariti con radioterapia dell'ipofisi. *Giorn di Psichiatria e di Neuropatologia* **60**: 45.

Barré JA (1931) Maladie de Dupuytren unilatérale et arthrite cervicale. *Presse Médic* **39**: 881.

Barthelemy (1912) A propos d'un cas de rétraction de l'aponévrose palmaire. *Revue Médicale de l'Est* **39**.

Baseggio N (1914) Sulla contrazione delle dita delle mani detta di Dupuytren. *La sicurezza e l'igiene nell'industria. Boll Assoc Industriali Ital per prevenire gli Infortuni del lavoro* **5**: 150.

Bastianelli R (1892) Sulla malattia di Dupuytren. *Boll Soc Lancisiana Ospedali di Roma* **12**: 173.

Baum W (1878) Zue Lehre von Dupuytren's permanenter Fingercontractur. *Zentralbl Chir, Jahr* **5**: 129.

Baum W (1879) De la rétraction permanente des doigts. *Arch gén Méd* **2**: 106.

Baumeyer F (1925) *Die Vererbung der Dupuytren'schen Contraktur.* Inaugural dissertation, München.

Bayer (1898) Zur operation von Sehnenund Muskelcontracturen. *Zentralbl Chir* **25**: 276.

Beard (1900) De la rétraction de l'apnoévrose plantaire. Thèse, Paris.

Beatty SR (1938) Roentgen-therapy of Dupuytren's contracture. *Radiology* **30**: 610.

Beck C (1919) *Ueber Palmarfaszienkontraktur.* Inaugural dissertation, Berlin.

Beck C (1924) *The Crippled Hand and Arm. A monograph on the various types of deformities of the hand and arm, as a result from abnormal development, injuries and disease.* Lippincott, London.

Becker (1907) Ueber Fibrolysinkuren. *Deutsche med Wochenschr* **33**: 1785.

Bejul AP, Kogan AV (1938) Falsa contrattura di Dupuytren. *Zentralorg Chir* **86**: 668.

Bellamy E (1882) Note on the treatment of contracted fingers. *Lancet* **ii**: 439.

Belot J. Traitement röntgenthérapique de la maladie de Dupuytren. *J Radiol Electrol* 476–77.

Bennett EH (1900) Dupuytren's contraction of the palmar fascia. *Lancet* **ii**: 24.

Bergel D (1936) Zur Frage der Dienst-beschädigung bei Dupuytren'scher Kontraktur. *Medizinische Welt* **10**: 16–18.

Berger P (1892) Traitement de la rétraction de l'aponévrose palmaire par une autoplastie. *Bull Acad Med Paris* **56**: 608.

Berger P (1893) Traitement de la rétraction de l'aponévrose palmaire par la transplantation d'un lambeau pédiculé, emprunté au tronc. *7th Congr Français de Chirurg, Paris, 3–8 April.*

Berger P (1896) Rétraction de l'aponévrose palmaire; autoplastie par la méthode italienne; résultats éloignés. *Bull Mém Soc Chirurg, Paris* **21**: 650.

Berger P (1900) Procédé opératoire pour le traite-ment de la rétraction limitée de l'aponévrose palmaire. *Rev Int Méd Chirurg* (cited by Mauclaire (1934)).

Bergmann (1907) Aetiologischer Beitrag zur Dupuytren'schen Fingerkontraktur. *Prager med Wochenschr* **45**: 582.

Bertrand JE (1894) Contribution à l'étude de la rétraction de l'aponévrose palmaire (maladie de Dupuytren); traitement par l'aponévréctomie. Thèse, Nancy.

Béyoul A (1927) Contrattura di Dupuytren: sua patogenesi (Russo). *Zentralorgan Chir* **36**: 842.

Béyoul A (1935) La maladie de Dupuytren. *Rev Chirurg* **54**: 351.

Bieganski W (1896) Die spontane Kontraktur der Finger (Retractio apon. palmaris) als ein trophischer Prozess centralen Ursprungs. *Deutsche med Wochenschr* **21**: 497.

Binda P (1912) Sulla contrattura di Dupuytren. *Gazzetta Med Ital* **63**: 21.

Bitot, Papin (1912) Rétraction bilatérale de l'aponévrose palmaire chez un tuberculeux. *J Méd Bordeaux* **30**: 478.

Black K (1883) Dupuytren's contraction in a female. *Lancet* **i**: 412.

Black K (1915) Dupuytren's contraction. *BMJ* **2825**: 326.

Blair VP (1924) The full thickness skin graft. *Ann Surg* **80**: 298.

Blum A (1882) *Chirurgie de la main*, 126–33. Asselin, Paris.

Bobbio L (1939) Sulla anatomia patologica e sull'etiopatogenesi della malattia del Dupuytren. *Giornale R Acad Med Torino* **102**.

Böcking H (1884) *Ueber Fascienkontrakturen.* Inaugural dissertation, Würzburg.

Böhme H (1933) *Zur Aetiologie der Dupuytren'schen Fingerkontraktur.* Inaugural dissertation, Freiburg in Br.

Bolli V (1902) Retrazione dell'aponevrosi palmare (malattia del Dupuytren) con iperidrosi delle mani. *Policlinico, Sez Pratica* **9**: 264.

Bordier (1883) Sur la rétraction diabétique de l'aponévrose palmaire. *J Therapie* **889**.

Borri L (1912) Retrazione dell'aponevrosi palmare. In: *Infortuni del lavoro sotto il rispetto medicolegale*, Vol. 2, 404. Soc Editr Libraria Milano.

Boulogne (1926) Rétraction symétrique des aponé-vroses palmaries par ectasie de l'aorte. *Bull Méd.*

Boulogne (1935) Deux observations concordantes pour une etiologie de la maladie de Dupuytren. *Rev Neurol* **63**: 991.

Bourgery JM, Jacob NA (1832) *Traité complet de l'anatomie de l'homme comprenant la médecine opératoire.* CA Delaunay, Paris.

Bouvier (1842) Rétraction des doigts. *Bul Acad Med* **8**: 129.

Bouygues J (1906) De la rétraction de l'aponévrose palmaire. *Archives génér de Médec* 2513.

Boyer (1826) Rétraction permanente des doigts. In: *Traité des Maladies Chirurgicales et des Operations qui leur Convennent, Vol.* XI, 55, Paris.

Boyer A (1826) *Traité des Maladies Chirurgicales*, Vol. II. Migneret, Paris.

Bradshaw (1911) A clinical lecture on a case of syringomyelie. In: Haenel, Lewandowsky, *Handbuch der Neurologie*, Vol. 2, 612. Springer, Berlin.

Braine J (1933) Maladie de Dupuytren. Résultat opératoire sept mois après l'intervention. *Presse Médicale* 41: 1889.

Braquehaye J (1897) Autoplastie dans la maladie de Dupuytren. *J Med Bordeaux* 14.

Brasch M (1900) Cit. senza indicazione bibliografica da Neutra. *Centralbl Nervenheilk Psychiatric* 551.

Braune WA, Trübiger A (1873) *Die Venen der menschlichen Hand.* Leipzig. (Cited by Grapow, 1887.)

Breitwieser O (1935) *Eine eigenartige Beobachtung von Dupuytren'scher Fingerkontraktur.* Inaugural dissertation, Würzburg.

Brodhurst (1868) Lectures on orthopaedic surgery. *Lancet.*

Brooks B (1930) Aneurysm of the axillary artery. A case of spontaneous aneurysm of the first portion of the axillary artery, associated with unilateral clubbing of the fingers and Dupuytren's contracture. *Zentralorg Chir* 52: 215.

Brown EA (1899) Dupuytren's contraction of the palmar fascia. *BMJ* 1107.

Bryant T (1872) *The Practice of Surgery, 1015–16.* Churchill, London. 1879, 3rd edn, 323–24.

Buch G (1905) Zur Pathologi und Aetiologie des Malum Dupuytren. *Deutsch Arch klinisch Med* 85: 89.

Buet (1832) Des diverses espèces de flexion permanente des doigts, et des moyens de les distinguer. *J Complémentaire des Sciences Médecales* 43: 172–77.

Bulley FA (1864) Contraction of the fingers. The result of chronic rheumatic affection. *Medical Times and Gazette* 2: 218–19.

Bunch JL (1913) Hereditary Dupuytren's contracture. *Br J Dermatol* 25: 279–83.

Bury JS (1882) Contraction of the palmar fascia. *BMJ* 1: 189.

Busch (1877) Operative Behandlung der Dupuytren'schen Fingerverkrümmung. *Verandl Deutsche Gesellsch Chir, 5th Congresso, Berlino*, 72.

Byford WH (1921) The pathogenesis of Dupuytren's contraction of the palmar fascia. *Medic Record* 100: 487.

Callomon F (1920) Induratio penis plastica. *Berliner klinisch Wochenschr* 57: 1092.

Cameron (1906) Kombination der plastischen Induration des Penis mit Dupuytren Finger-contractur (cited by Neumark (1906)).

Canestro C (1909) Malattia del Dupuytren da trauma diretto. Infortunio sul lavoro. *La Medicina degli Infortuni del lavoro e delle Malattie profession* 2.

Cannanus G (1543) *Musculorum Humani Corporis – Picturata Dissecto.* Ferrara.

Cardarelli A (1887) Sull'origino neuropatica del morbo di Dupuytren. *Atti dell'Associaz Medica Ital, 3rd Congr, Pavia.*

Cardi G (1909) Sulla patogenesi della malattia di Dupuytren. *Rivista di Patologia nervosa e mentale* 14: 361.

Carless A (1910) Dupuytren's contraction treated by fibrolysin. *Lancet* 240.

Carrel A (1921) Cicatrization of wounds. XII. Factors initiating regeneration. *J Exp Med* 34: 425–34.

Carter TA (1881) Dupuytren's contraction of the fingers. *BMJ* 2: 1014.

Caspari (1896) Ueber den neuropathischen Ursprung der Aponeurositis palmaris. *Arch Unfallheilk, Gewerbehyg Gewerbekrankheiten* 1: 143.

Cassirer Le nevrosi professionali. In: Leyden, Klemperer *La clinicia contemporanea*, Vol. 6, 728 (cited by Agosti (1910)).

Castellino P, Pende N (1915) Malattia di Dupuytren. In: *Patologia del simpatico*, 312. Vallardi, Milano.

Catterina A Contrattura delle dita del Dupuytren. *Trattato Italiano di chirurgia*, Vol. 6, 652. Vallardi, Milano.

Cayla A (1883) Diabète et rétraction de l'aponévrose palmaire. *J Hebdo Med* 20: 770.

Cénas L (1884) Troubles nerveux complexes des extrémités, consécutifs à une blessure du nerf cubital. *Rev Médecine* 4: 479.

Chalier A, Cordier V (1908) Rétraction de l'apronévroses plantaires et palmaires d'origine tuberculeuse. *Lyon Médical* 4: 195.

Charcot JM (1877) Rétraction de l'aponévrose palmaire. *Progrès Médic* 19.

Charcot JM (1890) *Oeuvres complètes*, Vol. 7. Paris (cited by Ebstein (1911)).

Charpentier A, Bailleul LC (1926) Sur le traitement de la maladie de Dupuytren. *Revue Neurologique* 33: 327.

Chassaignac E (1858) Rétraction de l'aponévrose palmaire traitée avec succès par l'excision. *Bull Soc Chirurg* 8: 506.

Chatagnon A, Soulairac A, Chatagnon C (1938) Maladie de Dupuytren chez une mélancolique. *Annales médico-psychologiques* 11: 238.

Chauffart (1886) Des affections rhumatismales du tissu cellulaire souscutanée. Thèse, Paris.

Chevrot F (1882) Recherches sur la rétraction de l'aponévrose palmaire et son traitement chirurgical. Thèse, Paris.

Chomel AF (1837) *Lécons de clinique médidicale*, Vol. 2, *Paris* (cited by Ebstein (1911)).

Christel (1904) Recensione del lavoro di Féré et Demanche: Rétraction de l'aponévrose palmaire consécutive à une fracture de l'avant-bras. *Zentralbl Chir* **31**: 344.

Ciampolini A (1926) Rapporti fra traumi e retrazioni dell'aponevrosi palmare. *La traumatologia del lavoro nei rapporti colla legge*, 529. Pozzi, Roma.

Ciampolini A (1932) Morbo di Dupuytren. *Il trauma nella etiogenesi delle malattie*, 59. Pozzi, Roma.

Ciarrocchi (1892) Sulla malattia di Dupuytren. *Bollettino della Società Lancisiana Ospedali di Roma*, **12**: 173. Artero, Roma.

Clavel (1930) Rétraction de l'aponévrose palmaire. *Lyon Médic* **72**: 313.

Cleland J (1878) On the cutaneous ligaments of the phalanges. *J Anat Physiol* **12**: 526.

Cline H (1777) Notes on pathology and surgery. Manuscript 28:185. St Thomas' Hospital Library, London.

Cline H (1787) Notes of Richard Whitfield (student) from a lecture by Henry Cline Senior. Manuscript 30, St Thomas' Hospital Library, London.

Cline H Jr (1808) Notes of John Windsor (student) from a lecture by Henry Cline Jr. Manuscript collection, John Rylands University Library of Manchester, Manchester, 486–89.

Coenen H (1918) Zur Frage der Dupuytren'schen Fingerkontraktur nach Verletzung des Ellen-Nerven. *Berliner klinisch Wochenschr* **55**: 419.

Coenen H (1918) Die Dupuytren'sche Fingerkontraktur. *Ergebnisse Chir Orthopädie* **10**: 1170.

Coenen H (1927) Zur traumatischen Genese der Dupuytren'schen Kontraktur. *Zentralbl Chir* **54**: 1248.

Coenen H (1935) Die Dupuytren'sche Fingerkontraktur. *Med Klinik Jahr* **31**: 1657.

Cokkalis P (1926) Dupuytren'sche Contractur der Palmar- und Plantaraponeurose. *Deutsch Zeitschr Chir* **194**: 256.

Collis E, Eatock R (1912) *Report of an inquiry on Dupuytren's contraction as a disease of occupation, with special reference to its occurrence among minders of lace machines*. Home Office, London.

Combault A (1924) Traitement des rétractions de l'aponévrose palmaire. *La Clinique* **19**: 114.

Conner PS Contrazione di Dupuytren delle dita. In: Ashurst G, *Enciclopedia internazionale di Chirurgia Traduz Ital*, Vol. 3, 29. Vallardi, Milano.

Constantinescu M, Tuchel V, Corâciu G (1938) Ueber einen Fall von angeborener doppelseitiger Dupuytren'scher Kontraktur. *Zentralbl Chir* **65**: 191.

Cooper A (1822) On dislocations of the fingers and toes – dislocation from contraction of the tendon. In: Cooper A, *A Treatise on Dislocations and Fractures of the Joints*. Longman, Hurst, Rees, Orme, Brown & Cox, London.

Cooper A (1837) *Ouvres chirurgicales* 122.

Costilhes J (1885) De la rétraction de l'aponévrose palmaire (maladie de Dupuytren). Thèse, Paris.

Couch H (1938) Identical Dupuytren's contracture in identical twins. *Can Med Assoc J* **39**: 225.

Coulon E (1896) Traitement de la rétraction de l'aponévrose palmaire. *Presse Médicale* **4**: 306.

Crévalew EA (1917) Sur la fréquence de la contracture de Dupuytren chez les malades psychiques. *Revue Neurologique* **I**: 207.

Croft J (1884) Dupuytren's contraction. *Lancet* **i**: 565.

Cruveilhier J (1841) *Vie de Dupuytren*. Béchet et Labé, Paris.

Cunéo (1932) Technique opératoire concernant la maladie de Dupuytren. *Presse Médicale* **40**: 399.

Czerny Marwedel (1901) Aerztliches Obergutachten, betreffend den ursächlichen Zusammenhang zwischen einer sogenannten Dupuytren'schen Contractur der rechten Hand und einer durch Betriebsunfall erlittenen Quetschung der rechten Schultergegend. Cited in *Monatschr Unfallheilk* **8**: 353.

Daeschler (1903) *Ueber die Dupuytren'sche Palmarfascien Kontraktur*. Inaugural dissertation, München.

D'Ambrosio A (1892) Retrazione dell'aponevrosi palmare; malattia di Dupuytren; contrattura di flessione delle dita della manno. (Lezione raccolta da A. Virdia). *Riforma Medica* **8**: 482.

Daniel JM (1891) Contractions of the palmar fascia. *Maritime Medical News* **3**: 48–51.

David V (1935) Etiologia traumatica della malatia di Dupuytren. *Zentralorgan Chirurg* **74**: 587.

Davis AA (1932) The treatment of Dupuytren's contractur. A review of 31 cases, with an assessment of the comparative value of different methods of treatment. *Br J Surg* **19**: 539.

Davis JS (1919) *Plastic Surgery, its Principles and Practice*. London (cited by Skoog (1948)).

Davis JS, Finesilver EM (1932) Dupuytren's contracture with a note on the incidence of the contraction in diabetes. *Archives of Surgery* **24**: 933.

De Lisi L (1913) Malattia di Dupuytren con sindrome di Benard-Horner. *Il Morgagni* **55**: 281.

De Nobele (1922) Quelques applications intéressants et peu utilisées de la radiumthérapie. *Scalpel* **75**: 570.

De Quervain F *Diagnostica chirurgica*, 594. Vallardi, Milano.

De Villaverde JM (1929) Algo sobre la supuesta patogenia de la enfermedad de Dupuytren: un caso de polineuritis con retracción de la aponeurosis palmar. *Medicina Ibera* **13**: 213.

Debrunner H (1934) Sippschaftstabelle einer Familie mit Dupuytren'scher Kontraktur. *Zeitschr orthopädisch Chirurgie* **62**: 321.

Deckner K (1938) Gleichzeitiges Vorkommen von muskulären Schiefhals und Dupuytren'scher Fingerkontraktur. *Zentralbl Chir* **65**: 1192.

Deckner K (1939) Die Dupuytren'sche Kontraktur als ein Beispiel für das Zusammenwirken von Erbanlage und Umwelt für die Ausbildung eines variablen Merkmals. *Zeitschr menschliche Vererbungs- und Konstitutionslehre* **22**: 734.

Deckner K (1939) Wesen und Behandlung der Dupuytren'schen Fingerkontraktur. *Therapie der Gegenwart* **80**: 69.

Decref J (1929) La enfermedad llamada de Dupuytren, o retracción de la aponeurosis palmar, puede ser considerada como un accidente del trabajo, o como una enfermedad professional. *El Siglo Medico* **76**: 569.

Dejerine J (1914) Maladie de Dupuytren. *Sémiologie des affections du système nerveux*, 1109. Masson, Paris.

Delaborde (1887) De l'induration plastique des corps caverneux. Thèse, Paris.

Delbet P (1899) Retraction de l'aponévrose palmaire. *Leçons de Clinique chirurgicale faites a l'Hôtel-Dieu*, 191. Steinheil, Paris.

Delchef (1935) Maladie de Dupuytren, aponévrectomie palmaire par double incision cutanée. *Scalpel* **80**.

Delherm (1925) Traitement röntgenthérapique de la maladie de Dupuytren. *J Radiol Electrol* **9**: 476–77.

Demerliac, Dupitout (1932) Sur un cas de rétraction de l'aponévrose palmaire consécutifs à une atteinte du nerf cubital droit avec syndrome de Cl. Bernard-Horner. *Revue Neurologique* **2**: 309.

Deneffe (1895) Sur la rétraction de l'aponévrose palmaire. *Annales de la Soc de Médec de Gand* (cited by Neutra (1901)).

Desplas B (1931) À propos du traitement chirurgical de la maladie de Dupuytren. *Bull Mém Soc Nat de Chirurg* **57**: 1409.

Desplas B (1932) Le traitement chirurgical de la maladie de Dupuytren. *Le Monde Médical* **42**: 795.

Desplas B (1934) À propos du traitement de la maladie de Dupuytren. *Bull Mém Soc Nat Chirurg* **60**: 1174.

Desplas B, Meillière J (1932) Sur une technique opératoire concernant la maladie de Dupuytren. *Bull Mém Soc Nat Chirurg* **58**: 424.

Desplas B, Portret (1934) Au sujet de la maladie de Dupuytren: technique chirurgicale et radiologique. *J Radiol Electrol* **18**: 57.

Desplats (1925) Traitement röntgenthérapique de la maladie de Dupuytren. *J Radiol Electrol* **9**: 476–77.

Després A (1877) Rétraction de l'aponévrose palmaire. *Bull Soc Anat* 9 March.

Després A (1880) Rétraction de l'aponévrose palmaire d'origine traumatique. *Gazzette Méd Paris* **2**: 202.

Devoto L (1925) Due casi di malattia di Dupuytren. *La Medicina del Lavoro* **16**: 75.

Devoto L (1925) La retrazione della palma della mano e della pianta del piede. *La Medicina del Lavoro* **16**: 407.

Doberauer G (1902) Ueber die Dupuytren'sche Fingerkontraktion. *Brun's Beiträge z klin Chir* **36**: 123.

Doyen E (1910) Rétraction de l'aponévrose palmaire. *Traité de Thérapeutique chirurgicale et de Technique opératoir*, Vol. 3, 468. Maloine, Paris.

Drehmann (1913) Zur Operation der Dupuytren'schen Fingerkontraktur. *Zentralbl Chir* **40**: 19.

Dreifus F (1883) Pathogénie et accidents nerveux du diabète sucré. Thèse, Paris.

Ducastaing R (1920) Tumeurs fibreuses de la paume de la main. *Paris Médic* **10**: 248.

Dudley HC (1939) Dupuytren's contraction. *Northwest Medicine* **38**: 138.

Duplay (1899) Rétraction de l'aponévrose palmaire. In: Depage, *Année chirurgicale*, Vol. 1, 1800 Bruxelles.

Dupuytren G (1831) Contracture du petit doigt et de l'anulaire de la main gauche dissipé complétement par le simple debridement de l'aponévrose palmaire. *Gazette Hop*.

Dupuytren G (1831) Contracture permanente des doigts avec mobilité de chaque articulation et impossibilité de l'extension. *Gazette Hop* 26 novembre.

Dupuytren G (1831) De la rétraction des doigts par suite d'une affection de l'aponévrose palmaire par MM. les docteurs Paillard et Marx. *Journal Universel et Hebdomadaire de Médecine et de Chirurgie Pratiques et des Institutions Médicales*, Paris. Reprinted in *Medical*

Classics 1939–1940, Vol. 4. Royal Society of Medicine, London.

Dupuytren G (1832) De la rétraction des doigts par suite d'une affection de l'aponévrose palmaire. Opération chirurgicale qui convient dans ce cas. *J Hébdo Méd* **5**: 348; **6**: 67.

Dupuytren G (1832) De la rétraction permanente des doigts et du diagnostic différential. *Lécons orales de clinique chirurgicale faites a l'Hôtel Dieu*, 473. Baillière, Paris.

Dupuytren G (1832) Rétraction permanente des doigts. *Gazette Méd Paris* **3**: 41.

Dupuytren G (1832) Rétraction permanente des doigts. In: Dupuytren G, *Leçons orales de clinique chirurgicale faites à l'Hôtel-Dieu de Paris*, 2–24. Germer Baillière, Paris.

Dupuytren G (1833) Flexion forcée de tous les doigts de la main droite. Rétraction présumée de l'aponévrose palmaire. Section des brides. *Gazette Méd Paris* **4**: 112.

Dupuytren G (1834) Contratture permanente delle dita in conseguenza di una malattia dell'aponevrosi palmare. *Lezioni verbali di clinica chirurgica pronunciate all'ospitale maggiore di Parigi, raccolte e pubblicate da una società di medici*, 11. Tip. P. Lampato, Venezia.

Dupuytren G (1834) Permanent retraction of the fingers, produced by an affection of the palmar fascia. *Lancet* **ii**: 222–25.

Durante F (1905) Malattie delle fascie. *Trattato di Patologia e Terap. chirugica gener. e speciale*, Vol. 2, 487. Soc Edit Dante Alighiere, Rome.

Durel L (1888) Essai sur la maladie de Dupuytren. Thèse, Paris.

Dusatti C (1936) Considerazioni patogenetiche su un caso di morbo di Dupuytren. *Minerva Medica* **27**: 79.

Dutto U (1927) *Due parole sul morbo di Dupuytren.* Tipogr Editrice Romana, Roma.

Dutto U (1928) Sul morbo di Dupuytren. *Malpighi, Gazzetta Medica di Roma* **54**: 198.

Ebstein W (1911) Zur Aetiologie der Dupuytren'schen Kontraktur. *Deutsch Arch klinische Med* **103**: 201.

Eckstein H (1922) Phalangresektion zu Beseitigung von Fingerkontraktur. *Zentralbl Chir* **49**: 547.

Ely LW (1926) Dupuytren's contraction. *Surgical Clinics of North America* **6**: 421.

Enderlen (1907) Dupuytren'sche Kontraktur; Exstirpation der Fascia palmaris; Deckung des Defektes mit gestielten Lappen aus dem Skrotum. *Korrespondenzbl Schweiz Aerzte* **9**.

Enderlen (1913) Dupuytren'sche Kontraktur. *München med Wochenschr* **60**: 217.

English TC (1902) A case of rupture of Dupuytren's contraction. *Lancet* **i**: 1104.

Eulenburg A (1863) Ueber die Kontraktur der Finger. *Deutsch Klinik* 494.

Eulenburg A (1864) Eine Bemerkungen ueber die flektierten Fingerkontrakturen. *Berliner klinisch Wochenschr* **22–23**.

Eulenburg A (1883) Neuritis des Nervus ulnaris in Zusammenhang mit Strangkontrakturen der Finger. *Neurologisch Zentralbl* **3**: 49.

Eulenburg A, Cenas (1883) Zusammenhang von Dupuytren'scher Fingerkontraktur mit Neuritis. *Neurologisch Zentralbl* **3**.

Evans HM, Burr GO (1928) Development of paralysis in the suckling young of mothers deprived of vitamin E. *J Biol Chem* **76**: 273–97.

Ewart (1883) Dupuytren's contraction in a female. *Lancet* **i**: 412.

Exner A (1921) Ueber Tuberkulose der Aponeurosis palmaris unter dem Bilde der Dupuytren'schen Fingerkontraktur. *Wiener klinisch Wochenschr* **34**: 252.

Façon E, Bruch, Vasilescu (1933) Considerations sur un cas de maladie de Dupuytren. *Bull Mém Soc Méd Hôp Bucarest* **15**: 12.

Fairbank HAT (1932) Dupuytren's contraction of the plantar fascia. *Proc Roy Soc Med London* **26**: 103.

Fasquelle A (1892) Contributions a l'étude du traitement chirurgical de la contracture de Dupuytren, dite rétraction de l'aponévrose palmaire. no. 1892/724, Thèse, Lyon.

Feindel E (1896) Névrite traumatique du cubital, déviation des doigts en coup de vent, rétraction de l'aponévrose palmaire. *Revue Neurologique* **4**: 537.

Féré CH (1897) Note sur la rétraction de l'aponévrose palmaire. *Revue de Chirurgie* **17**: 797.

Féré CH (1899) Note sur la rétraction de l'aponévrose plantaire. *Revue de Chirurgie* **19**: 272.

Féré CH (1903) Rétraction de l'aponévrose palmaire consécutive à une névrite blenorrhagique. *La Normandie Médicale*, 217.

Féré CH, Demanche R (1903) Note sur un cas de rétraction de l'aponévrose palmaire consécutive a une fracture de l'avantbras. *Revue de Chirurgie* **23**: 324.

Féré CH, Francillon M (1902) Note sur la fréquence de rétraction palmaire chez les aliénés. *Revue de Médecine* **22**: 539.

Fergusson W (1842) *A System of Practical Surgery.* Churchill Livingstone, London.

Fergusson W (1875) A system of practical surgery. *BMJ* **I**: 258.

Fernandez JC (1936) Enfermedad de Dupuytren: tratamiento quirúrgico. *Semana Médica* **44**: 260.

Ferrari G (1883) Retrazione delle dita mignolo anulare e pollice della mano sinistra. *Italia Medica, Genova* (edited by Neutra (1901)).

Ferrari G (1906) Considerazioni sopra un caso di malattia di Dupuytren guarito con cura medica locale. *Riforma Medica* **22**: 393.

Ferrarini M (1936) Morfogenesi dell'aponevrosi palmare. *Pathologica* **27**: 586.

Ferrarini M (1938) L'articolazione del polso. Ricerche anatomoembriologiche. *Archivio Ital di Anatomia e di Embriologia* **41**, 207.

Ferrarini M (1939) Sulla anatomia patologica e sulla etiopatogenesi della malattia del Dupuytren. *Giornale R Acad Med, Torino* **102**: 40.

Ferrarini M (1939) Sulla anatomia patologica e sulla etiopatogenesi della malattia del Dupuytren. *Arch Ital di Chirurgia* **57**: 1.

Ferrarini M (1940) Se la malattia del Dupuytren possa essere considerata quale una malattia professionale. *Rassegna di Medicina Industriale* **11**: 70.

Feuerstein G (1936) Ueber Erfahrungen mit der Strahlenbehandlung bei der Dupuytren'schen Kontraktur. *Wiener klinische Wochenschr* **49**: 1090.

Fildermann (1931) Présentation d'une malade atteint de la maladie de Dupuytren en bonne voie de guérison par l'hémocrinothérapie. *Bull Mém Soc Méd Hôp Paris* **4**: 115.

Fildermann (1933) Traitement de la maladie de Dupuytren. Hémocrinothérapie. *Presse Médicale* **41**: 548.

Fiori L (1910) La fibrolisina nella cura del morbo di Dupuytren. *Riforma Medica* **26**: 796.

Fischer H (1897) Contrattura cordoniforme di Dupuytren. *Trattato di Chirurgia speciale*, Vol. 2, 472. Soc Editr Libraria, Milano.

Fisher FR (1883) Dupuytren's contraction in a female. *Lancet* **i**: 412.

Fisher FR (1885) The treatment of Dupuytren's contraction of the palmar fascia. *BMJ* **1259**: 327.

Flatau E (1900) Dupuytren'sche Fingerkontraktur. In: Nothnagel *Specielle Pathologie u. Therapie*, Vol. 11, 172, *Neuritis und Polyneuritis*. Hölder, Wien.

Follin E, Duplay S (1888) Rétration de l'aponévrose palmaire. *Traité élémentaire de pathologie externe*, Vol. 7, 847. Masson, Paris.

Fort (1869) Des difformités congénites et acquises des doigts. *Thèse, Paris*.

Foucart (1889) Induration des tissus érectiles de la verge. *La France Médic* 618.

Fragola V (1915) Contributo clinico alla malattia del Dupuytren. *Rassegna di Studi psichiatrici* **5**: 53.

Frangenheim (1927) Zur traumatische Genese der Dupuytren'schen Kontraktur. *Zentralbl Chir* **54**: 1248.

Frank (1910) Dupuytren'sche Kontraktur; Radiusbruch; kein Zusammenhang. *Mediz Klinik* **6**.

Frankenthal L (1937) Deckung des Defektes der Hohlhandhaut durch die Kleinfingerhaut bei der Dupuytren'schen Kontraktur. *Zentralbl Chir* **64**: 211.

Fredet P, Moure P (1932) À propos de la maladie de Dupuytren. *Bull Mém Soc Nat Chirurg* **58**: 440.

Freund E (1934) Caso di contrattura di Dupuytren. *Giornale Veneto di Scienze Mediche* **8**: 513.

Freund L (1913) Die Strahlenbehandlung der fehlerhaften Narben und Keloide. *Wiener med Wochenschr* **63**: 2356.

Friedrich PL (1901) Dupuytren'sche Finger-kontraktur. In: Bergmann, Bruns, Mikulicz, *Handbuch d. praktische. Chirurgie* Vol. 4, 466. Stuttgart.

Frohse F (1906) Die Aponeurosis palmaris und digitalis der menschlichen Hand, mit besonderer Berücksichtigung ihrer Funktion. *Arch Anat Physiol* 101.

Froriep (1847) Zur Erläuterung de Palmarkontaktion der Finger. In: Henle, *Anatomie Chirurg Kupfeltafeln*, 356. Weimar.

Frund (1926) Hypoplasie der Hypophysis. *Zentralbl Chir* **53**: 1283.

Fullerton (1907) A case of Dupuytren's contraction treated by complete excision. *BMJ* **1**: 203.

Gabourd (1905) Rétraction d'origine tuberculeuse de l'aponévrose palmaires des 2 mains. *Lyon Médical* **49**.

Galdi F (1931) Retrazione dell'aponevrosi palmare o morbo di Dupuytren. *Trattato Ital di Medic Interna*, Vol. 2, 1218. Soc Editr Libr, Milano.

Gangolphe M (1891) Traitement de la rétraction de l'aponévrose palmaire par les sections multiples sous-cutanées. *Lyon Médical* 577.

Garrod AE (1893) On an unusual form of nodule upon the joints of the fingers. *St Bartholomew's Hospital Report* **29**: 157–61.

Geck AO (1889) *Ueber die Dupuytren'sche Fingerkontraktur*. Inaugural dissertation, Bonn.

Gemmel (1899) Drei Fälle doppelseitiger symmetrischer Contractur der Palmaraponeurose (Dupuytren) im Anschluss an Gicht. *Deutsch med Wochenschr* **18**: 286.

Gemmel (1902) Weitere Beobachtungen betreffend das symmetrische Aufreten der Kontraktur der Palmaraponeurose (Dupuytren) im Anschluss an Gicht und harnsäure Diathese. *Deutsch med Zeitung.*

Gerdy (1844) Rétraction des tissus albuginés. *Bull Acad Roy Méd* **9**: 766.

Gerdy (1853) *Traité de chirurgie* Vol. 2, 62.

Gerritzen P (1935) Die Aetiologie der Dupuytren'schen Kontraktur und ihre Beziehung zu Beruf und Trauma. *Monatschr Unfallheilk Versicherungsmed* **42**: 545.

Gerritzen P (1936) Operationserfolge der Dupuytren's-chen Kontraktur unter Berücksichtigung der unfallweisen Entstehung. *Zentralbl Chirurg* **63**: 161.

Gersuny R (1884) Operation bei Kontraktur der Palmaraponevrose. *Wien Med Wochenschr* **34**: 969.

Gianasso AB (1908) Su un craso di morbo di Dupuytren. *Riforma Medica* **24**: 403.

Gibbon JH (1922) Operation for Dupuytren's contracture. *Ann Surg* **75**: 505.

Gibney (1883) Adam's operation for Dupuytren's finger contraction. *Medical Record* **23**, **24**: 134.

Gilbeau W (1934) *Dupuytren'sche Kontraktur und Unfall.* Inaugural dissertation, Bonn.

Gilbert (1913) Sur un mémoire de M. Léopold Lévi concernant la rétraction de l'aponévrose palmaire et le traitement thyroïdien. *Bull Mém Acad Méd Paris* **69**: 23.

Gill AB (1919) Dupuytren's contracture, with a description of a method of operation. *Ann Surg* **70**: 221.

Gill AB (1922) End results of operation for Dupuytren's contracture. *Ann Surg* **75**: 503.

Gill AB (1938) Dupuytren's contracture. *Ann Surg* **107**: 122.

Gilmour J (1934) Dupuytren's contraction. *BMJ* **3854**: 926.

Girdwood R (1916) An unusual case of Dupuytren's contracture. *BMJ* **2915**: 650.

Gold (1926) Behandlung der Dupuytren'schen Kontraktur. *Zentralbl Chir* **53**: 724.

Golebiewski (1894) Ueber die Bedeutung der Gewerbehygiene und Statistik für die Socialgesetzgebung Deutschlands. *Monatschr Unfallheilk* **10–11**: 297.

Gonzales Aguilar J, Sala de Pablo J (1936) El tratamiento de la enfermedad de Dupuytren. *La Medecina Ibera* **30**: 969.

Gosselin (1877) Flexion incomplète et permanente de l'auriculaire due `a l'existence d'une bride fibreuse. *Gazette Hôp* **50**: 649–50.

Goyrand G (1833) Recherches sur la rétraction permanente des doigts. *Bull Mém Acad Méd* **3**: 489.

Goyrand G (1834) De la rétraction permanente des doigts. *Gazette Méd Paris* **3**: 219.

Goyrand G (1835) Nouvelles recherches sur la rétraction permanente des doigts, suivi du rapport à l'Académie (avril 1834). *Gaz Méd Paris* **4**: 205.

Gräff S (1930) Ueber Dupuytren'sche Finger-kontraktur. *Zentralbl Chirurg* **18**: 1102.

Grapow M (1887) Die Anatomie and physiologische Bedeutung der Palmaraponeurose. *Arch Anat Physiol* **143**: 2–3.

Grayson J (1940) The cutaneous ligaments of the digits. *J Anat* **75**: 164.

Greenberg L (1939) Dupuytren's contracture of palmar and plantar fasciae. *J Bone Joint Surg* **21**: 785.

Grieg DM (1917) A case of congenital Dupuytren's contraction of the fingers. *Edinburgh Med J* **19**: 384.

Griessmann Br (1918) Ein Fall von gebesserter Dupuytren'scher Kontraktur. *Münchener med Wochenschr* **65**: 1083.

Griffith E, Albutt C, Ruegg, Legge M (1913) *Minutes of evidence of the departmental committee, appointed to inquire, and report on Dupuytren's contraction.* Eyre and Spottiswood, London.

Gualdi C (1904) Morbo di Dupuytren e siringomielia. *Rivista critica di Clinica Medica* **5**: 477.

Guarraccino G (1886) La malattia di Dupuytren: retra-zione dell'aponevrosi palmare. *Riforma Medica* **2**: 453.

Gubern – Salisachs L (1933) Consideraciones acerca de la etiologia de la enfermedad de Dupuytren. *Revista de Cirugia de Barcelona* **3**: 81.

Guérin G (1833) Commentaires sur la rétraction permanente des doigts. *Gazette Med Paris* **1**: 111–13.

Guérin J (1842) Rétraction des doigts. *Bull Acad Méd* **8**: 129.

Guérin J (1843) Rétraction de l'aponévrose palmaire traité par les bandalettes de diachylon. *J univers hébdom Méd Chirurg pratique* **14**: 243.

Guérin J (1885) *Progrès Médical* **43**.

Guinebault P (1897) Contribution a l'étude de la rétraction de l'aponéurose palmaire. Thèse, Paris.

Gurlt E (1896) Finger. In: Eulenburg, *Realencyklopädie der gesammten Heilkunde*, 3rd edn, Vol. 9, 521.

Haberland HFO (1931) Zur Behandlung der Dupuytren'schen Kontraktur. *Zentralbl Chir* **58**: 1533.

Hanke H (1936) Fingerspitzennekrose nach in Lokalanästhesie ausgeführter Operation wegen Dupuytren'scher Kontraktur. *Der Chirurg* **8**: 684.

Hardie J (1884) Contraction of the palmar fascia. *BMJ* **1218**: 859.

Hardie J (1885) On the treatment of Dupuytren's contracture of the fingers. *Zentralbl Chir* **12**: 115.

Hardie J (1885) The treatment of Dupuytren's finger-contraction. *BMJ* **1265**: 681.

Hare (1883) Dupuytren's contraction in a female. *Lancet* **i**: 412.

Harper WJ (1935) Distribution of palmar aponeurosis in relation to Dupuytren's contraction of the thumb. *J Anat* **69**: 193.

Hartmann (1909) Rétraction de l'aponévrose palmaire (Dupuytren) traitée par ionisation salicylée. *Bul Mém Soc Nat Chirurg, Paris* **34**: 742.

Hartmann (1928) Retraction de l'aponévrose palmaire. *Policlinico, Sez Prat* **35**: 1855.

Hawkins C (1835) Contraction of the fingers. *London Med Gazette* **15**: 814–15.

Hawkins C (1844) On contraction of the fingers of both hands. *London Med Gazette* **34**: 277–78.

Hedges CHE (1897) The relation of gout and rheumatism to Dupuytren's contraction of palmar fascia. *St Bartholomew's Hosp Reports* **32**: 119.

Heitz-Boyer (1929) A propos de l'action disséquante du bistouri à haute fréquence: cure radicale d'une rétraction de l'aponévrose palmaire. *Bull Soc Nat Chirurg Paris* **55**, 1305.

Helferich (1880) *Kontraktur der Fascia palmaris beider Hände.* Aerzliches Internat Blätter, München (cited by Neutra (1991)).

Helmuth WT (1887–88) *Contraction of the palmar fascia.* Report of Helmuth House, New York **2**: 47.

Henckel KO (1923) *Beiträge zur Klinik der Dupuytren'schen Fingerkontraktur.* Inaugural dissertation, München.

Henrard (1925) Traitement röntgenthérapique de la maladie de Dupuytren. *J Radiol Electrol* **9**: 476–77.

Herzberg M (1926) Endokrine Faktoren und chronischer Gelenkrheumatismus. *Zeitschr klinische Med* **103**: 507–29.

Hesse (1931) Zur Behandlung der Dupuytren'schen Krankheit. *Zentralbl Chir* **24**: 1532–33.

Heuser K (1905) Beitrag zur Frage der Dupuytren'schen Kontraktur und Unfall. *Münchener med Wochenschr* **52**: 1844.

Heuyer G (1927) Maladie de Dupuytren. In: Roger, Widal, Teissier, *Nouveau Traité de Médecine*, Vol. 21, 542. Masson, Paris.

Heyfelder J (1845) *Die Contractura digiti minimi manus sinist, aponeurotica.* Das Chirurgische und Augenkranken-Clinicum der Universität Erlangen, 32–33.

Hilger (1926) Dupuytren'sche Fingerkontraktur. *Münchener med Wochenschr* **73**: 86.

Hirsz (1937) Induramento iperplastcio del pene e retrazione palmare di Dupuytren. *Warszawskie Czasopisno Lekarskie* **14**.

His W (1921) Wesen und Formen der chronischen Arthritiden. *Berliner klinisch Wochenschr* **58**: 1525.

Hodson JWB (1908) A case of Dupuytren's contraction cured by hypodermic injections of fibrolysin. *Lancet* **i**: 106.

Hoffa A (1894) Die Dupuytren'schen Fingercontracturen. *Lehbuch der orthopädischen Chirurgie*, 488. Enke, Stuttgart.

Hoffa A (1898) Ein Beitrag zu der Erkrankungen der Plantarfascie. *Zentralbl Chir* **25**: 166.

Hohmann G (1936) Zur orthopädischen Behandlung der Dupuytren'schen Fingerkontraktur. *Münchener med Wochenschr* **83**: 2088.

Holfelder (1931) cited by Perussia (1934) coll'indicazione: Lazarus, *Tratt di Radioterapia München.*

Homans J (1887) A case of contracted fingers (Dupuytren's contraction) successfully operated upon, after the method of Adams. *Boston Med J* 24 February.

Homans J (1938) Dupuytren's contracture. *Ann Surg* **107**: 127.

Horák (1914) Sulla malattia di Dupuytren. *Zentralbl Chir* **41**: 78.

Horand R (1908) A propos de la camptodactylie. *Gazette Hop* **81**: 231.

Horodynski (1919) Morbus Dupuytreni. *Zentralbl Chir* **46**: 192.

Horwitz A (1920) Zur Behandlung von Narbenkotrakturen. *Zentralbl Chir* **47**: 920.

Houel (1877) Rétraction de l'aponévrose palmaire. *Progrès Médical* **19**.

Hough JH (1883) Dupuytren's contraction of the fingers. *Lancet* **i**: 15.

Howell BW (1831) Dupuytren's contraction. *Lancet* **221**: 269.

Howse HG (1892–93) A case of Dupuytren's contraction affecting both hands. *Clin J* **1**: 307–308.

Hueter C (1882) Cicatrizielle und neuromyogene Contracturen der Fingergelenke. *Grundriss der Chirurgie*, Vol. 2, 848. Vogel, Leipzig.

Hugonot G, Friess E (1932) Ulcère gastrique associé à une maladie de Dupuytren. Hypocalcémie et insuffisance parathyroïdienne. Traitement par la parathormone. *Lyon Médical* **64**: 465.

Humphry (1884) Dupuytren's contraction. *Lancet* **i**: 565.

Hutchinson J (1886) Simulation by muscular action of

Dupuytren's contraction of palmar fascia. *BMJ* **1328**: 1097.

Hutchinson J (1886) Dupuytren's induration of palmar and plantar fascia without material contraction. *BMJ* **1329**: 1158.

Hutchinson J (1893) On curving of the penis. *Arch Surg* **5**: 329.

Hutchinson J (1897) On the juvenile form of the Dupuytren's contraction. *Arch Surg* **8**: 20–21.

Hutchinson J (1913) Note on a improved method of operation in Dupuytren's contraction of the fingers. *Proc Roy Soc Med* **6**: 267.

Hutchinson J (1917) Hunterian lecture on Dupuytren's contraction of palmar fascia; Dupuytren's life and works. *Lancet* **192**: 285.

Iardini A (1906) Maladie de Dupuytren et artériosclerose médullaire. *Nouvelle J conogr de la Salpetrière* **19**: 552.

Iardini A (1907) Morbo di Dupuytren e arteriosclerosi midollare. *Il Morgagn,* **49**: 256.

Iklé C (1928) Zur Histologie und Pathogenese der Dupuytren'schen Kontraktur. *Deutsch Zeitschr Chir* **212**: 106.

Iklé C (1930) *Zur Histologie und Pathogenese der Dupuytren'schen Kontraktur.* Inaugural dissertation, Bern.

Imber I (1936) Sulla contrattura di Dupuytren a carattere famigliare. *Note e Riviste di Psichiatria* **65**: 209.

Imbert L, Oddo C, Chavernac P (1913) *Guide pour l'évaluation des incapacités,* 788. Masson, Paris.

Iversen J (1909) *Über die traumatische Entsehung der Dupuytrenschen Kontraktur u. deren Lokalisation am Daumen.* Inaugural dissertation, Kiel (cited by Skoog (1948)).

Jaccoud (1874) *Clinique Médic de la Charité* (cited by Canestro (1909)).

Jaerisch M (1898) *Ueber Dupuytren'schen Finger-kontrakturen.* Inaugural dissertation, Halle.

Janssen P (1902) Zur Lehre von der Dupuytren'schen Fingerkontraktur, mit besonderer Berücksichtigung der operativen Beseitigung und der pathologischen Anatomie dés Leidens. *Langenbeck's Arch klinisch Chirurg* **67**: 761.

Janssen P (1927) Zur traumatischen Genese der Dupuytren'schen Kontraktur. *Zentralbl Chir* **54**: 1247.

Janssen P (1933) Erblichkeit der Dupuytren'schen Fingerkontraktur. *Zentralbl Chir* **60**: 2214.

Jarjavay cited without bibliographical references in Guarraccino G, Testi A, Tranquilli E and Tricomi E.

Jeanpierre (1882) Considérations sur la rétraction de l'aponévrose palmaire. Thèse, Paris.

Jelliffe SE (1932) Dupuytren's contracture and the unconscious. A preliminary statement of a problem. *Zentralbl Neurol Psychiatrie* **63**: 33.

Jellinek S (1906) Zur kausalen Thiosinamin-behandlung des Malum Dupuytren. *Wiener klinisch Wochenschr* **19**: 869.

Jemmel (1902) *Deutsche Mediz Zeitung* (cited by Testi (1902, 1095)).

Jentsch F (1937) Zur Erblichkeit der Dupuytren'schen Kontraktur. *Zentralbl allg Pathol* **68**: 29.

Jobert (1849) *Gazette Hop* 104 (cited by Vogt (1881)).

Jobert de Lamballe AJ (1849) Sur la flexion permanente des doigts. *Gazette Hop* **3s 1**: 415–16.

Jobert, Blandin (1846) *Annales de Thérapie* (cited by Vogt (1881)).

Jochnan W (1935) *Ueber Vorkommen und Bedeutung der Dupuytren'schen Kontraktur bei Nervenkrankheiten.* Inaugural dissertation, Basel.

Joly (1914) Maladie de Dupuytren. *Annales de la Policlinique centrale de Bruxelles* **14**.

Jones R (1913) *Minutes of evidence of departmental committee appointed to inquire and report on Dupuytren's contracture.* Eyre and Spottiswood, London.

Jonesco (1920) Rétraction de l'aponévrose palmaire à la suite de plaies de guerre intéressant le nerf cubital. *Revue Neurologique* **11**: 1176.

Jorge JM (1926) Rétraction palmaire congénitale. *Revue d'Orthopedie,* **13**: 97.

Jovanovitch (1936) Traitement de la maladie de Dupuytren. *Revue Méd militaire Beograd* 7.

Julinsberg cited without bibliographical references in Binda P.

Julliard CH (1908) Infortunio sul lavoro e retrazione dell'aponevrosi palmare. *La Medicina degli Infortuni del lavoro e delle Malattie professionali* **1**: 3.

Jumentié J (1920) Cas curieux de rétraction de l'aponévrose palmaire. *Revue neurologique* **11**: 1176.

Jung A, Chinassi Hakki A (1932) Études sur la calcémie. Cent dosages du calcium sérique dans divers états pathologiques: affections osseuses, sclérodermie, rétraction de l'aponévrose palmaire etc. *Revue Chirurg* **51**: 537.

Kaern H (1912) Due casi di contrattura di Dupuytren verificatasi in seguito ad infiammazione acuta dell'aponevrosi palmare. *Zeitschr Chir* **39**: 903.

Kanavel AB (1917) *Missouri State Med Assoc,* August.

Kanavel AB, Koch SL, Mason M. (1929) Dupuytren's contraction with a description of the palmar fascia, a review of the literature, and a report of twenty-nine surgically treated cases. *Surg Gynecol Obstet* **48**: 145.

Kaplan EB (1938) The palmar fascia in connection with Dupuytren's contracture. *Surgery* **4**: 415–22.

Kaplan EB (1939) Operation for Dupuytren's contracture based on anatomy of palmar fascia. *Bull Russian Med Soc New York*, 78.

Kappelmeyer E (1929) Dupuytren'sche Finger-kontraktur mit Humanolinjektionen behandelt. *Münchener Med Wochenschr* **76**: 562.

Karlberg W (1935) Zur Anatomie der palmaraponeurose. *Anatomischer Anzeiger* **81**: 149–59.

Kartschikian SI (1927) Dupuytren'sche Kontraktur und Erblichkeit. *Zeitschr orthopäd Chirurg* **48**: 36.

Katzenstein (1895) *Zur Tenotomie bei Fingerkontraktur.* Inaugural dissertation, Kiel.

Kaufmann C (1919) Die Funktions-störungen der Hand. *Handbuch der Unfallmedizin*, 4th edn, Vol. 1, 639. Enke, Stuttgart.

Kayawa Y (1910) Die kurzen Muskeln und die langen beuge-Muskeln der Saügetierhand. *Anatomische Hefte* **42**.

Kayawa Y (1924) Musculus palmaris brevis. Ein Tretballenmuskeln beim Menschen (ein vergleichend-anatomische Studie). *Anatomische Anzeiger* **58**.

Keen WW (1882) The etiology and pathology of Dupuytren's contraction of the fingers. *Philadelphia Med Times* **12**: 370.

Keen WW (1903) Sucessful intraneural infiltration of the median and ulnar nerves during an operation for Dupuytren's contraction. *Am J Med Sci* **6**: 704.

Keen WW (1906) A new method of operating on Dupuytren's contraction of the palmar fascia together with the successful use of neural infiltration in such operations. *Am J Med Sci* **131**.

Kellock TH (1907) Multiple fibrous nodules in the hand with Dupuytren's contraction. *Lancet* **172**: 427.

Kemmer W (1913) *Wesen und Behandlung der Dupuytren'schen Kontraktur.* Inaugural dissertation, München.

Kingsbury GC (1891) Traumatic contraction of fingers treated during hypnosis. *Lancet* **i**: 876.

Kinzel H (1927) *Dupuytren'sche Kontraktur an Hand und Fuss.* Inaugural dissertation, Breslau.

Kirby J (1849) On an unusual affection of the penis. *Dublin Med Press* **22**: 209–10.

Kirby J (1850) Afféction particulière du penis. *Gazette Méd Paris* 676.

Kirmisson (1895) Retrazione dell'aponevrosi palmare. In: Duplay, Reclus, *Tratt di Chirurgia*, Vol. 8, 238. UTET.

Kisgen (1889) *Ueber Dupuytren'sche Fingerkontrakturen infolge narbiger Retraktion der Aponevrosis palmaris.* Inaugural dissertation, Würzburg.

Klapp R (1914) Contratture desmogene delle dita. In: Wallstein, Wilms, *Tratt di Chirurgia*, Vol. 3, 69. UTET.

Kleinschmidt O (1937) La contrattura delle dita di Dupuytren. *Tratt di operazioni chirurgiche*, Vol. 1, 227. Vallardi, Milano.

Knott J (1900) Dupuytren's contraction of the palmar fascia. *Lancet* **ii**: 24.

Knott J (1901) On Dupuytren's contraction of the palmar fascia. *Hildebrand's Jahersber Fortschr Gebiete Chir* **7**: 1049.

Koch H (1907) Dupuytren'sche Fingerkontrakur und Fibrolysineinspritzungen. *Münchener Med Wochenschr* **54**: 1104.

Koch SL (1933) Dupuytren's contraction. *J Am Med Assoc* **100**: 878.

Kocher T (1887) Behandlung der Retraktion der Palmaraponeurose. *Centralbl Chirurg* **14**: 482–87, 497–502.

Kohlmayer H (1935) Zur Frage der traumatischen Entstehung der Dupuytren'schen Finger-kontraktur. *Zentralbl Chir* **62**: 1928.

Kölliker TH (1905–7) Die desmogene Kontraktur (Dupuytren'sche Kontraktur) der palmarapo-neurose. In: Joachimsthals' *Handbuch der orthopädisc, Chirurgie*, Vol. 2, 43. Fischer, Jena.

König E (1940) Die Dupuytren'sche Kontraktur. *Med Klinik* **36**: 568.

König F Retrazione dell'aponevrosi palmare. In: *Trattato di Chirurgia Speciale*, 4th edn, Vol. 3, 198. Vallardi, Milano.

Korf K (1930) *Epithelcysten enstanden nach Humanolinjection bei Dupuytren'scher Fingerkontraktur.* Inaugural dissertation, Erlangen.

Koster S (1935) Un cas intéressant de rétraction bilatérale de l'aponévrose palmaire de Dupuytren. *Revue Neurologique* **63**: 281.

Koster S (1935) Caso non comune di contrattura di Dupuytren della fascia palmare di ambo le mani. *Neederlandsch tijdschrift voor Geneeskunde* **79**: 674.

Krecke (1913) Dupuytren'sche Kontraktur. *Münchener med Wochenschr* **60**: 2091.

Krigar K (1931) *Die Dupuytren'schen Fingerkontraktur.* Inaugural dissertation, Frankfurt.

Krinke J (1935) Cura cruenta ed incruenta della malattia di Dupuytren. *Zentralorgan Chir* **74**: 587.

Krogius A (1920) Neue Gesichspinkte zur Aetiologie der Dupuytren'schen Fingerkontraktur. *Zentralbl Chir* **47**: 914.

Krogius A (1922) Studii ed osservazioni sulla patogenesi della contrattura delle dita di Dupuytren. *Zentralbl Chir* **49**: 1489.

Krogius A (1922) Studii ed osservazioni sopra la patogenesi della contrattura delle dita di Dupuytren. *Zentralorg Chir* **15**: 381.

Kühn E (1937) *Die Dupuytren'sche Fingerkontraktur.* Inaugural dissertation, Düsseldorf.

Kurtzahn H, von Bulow W (1926) Praktische Erfahrungen mit einigen narbenlösenden Mitteln. *Deutsche Zeitschr Chir* **198**: 42.

Labbé M, Bourguignon G, Justin-Besançon L, Nepveux F (1934) Un cas de rétraction poly-aponévrotique (maladie de Dupuytren). Etudes des troublehumoraux et de la chronaxie. *Rev Rhum* **2**: 130.

Labeau (1909) Rétraction de l'aponévrose palmaire guérie par la radiotherapie. *Presse Médicale* **17**: 590.

Lacroix (1868) Considérations sur la flexion permanente des doigts. Thèse, Paris.

Lafora G (1916) La malattia di Dupuytren e la sua etiologia radicolitica o nevritica. *Revista clinica, Madrid* **7**: 451.

Laigne-Lavastine (1924) *Pathologie du Sympatique,* 529. Alcan Édit, Paris.

Laignel-Lavastine, Courbon P (1916) Campto-dactylie, causalgie et inversion du réflexe tricipital par lésion de la VII paire cervicale. *Neurologique* **6**: 927.

Laignel-Lavastine, Nogues G (1918) Maladie de Dupuytren unilatérale par lésion traumatique légère du cubital. *Presse Médicale* **26**: 278.

Laignel-Lavastine, Bonnard R, Gaultier M (1934) Syndrome de Cl. Bernard–Horner traumatique avec maladie de Dupuytren et anxiété parossystique par aérophagie. *Revue Neurologique* **62**: 784.

Lamarque (1925) Traitement röntgenthérapique de la maladie de Dupuytren. *J Radiol Electrol* **9**: 476–77.

Lambotte (1911) Un cas heureux d'intervention pour rétraction progressive de l'aponévrose palmaire. *Ann Soc Belge Chirurg* **11**: 201.

Lancereaux E (1883) Traité de l'herpétisme, 179. Paris.

Lancereaux E (1885) Phlegmasies prolifératives de l'aponévrose palmaire. *Traité d'anatomie pathologique,* Vol. 3, 324. Delahaye, Paris.

Lane WA (1886) Flexions of the fingers: Dupuytren's and some senile changes in joints. *Guy's Hospital Reports* **28**: 53.

Lange (1885) Zur Aetiologie der Dupuytren'schen Fingerkontraktur. *Virchow's Archiv* **102**: 220.

Langemak (1907) Zur Thiosinaminbehandlung der Dupuytren'schen Fascienkontraktur. *Münchener Med Wochenschr* **54**: 1380.

Langenbeck (1863) *Deutsche Klinik* **50**: 495.

Langhans (1887) in: Kocher TH, Behandlung der retraktion der Palmaraponeurose. *Zentralbl Chir* **14**: 481.

Laranza (1893) Rétraction de l'aponévrose palmaire améliorée par les boues de Dax. *J Méd Bordeaux,* 20 May.

Largillière L (1878) Essai sur la rétraction de l'aponévrose palmaire. Thèse, Paris.

Laurent O Retrazione dell'aponevrosi palmare. *Trattato di Anatomie clinica, Terapia chirurgica e Tecnica operatoria,* 3rd edn, 636. Vallardi, Milano.

Lavenant A (1920) Rétraction de l'aponévrose palmaire à la suite de plaies de guerre interessant le nerf cubital. *Revue Neurologique* **11**: 1176.

Lavenant A, Jonescu (1920) Sur deux cas de rétraction de l'aponévrose palmaire, à la suite de plaies de guerre intéressant le nerf cubital. *Revue Neurologique* **11**: 1176.

Lavenant A, Zislin J (1911) L'induration plastique des corps caverneux. *Ann malad organ genito-urin* **29**: 2088.

Lawrie WD (1907) A case of Dupuytren's contraction treated with fibrolysin. *Lancet* **172**: 882.

Lazarus P (1931) *Handbuch der Strahlentherapie,* Vol. 2. Bergmann, München.

Le Bec (1887) Rétraction de l'aponévrose palmaire; dissection de la bride fibreuse. *Gazette des Hop* **60**: 488.

Le Becq P (1928) Note sur la maladie de Dupuytren. Thèse, Paris.

Le Dentu Art: Main. *Diction de médec et de chir pratiques,* Vol. 21, 360.

Le Roy Steinberg C (1941) Vitamin E in the treatment of primary fibrositis. *Am J Med Sci* **201**: 347–49.

Lebon (1910) *Policlinico, sez prat* **17**: 1332.

Lechelle P, Baruk H, Donedy D (1927) Association de sclérodermie et de maladie de Dupuytren chez un spécifique. *Gazette Hop* **100**: 816.

Lecorché (1884) *Traité théorique et pratique de la goutte,* 369. Paris.

Ledderhose G (1894) Ueber Zerreisungen der Plantarfascie. *Arch Klin Chir* **48**: 853.

Ledderhose G (1897) Zur Pathologie der Aponevrose des Fusses und der Hand. *Arch Klin Chir* **55**: 694.

Ledderhose G (1920) Die Aetiologie der Fasciitis

palmaris (Dupuytren'scher Kontraktur). *Münchener med Wochenschr* **67**: 1254.

Legueu F, Juvara E (1892) Des aponévroses de la paume de la main. *Bull Soc Anat Paris* **6**: 383.

Lemoine-Maudet J (1832) Dissertation sur la rétraction permanente des doigts, ayant pour cause la rétraction de l'aponévrose palmaire. no. 1832/141, Thèse, Paris.

Lengemann (1903) Unblutige Behandlung der Dupuytren'schen Fingerkontraktur. *Zentrabl Chir* **30**: 985.

Lengemann P (1904) Zur Thiosinamin – Behandlung von Kontrakturen. *Deutsch med Wochenschr* **30**: 463.

Lepicard (1889) Nerveux et arthritiques. Thèse, Paris.

Leriche R (1940) Les algies diffusantes post-traumatiques. In: Leriche R, ed., *La chirurgie de la douleur*, 129–50. Masson, Paris.

Leriche R, Jung A (1930) Sur les relations de la rétraction de l'aponévrose palmaire, de l'hypo-calcémie et de l'insuffisance parathyroïdienne. *Presse Médicale* **38**: 1641.

Lévi L (1913) La rétraction de l'aponévrose palmaire et le traitement thyroïdien. *Bull Acad Méd* **69**: 23.

Lexer E (1907) Contrattura delle dita di Dupuytren. *Tratt di chirurgia generale*, Vol. 2, 222. Soc Editr, Libraria, Milano.

Lexer E (1931) *Die gesamte Wiedereherstellungschirurgie*, 2nd edn. Leipzig.

Licciardi S (1907) Un caso di morbo del Dupuytren. *Gazz Osped Clin* **28**: 1550.

Licciardi S (1912) Il morbo di Dupuytren. *Tommasi* **7**: 232.

Little Deformity from disease of the palmar fascia. In: Holmes, *A System of Surgery*, Vol. 3, 697 (cited by Vogt (1881)).

Lockwood CB (1885) Contracted fingers. *BMJ* **1299**: 967.

Lockwood CB (1890) Treatment of Dupuytren's finger contraction. *BMJ* **1526**: 722.

Lockwood CB (1893) Contraction of palmar fascia of gouty origin. *Lancet* **71**: 1386.

Lotheissen G (1900) Behandlung der Dupuytren'schen Kontraktur. *Wiener klinisch Wochenschr* **13**: 701.

Lotheissen G (1900) Zur operativen Behandlung der Dupuytren'schen Kontraktur. *Zentralabl Chirurg* **27**: 761.

Löwensberg (1906) *Ueber die Aetiologie der Dupuytren'schen Kontraktur.* Inaugural dissertation, Würzburg.

Löwy E (1923) Ein Beitrag zur Heredität der Dupuytren'schen Kontraktur. *Zentralbl inn Med*, **44**: 51.

Lubinau cited in Savarese E.

Lucas-Championnière (1888) Rétraction de l'aponévrose palmaire. *Bull Soc Chirurg* **14**: 265.

Lucke cited without bibliographical references in Friedrich PL and Canestro C.

Lund M (1941) Dupuytren's contracture and epilepsy. *Acta Psychiatr Scand* **16**: 465–82.

Lunedei A (1932) Morbo di Dupuytren. In: Ceconi A, *Trattato di Medicina interna*, Vol. 5, 740. Ediz Minerva Med, Torino.

Lusena G (1926) *Trattato di Traumatologia clinica*, 897. UTET, Torino.

Luzzatto M (1900) Sopra un caso di malattia di Dupuytren. *Boll Soc Lancisiana degli Ospedali di Roma* **20**: 182.

Lyle M (1922) The treatment of hand contracture. *Ann Surg* **76**: 121.

Macaggi D (1933) Veri e pseudo – Dupuytren in rapporto alla discussa etiogenesi traumatica di tale malattia. *Policlinico Sez Chir* **40**: 743.

Macready I (1890) On the treatment of Dupuytren's contraction of the palmar fascia. *BMJ* **1521**: 411.

MacWilliams CL (1904) Dupuytren's finger contraction. *New York State J Med* **80**: 673.

Madelung OW (1875) Die Aetiologie und die operative Behandlung der Dupuytren'schen Fingerverkrümmung. *Berlin-Klin Wochenschr* **12**: 191.

Madelung OW (1876) *The Causes and Operative Treatment of Dupuytren's Finger Contraction.* London (cited by Neutra (1901, 1903)).

Madelung OW (1878) Ueber die Operation der Dupuytren'schen Fingerverkrümmung. *Zentralbl Chir* **5**: 77.

Madelung OW (1886) Ueber eine der Dupuytren'schen Palmarkontraktur entsprechende Erkrankung der Planta. *Zentralbl Chir* **13**: 758.

Magnus G (1937) Beziehung zwischeri eiterigen Prozessen im Bereich des Armes und einer später beobachteten Dupuytren'schen Kontraktur. *Münchener Med Wochenschr* **84**: 1106.

Mailland (1905) Tuberculose infiammatoire, rétraction de l'aponévrose palmaire (maladie de Dupuytren) d'origine tuberculeuse. *Zentralbl Chir* **32**: 988.

Mainzer (1906) Ein Fall von Dupuytren'scher Kontraktur mit spinaltraumatische Aetiologie. *Münchener Med Wochenschr* **52**: 2155.

Maire R (1932) Contribution à l'étiologie nerveuse de

certaines rétractions de l'aponévrose palmaire. La maladie de Dupuytren d'origine nerveuse. Thèse, Paris.

Maisonneuve (1840) Post-mortem report. *Bull Soc Anat Paris* **15**: 77.

Malgaigne IF (1862) Déviations des doigts. *Leçons d'Orthopedie professées a la Faculté de Médecine de Paris*, 7. Delahaye, Paris.

Mangiavillani G (1896) Sopra un caso di retrazione dell'aponevrosi palmare. *Riforma Medica* **12**: 254.

Manson JS (1931) Heredity and Dupuytren's contraction. *BMJ* **3678**: 11.

Marchand (1938) Maladie de Dupuytren chez une mélancolique. *Ann médico-psycholog* **96**: 245.

Maréchal (1899) La rétraction de l'aponévrose palmaire chez les diabétiques. *Semaine Méd* **19**: 222.

Margarot, Castagné, Lafon (1933) Kératose palmaire, maladie de Dupuytren et syndrome sympathique cervicale postérieur. *Presse Médicale* **41**: 146.

Marion G (1917) Rétraction de l'aponévrose palmaire. *Manuel de Technique chirurgicale*, 4th edn, 102, 1070. Maloine, Paris.

Markovitz (1934) *Trattato di Röntgenterapia* (cited by Anzilotti (1935)).

Markus Antonius J (1927) *Untersuchungen über histologische und klinische befunde bei Dupuytren'scher Fingerkentraktur.* Inaugural dissertation, Tübingen.

Martenstein H (1921) Induratio penis plastica und Dupuytren'sche Kontraktur. *Medic Klinik* **17**: 44.

Marwedel P (1927) Zur traumatischen Genese der Dupuytren'schen Kontraktur. *Zentralbl Chirurg* **54**: 1246.

Masciotra AA (1925) Enfermedad de Dupuytren por causa traumatica. Estudio pericial. *La Semana Medica* **32**: 1615.

Maslieurat-Lagémard GE (1839) De l'anatomie descriptive et chirurgicale des aponévroses et des membranes synoviales de la main, de leur application à la thérapeutique et à la médecine opératoire. *Gazette Med Paris* **7**: 273–80.

Maslieurat-Lagémard GE (1840) Post-mortem report. *Bull Soc Anat Paris* **15**: 106.

Mason ML (1939) Dupuytren's contracture: plastic surgery of hands. *Surg Clinics of North America* **19**: 227.

Massarotti G (1928) Su di un caso di morbo di Dupuytren. *Giornale di Medicina militare* **76**: 600.

Mathieu, Josef (1922) Maladie de Dupuytren bilatéral. *Revue Médicale de l'Est* **50**.

Mauclaire PL (1913) Chirurgie générale et chirurgie orthopédique. In: Le dentu et Delbet, *Nouveau Traité de chirurgie*, Vol. 33, 128. Baillière, Paris.

Mauclaire PL (1934) Traitement chirurgical de la maladie de Dupuytren. *Bull Mém Soc Nat Chirurg Paris* **60**: 1174.

Maurer G (1936) Zur Lehre der Dupuytren'schen Palmarfascienkontraktur und ihre Behandlung. *Deutsche Zeitschr Chirurg* **246**: 685.

Mazzoni E (1934) Sul morbo di Dupuytren. *Gazz Osped e Cliniche* **55**: 1323.

Megis (1887) Maladie de Dupuytren. Paralysie générale. Arthritisme. *Gazette Méd Paris* (cited by Kölliker (1905–7)).

Meillet (1874) Des deformations permanentes de la main au point de vue de la séméiologie médicale. Thèse, Paris.

Mellin (1904) Thiosinaminjektionen bei Narbenkontrakturen. *Zentralbl Chir* **51**: 1471.

Mende (1919) Ein Fall von Dupuytren'scher Kontraktur nach einmaligen Trauma. *Mediz Klinik* **46**: 1172.

Menjaud AL (1861) De la rétraction spontanée et progrèssive des doigts dans les rapports avec la goutte et le rheumatisme goutteux. Thèse, Paris.

Mercari (1904) *Nuovo Raccoglitore Medico* (cited by Castellino Pende (1915)).

Merker (1897) *Die Dupuytren'sche Fingerkontraktur.* Inaugural dissertation, Berlin.

Merle P (1909) Maladie de Recklinghausen et rétraction de l'aponévrose palmaire. *Gazette Hop* **82**: 365.

Meyer W (1888) *New York Med Record* (cited by Antonioli (1927)).

Meyerding HW (1935) Dupuytren's contracture. *Proc Staff Meetings Mayo Clinic* **10**: 694.

Meyerding HW (1936) Dupuytren's contracture. *Arch Surg* **32**: 320.

Meyerding HW, Krusen FH (1936) Physical therapy in treatment of Dupuytren's contracture. *Physiotherapy Review* **16**: 42.

Meyerding HW, Overton LM (1935) Bilateral Dupuytren's contracture. *Proc Staff Meetings Mayo Clinic* **10**: 801.

Meyerding HW, Black JR, Broders AC (1936) The etiology and pathology of Dupuytren's contracture. *Surg Gynecol Obstet* 582–90.

Meyerding HW, Black JR, Broders AC (1941) The etiology and pathology of Dupuytren's contracture. *Surg Gynecol Obstet* **72**: 582–90.

Michaux J, Lamache A, Picard J (1925) La rétraction de l'aponévrose palmaire dans le saturnisme. *Presse Médicale* **33**: 702.

Miller AG (1893) Epilepsy and contraction of palmar fascia. *Lancet* **71**: 1203.

Mills CK (1884) A case of Dupuytren's contractions of the fingers. *Cincinnati Med News* (cited by Tranquilli (1892)).

Mingazzini (1905) Sulla patogenesi della malattia di Dupuytren. *Lavori Congressi Med Int, Roma* 233.

Momburg F (1920) Die Behandlung der Dupuytren'schen Fingerkontraktur. *Deutsche Med Wochenschr* **46**: 602.

Monier-Vinard, Delherm cited without bibliographical references in Palmer RG.

Monod CH, Vanverts J (1904) Retrazione dell'-aponevrosi palmare. *Trattato di Tecnica operatoria*, Vol. 1, 532. Soc Editr Libraria Milano.

Moore EJ (1898) *Orthopedic Surgery* (cited by Salaghi (1902)).

Moorhead (1910) Injury and Dupuytren's contraction. *Post-Graduate Med J* **24**: 789.

Morel Lavallée (1844) De la rétraction permanente des doigts. Thèse, Paris.

Morestin (1896) Rétraction de l'aponévrose palmaire. *Bull Soc Anat* **1**: 32.

Mori A (1928) Della malattia di Dupuytren e dei suoi rapporti etiopatogenetici col lavoro manuale. *Atti des 7° Congr Nazla di Medicina del Lavoro, Parma Modena Carpri*, 24–26 October 1927. Tip Cordani, Milano.

Moser E (1894) *Ueber die Dupuytren'sche Finger-kontraktur und deren Operation.* Inaugural dissertation, Berlin.

Moser E (1936) Einiges ueber Dupuytren'sche Fingerkontraktur. *Zentralbl Chir* **63**: 149.

Moure (1932) A propos de la maladie de Dupuytren. *Presse Médicale* **23**: 438.

Moure (1934) A propos de la maladie de Dupuytren. *Presse Médicale* **42**: 1885.

Moure P (1932) A propos de la maladie de Dupuytren. *Bull Mem Soc Nat Chir* **63**: 149.

Müller W (1930) Ueber Dupuytren'scher Finger-kontraktur. *Zentralbl Chir* **57**: 1103.

Muskat (1933) Dupuytren'sche Kontraktur und Beruf. *Zentralbl Chir* **40**: 987.

Myrtle AS (1881) Dupuytren's contraction of the fingers. *BMJ* **2**: 894.

Myrtle AS (1882) Contraction of palmar and plantar fasciae. *BMJ* **1**: 48.

Myrtle AS (1885) The treatment of Dupuytren's contraction of the palmar fascia. *BMJ* **1260**: 378.

Nalivkin L (1937) Sopra la contrattura di Dupuytren. *Zentralorgan Chir* **85**: 251.

Nélaton A (1859) Flexion permanente des doigts dépendant de la rétraction de l'aponévrose palmaire. *Élémens de Pathologie chirurgicale*, Vol. 5, 937. Germer-Baillière, Paris.

Nélaton A (1910) Rétraction de l'aponévrose palmaire. *Bull Mém Soc Chirurg, Paris* **36**: 319.

Neumark H (1906) Plastische Induration des Penis und Dupuytren'sche Kontraktur. *Berliner klinisch Wochenschr* 1483.

Neumark H (1906) *Plastische Induration des Penis.* Inaugural dissertation, Leipzig.

Neutra W (1901) Beitrag zur Aetiologie der Dupuytren'schen Fingerkontraktur. *Wiener klinisch Wochenschr* **14**: 907.

Neutra W (1901) Ueber die Dupuytren'sche Kontraktur, mit besonderer Berücksichtigung ihrer Beziehungen zu den inneren Erkrankungen. *Zentralbl Granzgebiete Med Chirurg* **4**: 737.

Neutra W (1903) Zwei Fälle von Dupuytren'scher Fingerkontraktur bei Tabes, resp. Tabes mit multipler Sklerose. *Wiener klinisch Wochenschr* **16**: 42.

Nicaise (1873) De troubles trophiques des tendons extenseurs de la main et de leurs gaînes, consecutifs aux paralysies du nerf radial. *Gazette Méd Paris* **2**: 458.

Nicaise (1874) Flexion permanent des doigts. *Bull Soc Anat Paris* (cited by Neutral (1901, 1903)).

Nichols JB (1899) A clinical study of Dupuytren's contraction of the palmar and digital fascia. *Am J Med Sci* **27**: 285.

Nichols JB (1899) The hystologie of Dupuytren's contacture of the palmar fascia. *Med News* **75**: 491.

Nicolesco I, Hornet T, Runcan V (1933) A propos de la maladie de Dupuytren. *Revue Neurologique* **1**: 283.

Niedergang (1911) Fibrome fasciculé de la main. *Bull Mém Soc Anat Paris* **10**: 706.

Niederland W (1932) Dupuytren'sche Kontraktur und Beruf. *Archiv Gewerbepathol Gewerbehygiene* **3**: 23.

Niederland W (1933) Die traumatische Aetiologie der Dupuytren'scher Kontraktur. *Arch orthopäd UnfallChirurg* **32**: 651.

Niederland W (1933) Dupuytren'sche Fingerkontraktur als Unfallfolge. *Mediz Klinik* **29**: 614.

Niederland W (1933) Dupuytren'sche Kontraktur und Beruf. *Medizinische Welt* **7**: 126.

Niederland W (1933) Dupuytren'sche Kontraktur und Beruf. *Zentralbl Chir* **60**: 985.

Niederland W (1935) Zur Frage der Dupuytren'schen Fingerkontraktur. *Zentralbl Chir* **62**: 2238.

Niederland W (1936) Die Dupuytren'sche Finger-kontraktur als Berufskrankheit. *Jahreskurse ärztl Fortbildung* **27**: 60.

Niehues (1927) Die traumatische Entstehung der Dupuytren'schen Fingercontractur. *Aerztliche Sachverständig – Zeitung* **33**: 250.

Nijkerk M (1939) Iontophoresis in treatment of keloids, Dupuytren's contracture and scleroderma. *Neederlandsch tijdschrift vor Geneeskunde* **83**: 5135.

Nippert (1929) Konstitution, Stoffwechsel und Dupuytren'sche Kontraktur. *Deutche Zeitschtr Chirurg* **216**: 289.

Noica D, Parvulescu N (1932) Patogenesi della malattia di Dupuytren. *Revista Sanitaria Militara, Bucarest* **31**: 3.

Noica D, Parvulescu N (1932) Sur l'étiologie nerveuse de la maladie de Dupuytren. *Revue Neurologique* **1**: 703.

Noica D, Arama O, Parvulescu N, Lupulescu J (1936) Nuovi dati sulla patogenesi della contrattura di Dupuytren. *Revista Sanitaria Militara, Bucarest* **35**: 512.

Noica D, Arama O, Lupulescu J, Stroesco G (1937) Contrattura di Dupuytren bilaterale dovuta a lesione del nervo cubitale al terzo distale dell'antibraccio. *Romania Medicale* **15**: 261.

Nole cited without bibliographical references in Tichet H.

Norsa G (1934) Retrazione dell'aponevrosi palmare e sclerodermia. *Gazz Ospedali Cliniche* **55**: 1285.

Occhini F Aponevrotomia. *Trattato di Medicina operatoria*, 2nd edn, Vol. 2, 97. Vallardi, Milano.

Oehlecker F (1930) Demonstration für Dupuytren'schen Fingercontractur. *Zentralorgan Chir* **50**: 122.

Oehlecker F (1930) Ueber Dupuytren'sche Fingerkontraktur. *Brun's Beiträge klinisch Chirurg* **149**: 333.

Oehlecker F (1930) Ueber Dupuytren'sche Fingerkontraktur. *Zentralbl Chir* **18**: 1102.

Ollier A (1929) Puede considerarse la contractura de Dupuytren accidente del trabajo? *Ars Medica* **5**: 96.

Oppenheim H (1904) Contrattura palmare di Dupuytren. In: *Trattato delle Malattie nervose*, 3rd edn, Vol. 1, 413. Soc Editr Libraria Milano.

Orbach E (1932) Ueber die Therapie der Dupuytren'schen Fingerkontraktur. *Med Welt* **6**: 955.

Orbach E (1934) Die funktionelle Behandlung der Dupuytren'schen Fingerkontraktur. *Archiv orthop Unfall – Chirurg* **34**: 572.

Orel H (1931) Kleine Beiträge zur Vererbung-swissenschaft. *Zentralbl allg Path path Anat* **52**: 165.

Oshinsky S (1928) *Behandlung der Dupuytren'schen Kontraktur*. Inaugural dissertation, Berlin.

Paalzow (1899) Die Aponeurositis palmaris der Schumacher. *Monatschr Unfallheilleunde* **6**: 13.

Pacifico A (1930) Sindrome radicolare ed ipertrofia delle apofisi trasverse della VII vertebra cervicale. *Riv Patologia Nervosa e Mentale* **35**: 297.

Pacifico A (1938) Importanza di alcuni processi morbosi del rachide cervicale nella patogenesi della sindrome di Dupuytren. *Rassegna di Neurologia vegetativa* **1**: 34.

Padula F (1903) Morbo del Dupuytren. In: *Anatomi chir degli Arti*, Vol. 1, *Arto Super*, 506. Soc Ed Dante Alighieri, Roma.

Paget I (1875) On the minor signs of gout in the hands and feet. *BMJ* **751**: 665.

Paillard, Marx (1831) *J univ hébdom* **5**: 349.

Palmen AJ (1932) Die Sageplastik, eine unter anderen für Dupuytrensche Fingerkontraktur und Syndactylie geeignete Schnittführung. *Zentralbl Chir* **59**: 1377.

Palmer RG (1932) Rupture, par un retour de manivelle, d'une bride aponévro-cutanée de maladie de Dupuytren. *Ann Anat pathol Anat chirurg* **9**: 441.

Palmer RG (1933) Maladie de Dupuytren: rétraction de l'aponévrose palmaire. *Gazette Hop* **106**: 1369.

Pancrazio F (1933) Affezioni reumatiche e parareumatiche. *La specializzazione delle Terme di Viterbo*, 172. Ediz OND, Roma.

Papanti P (1929) Il morbo di Dupuytren nei rapporti col lavoro e considerazioni sulla etiologia. *Comunicaz all'8° Congr Med Lavoro, Napoli*.

Pardo Castello V (1932) Contraction of palmar aponeurosis (Dupuytren's disease). *Acta Dermato-venereologica* **13**: 649.

Parhon C, Goldstein M (1902) Sur un cas de pellagre accompagné de la rétraction de l'aponévrose palmaire. *Revue Neurologique* **10**: 555.

Parhon C, Goldstein M (1905) Sur un noveau cas de pellagre accompagné de la rétraction de l'aponévrose palmaire. *Revu Méd* **25**: 620.

Parhon C, Toupa A (1920) Sur deux cas de rétraction de l'aponévrose palmaire à la suite de plaies de guerre intéressant le nerf cubital. *Revue Neurologique* **11**: 1176.

Partridge (1854) Cast of the left hand of a middle-aged man and also a dissection of the same hand to show a contraction of the little finger. *Trans Pathol Soc London* **5**: 343.

Partsch (1933) Therapie der Dupuytren'schen Fingerkontraktur. *Zentralbl Chir* **60**: 2215.

Pascalis G (1913) Note sur deux cas de maladie de Dupuytren. *Bull Mém Soc Anat Paris* **15**: 285.

Paulian D (1926) Contribution à l'étude de la rétraction de l'aponévrose palmaire. *Revue Neurologique* **1**: 74.

Payr E (1922) Pepsin und Trypsin zur Narbenerweichung. *Zentralbl Chir* **49**: 1024.

Payr E (1922) Praktische Erfahrungen mit der Pepsin-Pregl-Lösung zur Narbenerweichung und Wiederbildung von Gleitgewebe usw. *Arch Klinisch Chirurg* **121**: 106.

Payr E (1922) Ueber eine keimfreie, kolloidale Pepsinlösung zur Narbenerweichung, Verhütung und Lösung von Verklebungen. *Zentralbl Chir* **49**: 2.

Peiser A (1917) Freie Fettransplantation bei der Behandlung der Dupuytren'schen Finger-kontraktur. *Zentralbl Chir* **44**: 6.

Perdrizet (1904) Rétraction de l'aponévrose palmaire d'origine tuberculeuse. Thèse, Lyon.

Perez G (1938) Malattia di Dupuytren. *Trattato di Patologia chirurgica*, Vol. 3, 277. Stamperia Reale, Roma.

Perrero E (1904) Contributo anatomopatologico alla conoscenza del morbo di Dupuytren. *Giornale R Acad Med Torino* **67**: 456.

Perrero E (1904) Contributo anatomopatologico alla patogenesi del morbo di Dupuytren. *Comunicaz al 12° Congr Soc Freniatrica Ital, 8 seduta, Genova.*

Perrero E (1905) Contributo alla patogenesi del morbo di Dupuytren. *Archiv Psichiatria, Neuropatologia, Antropologia criminale a Medicina legale* **26**: (Neuropatologia) 467.

Perséguers (1923) La maladie de Dupuytren. Thèse, Bordeaux.

Perussia F (1934) Il morbo di Dupuytren. *Trattato di Röntgen- e di Curieterapia*, Vol. 2, 774. Treves, Milano.

Peugnier P, Joly (1923) Rétraction de l'aponévrose palmaire guérie par la radiothérapie pénétrante. *Bull Acad Méd Paris* **89**: 35.

Picard I (1927) Quelques données sur la maladie de Dupuytren. *Vie Médicale* **8**: 225.

Picard I (1938) Maladie de Dupuytren chez une melancolique. *Ann médico-psychologiques* **9**: 245.

Picaza S (1938) Historia de la medicina; los grandes maestros de la cirugìa: el Baròn de Dupuytren. *Rev med Habana* **43**: 9.

Piéchaud, Laranza (1895) Rétraction de l'aponévrose palmaire traitée et améliorée par l'application locale de boues thermales. *Bull Mém Soc Méd Chir, Bordeaux.*

Pieraccini G (1906) Malattia del Dupuytren. In: *Patologia del lavoro e terapia sociale*, 577. Soc Editr Libraria Milano.

Pieri G (1920) Plastica cutanea per la retrazione cicatriziale delle dita. *Chirurgia Organi Movimento* **4**: 303.

Pierre J (1882) Sur la rétraction de l'aponévrose palmaire. Thèse, Paris.

Pilon A (1936) Deux obsérvations sur la maladie de Dupuytren. *J Hôtel-Dieu Montréal* **5**: 75.

Pistolese F (1921) Contributo su la contrattura palmare di Dupuytren. *Studium (Riv Scienza Med)* **11**: 138.

Pitaud P (1909) Opération sans suture, sans autoplastie dans le traitement chirurgical de la rétraction de l'aponévrose palmaire. Thèse, Paris.

Pitha, Billroth (1873) Retrazione dell'aponevrosi palmare. *Enciclopedia di Patologia chirurgica generale e speciale*, Vol. 1, 136. Pasquale, Napoli.

Plater F (1614) *Observationes in Hominis Affectibus*, Vol. 3. König and Brandmyller, Basel.

Plater F (1624) Plateri Felicis observationum in hominis affectibus ecc.; liber primus. *Basileae*, 149.

Poinso R, Recordier M, Sarradon P (1935) Algies post-zonateuses avec troubles de la pigmentation cutanée; rétraction bilatérale de l'aponévrose palmaire. *Marseille Méd* **72**: 20.

Poirier P, Charpy A (1899) *Traité d'anatomie humaine*, Vol. 2. Masson, Paris.

Polaillon (1886) Induration plastique du pénis – rétraction de l'aponévrose. *L'Union Médicale de Paris* **42**: 1–3.

Polaillon (1887) Main: *Dictionnaire éncyclopèdique des Sciences Méd.* Union Médicale.

Policaro RD (1937) Su di un caso di induratio penis plastica associata a retrazione dell'aponevrosi palmare o malattia del Dupuytren. *Giornale Med Alto Adige* **15**: 13.

Pommé B, Tricault G, Lubineau J (1931) Au sujet d'une étiologie possible du syndrome de la maladie de Dupuytren. *Revue Neurologique* **38**: 633.

Poncet A (1904) Rhumatisme tuberculeux abarticulaire; rétraction de l'aponévrose palmaire d'origine tuberculeuse. *Ann Chir Orthopéd* **3**.

Poncet A (1909) Rétraction bilatérale de l'aponévrose palmaire d'origine tuberculeuse. *Bull Mém Soc Chirurg* **467**: 1909.

Poncet A (1911) Rétraction bilatérale de l'aponévrose palmaire (rétraction d'origine tuberculeuse). *Gazette Hop* **84**: 592.

Portius W (1936) *Untersuchungen zur Frage der Dupuytren'schen Fingerkontraktur und des muskulären Schiefhalses.* Inaugural dissertation, Kiel.

Portret, Desplas (1933) Au sujet de la maladie de Dupuytren: technique chirurgicale et radiologique. *Presse Médicale* **41**: 257.

Post C (1876) On contraction of the palmar fascia, and of the sheats of the flexor tendons. *Arch Clin Surg* (August).

Powers H (1931) New light on cause of Dupuytren's contracture and possibility of its treatment by physiotherapy. *Am J Physic Therapy* **8**: 239.

Powers H (1934) Dupuytren's contracture 100 years after Dupuytren: its interpretation. *J Nervous Mental Dis* **80**: 386.

Pozzi (1877) Rétraction de l'aponévrose palmaire. *Progrès Médical* **19**.

Pozzilli P (1908) Contributo clinico alla malattia di Dupuytren. *Gazzetta Osped Cliniche* **29**: 978.

Previtera A (1933) Morbo di Dupuytren e terapia paratiroidea. *Atti Soc Ital Chirurgia 40 Congr, Pavia*, 578.

Pribram A (1902) Die Dupuytren'sche contractur. In: Nothnagel, *Spez Pathologie und Therapie, Vol. 7*, 144 (*cronischer Gelenkrheumatismus und Osteoarthritis deformans*). Hölder, Wien.

Quenu (1918) Société de Chirurgie séance du 24 juin 1918. In: Palmer RG (1933) Maladie de Dupuytren: rétraction de l'aponévrose palmaire. *Gazette Hop* **106**: 1369.

Rahm H (1922) Die Morestin'sche Plastik bei Fingerkontrakturen. *Brun's Beiträge klinisch Chirurgie* **127**: 214.

Ramstedt (1933) Zur Operation der Dupuytren'schen Fingerkontraktur. *Zentralbl Chir* **60**: 2214.

Redard P (1892) Rétraction de l'aponévrose palmaire. *Traité pratique de chirurgie orthopédique*, 488. Doin, Paris.

Reeves HA (1881) Remarks on the contraction of the palmar and plantar fascia. *BMJ* **2**: 1649.

Reeves HA (1885) The rapid cure of Dupuytren's contraction by excision. *BMJ* **1262**: 481.

Régis (1887) Maladie de Dupuytren, paralysie générale, arthritisme. *Gazette Méd Paris* (décembre) 582.

Regnault F (1931) Sur le début de la maladie de Dupuytren par la cellulite. *Gazette Hop* **104**: 555.

Reichel (1916) Dupuytren'schen Fingerkontraktur als Folge von Verletzung des Nervus ulnaris. *Deutsche Zeitsch Chir* **138**: 466.

Reichel (1925) Zur Aetiologie der Dupuytren'schen Fingerkontraktur. *Zentralbl Chir* **52**: 713.

Reichel (1931) Zur Aetiologie der Dupuytren'schen Fingerkontraktur. *Deutsche Zeitschr Chirurg* **230**: 291.

Reichel E (1937) Zur Operation der Dupuytren'schen Kontraktur. *Zentralbl Chir* **64**: 1570.

Reichel E (1939) Zur Aetiologie der Dupuytren'schen Kontraktur. *Wiener klinische Wochenschr* **52**: 315.

Reid I (1836) Permanent flexion of the fingers from shortening and thickening of the palmar aponeurosis. *Edinburgh Med Surg J* **46**: 74.

Rémy C (1877) Endocardite végétante des valvules mitrale et tricuspide – rétraction de l'aponévrose palmaire par traumatisme. *Bull Soc Anat Paris* **4s 2**: 275–77.

Rey I (1927) Die orthopädische Behandlung der Hand- und Fingerkontrakturen. *Zeitschr orthop Chir* **48**: 21.

Reynes (1919) Maladie de Dupuytren et sclérose rétractile des coulisses synovio-tendineuses. *Gazette Hop* **92**: 1154.

Richer P (1877) Rétraction de l'aponévrose palmaire. *Bull Mém Soc Anat, Paris* **2**: 124.

Richon, Kissel, Simonin I (1933) Maladie de Dupuytren et troubles nerveux associés. *Revue Méd l'Est* **61**: 231.

Rickel R cited without bibliographical references in Ebstein W.

Riedinger (1898) Bemerkungen zum Knochenbefund in der Plantarfascie. *Zentralbl Chir* **25**: 693.

Riedl L (1939) 30 beobachtete Fälle Dupuytren'schen Kontraktur in der zeit von 1932 bis 1938. *Zentralbl Chir* **66**: 1093.

Ringel (1930) Ueber Dupuytren'scher Fingerkontraktur. *(Discussione) Zentralbl Chir* **57**: 1103.

Rinné (1888) Ueber eine seltene Aetiologie der Dupuytren'schen Fingerkontraktur. *Deutsche Med Wochenschr* **14**: 761.

Ritter C (1930) Dupuytren'sche Fingerkontraktur. *Zentralbl Chir* **22**: 1356.

Ritter C (1930) Zur operativen Behandlung der Dupuytren'schen Fingerkontraktur. *Deutsche Zeitschr Chirurg* **227**: 544.

Roasenda G (1926) Malattia di Dupuytren e fisiopatia (Malattia di Dupuytren di origine simpatica). *Minerva Medica* **6**: 768.

Roasenda G (1939) Sulla anatomie patologica e sull'etiopatogenesi della malattia del Dupuytren. *Giornale R Acad Med Torino* **102**.

Rocher cited without bibliographical references in Testi A.

Rodrigues, Villegas R, Brachetto, Brian D (1930)

Rétracción de la aponeurosis palmar superficial: enfermedad de Dupuytren. *Bol trabaj Soc cirugìa Buenos Aires* **14**: 809.

Roeckel (1883) Dupuytren's contraction in a female. *Lancet* **i**: 412.

Roedelius E (1930) Fingergangrän nach Operation Dupuytren'scher Kontrakturen. *Zentralbl Chir* **57**: 936.

Roepke (1911) Dupuytren'sche Fingerkontraktur. *Münchener Med Wochenschr* **58**: 1108.

Rogues de Fursac (1892) Traitement de la rétraction de l'aponévrose palmaire par l'autoplastie (méthode italienne modifiée). Thèse, Paris.

Ronneaux G, Desgraz H (1933) Jonotherapie et maladie de Dupuytren. *Présse Médicale* **41**: 548.

Roos J (1926) Zur Frage der Fettgewebsverflüssigung und der Narbenerweichung. Experimentelle Studien über Pepsinwirkung. *Zentralbl Chir* **52**: 2136.

Roque PE (1872) De la rétraction de l'aponévrose palmaire. no. 1872/414, Thèse, Paris.

Rosch (1891) *Ueber die Dupuytren'sche Fingerkontrakur. Beiträge zur Kasuistik der Fingerkontrakturen und ihrer Therapie.* Inaugural dissertation, Strassburg.

Rosemburg G (1926) Dupuytren'sche Contractur und Unfall. *Monatschr Unfallheilk Versicherungsmediz* **33**: 97.

Roth PB (1919) Dupuytren's contraction in a young man following injury. *Proc Roy Soc Med* **13**: 227.

Roth PB (1928) Dupuytren's contracture, after operation. *Proc Roy Soc Med* **21**: 10.

Roudnew (1909) Maladie de Dupuytren. *Nouvelle Iconogr Salpétrière* **22**: 267.

Rouillard J, Schwob RA (1931) Rétraction des aponévroses palmaires et plantaires; coexistence des gros troubles sensitifs du type syringomiélique. *Bull Mém Soc Hop Paris* **347**: 712.

Roussy G, Levy G, Rosenrauch C (1932) L'origine médullaire de certaines rétractions de l'aponévrose palmaire. *Ann Méd* **31**: 21.

Routier (1908) Rétraction de l'aponévrose palmaire. Opération sans suture sans autoplastie. *Bull Mem Soc Chirurg Paris* **34**: 860.

Routier (1913) Rétraction de l'aponévrose palmaire; opération sans suture, sans autoplastie. *Bull Mém Soc Chirurg* **9**: 387.

Rubénovitch (1938) Maladie de Dupuytren chez une mélancolique. *Ann médico-psycologiques* **96**: 245.

Rugh IT (1922) Operation for Dupuytren's contracture. *Ann Surg* **75**: 505.

Ruiz Moreno A (1936) Enfermedad de Dupuytren y dedo a resorte. *Semana Médica* **43**: 939.

Russ R (1908) The surgical aspects of Dupuytren's contraction. *Am J Med Sci* **135**: 856.

Sabatier (1849) Causes diagnostic et traitement de la flexion permanente des doigts. Thèse, Paris.

Sachs O (1907) Beiträge zur Pathologie der Induratio penis plastica. *Archiv Dermatol Syphilis* **85**: 53.

Sachs O (1911) Plastische Induration des Corpus cavernosum Penis. *Handbuch Geschlechtskrank.* Hölder, Wien.

Sajdova V (1932) Etiology of Dupuytren's contracture, with report of case. *Revue Neurol Psychiatr* **29**: 188.

Sajdova V (1933) Contracture de Dupuytren. *Revue Neurologique* 187.

Salaghi M (1902) Contributo allo studio della retrazione dell'aponevrosi palmare (contrattura di Dupuytren). 4° *Congr Pediatrico Ital, Firenze, 1901*, 375. Tip Nicolai, Firenze.

Salaghi M (1902) Della contrattura di Dupuytren o retrazione dell'aponevrosi palmare. *Archivo di Ortopedia*, **19**: 32.

Salaghi M (1902) Sulla contrattura di Dupuytren o retrazione dell'aponevrosi palmare. *Rivista Critica Clin med* **3**: 550.

Salvolini U (1907) Morbo di Dupuytren contributo anatomopatologico. *Annuario del Manicomio provinc di Ancona*, Vol. 4–5, 1906–07, 93. Tip Economica, Ancona.

Sand (1907) *La simulation et l'interpretation des accidents du travail*, 190. Paris (cited by Mori (1928)).

Sanson JL (1834) Rapport sur le mémoire de Goyrand. *Mem Acad R Med* **4**: 497–500.

Sanson JL (1834) Rapport sur le mémoire du Dr G Goyrand 'Nouvelles recherches sur la rétraction permanente des doigts' *Mem Acad R Med* **3**: 496–500.

Sanson JL, Breschet G (1834) Rapport sur le mémoire de Goyrand. *Gaz Med Paris* **2**: 219.

Sauerbruch F (1933) Dupuytren'sche Kontraktur und Beruf. *Zentralbl Chir* **40**: 988.

Sauerbruch F, Dankelmann A (1938) Zur chirurgichen Behandlung einiger Typen von Fingerkontrakturen. *Arch Ital Chirurg* **54**: 502.

Savarese E (1894) La malattia di Dupuytren. *Clinica chirurgica* **11**: 583.

Savory W (1894) A lecture on gout in some of its relations with surgery. *Lancet* **i**: 75.

Schaefer V (1933) Die traumatische Aetiologie der Dupuytren'scher Kontraktur. *Arch orthopäd Unfall – Chirurg* **32**: 651.

Schaefer V (1936) Die Genese der Dupuytren'schen Kontraktur. Die Bedeutung der Anlage, des kronischen Trauma und des Unfalles. *Zentralbl Chir* **63**: 1712.

Schaeffer E (1902) Ueber subkutane Muskelrisse und deren Folgezustände nebst Bemerkungen ueber die Aetiologie der Dupuytren'schen Strangkontraktur. *Vierteljahrschr Mediz Sanitäatsw* **23**: 268.

Schlesinger H (1901) *Die Syringomyelie*, 2nd edn. Wien.

Schlesinger H (1901) Syringomyelie mit seltener Symptomen. *Neurol Centralbl* **20**: 826.

Schlosser (1932) Dupuytren'sche Erkrankung begünstigt durch Diabetes mellitus. *Münchener Med Wochenschr* **79**: 1238.

Schmidt (1889) *Ueber die Dupuytren'sche Palmarfascienkontraktur*. Inaugural dissertation, Würzburg.

Schmidt G (1935) *Ein Beitrag zu den Ergebnissen der Behandlung bei Dupuytren'scher Kontraktur*. Inaugural dissertation, Berlin.

Schmieden V, Ficher AW, Ufreduzzi O (1938) Estirpazione dell'aponevrosi palmare. *Manuale di operazioni chirurgiche*, 3rd edn, 214. UTET, Torino.

Schnitzler O (1934) Ueber den Einfluss der Brufsarbeit auf die Entwicklung der Dupuytren'schen Kontraktur. *Münchener Med Wochenschr* **80**: 1558.

Schnitzler O (1935) Bedeutung von Berufs- und Sportsschäden bei Morbus Dupuytren. *Münchener Med Wochenschr* **82**: 248.

Schoenals (1919) *Die Dupuytren'sche Fingerkontraktur*. Inaugural dissertation, Berlin.

Scholle W (1930) Ueber die Dupuytren'sche Finger-kontraktur unter besonderer Berücksichtigung ihres Vorkommens bei Jugendlichen. *Deutsche Zeitschr Chirurg* **223**: 328.

Schönborn C (1870) Eine neue Maschine zur allmäligen Streckung von Contracturen der Finger. *Langenbeck's Arch klinisch Chirurg* **12**: 371.

Schörcher F (1937) Die Kontraktur der Palmara-poneurose: Dupuytren'sche Fingerkontraktur. *Münchener Med Wochenschr* **84**: 873.

Schröder CH (1933) Erblichkeit der Dupuytren'schen Kontraktur. *Zentralbl Chir* **60**: 2214.

Schröder CH (1934) Berufsarbeit und Trauma bei der Dupuytren'schen Kontraktur. *Deutsch Zeitschr Chirurg* **244**: 140.

Schröder CH (1934) Der Erbgang der Dupuytren'schen Kontraktur. *Zentralbl Chir* **61**: 1056.

Schröder CH (1934) Der Erhgang der Dupuytren's-chen Kontraktur. *Zentralbl Chir* **61**: 1193.

Schröder CH (1934) Dupuytren'sche Kontraktur und Trauma. *Arch orthop unfall-Chirurg* **35**: 125.

Schröder CH (1935) Dupuytren'sche Kontraktur und Trauma. *Zentralbl Chir* **62**: 59.

Schröder CH (1937) Die Vererbung der Dupuytren'sche Fingerkontraktur. *Monatschr Unfallheilk* **44**: 162.

Schubert A (1923) Die Aetiologie der Dupuytren'schen Contractur. *Deutsch Zeitschr Chirurg* **177**: 362.

Schubert A (1927) Dupuytren'sche Kontraktur und Unfall. *Med Klinik* **23**: 549.

Schule cited without bibliographical references in Policaro RD.

Schulthess (1888) *Ein Beitrag zur pathologischen Anatomie der Dupuytren'schen Palmarfascienkontraktur*. Inaugural dissertation, Nördlingen.

Schulz H (1879) *Zur Aetiologie der Verkrümmung des 4 Fingers*. Inaugural dissertation, Marburg.

Schulz H (1888) Aetiologie der Dupuytren'schen Fingerkontraktur. *Deutsch med Wochenschr* **14**: 761.

Schuster P (1913) Zur Differentialdiagnose der Fingerkontrakturen. *Berliner klinisch Wochenschr* **25**: 1161.

Schwalbach (1908) Dupuytren'sche Kontraktur. *Zentralbl Chir* **35**: 652.

Sciamanna E (1893) Malattia di Dupuytren. In: Cantani, Maragliano, *Trattato Ital di patologia e terapia medica*, Vol. 2, 89. Vallardi, Milano.

Sédillot CH, Legouest L (1870) Aponévrotomie. *Traité de Médecine opératoire*, Vol. 1, 627. Baillière, Paris.

Senator H (1898) Zwei Fälle von Tabes dorsalis. Tabesfus und Tabes mit Dupuytren'scher Sehnenkontraktur. *Berliner klinisch Wochenschr* **35**: 633.

Serstov F (1929) È la contrattura di Dupuytren una malattia del lavoro. *Zentralorgan Chir* **46**: 534.

Sevestre A (1867) Note sur un cas de rétraction permanente des doigts. *J Anat Physiol norm patholog* **4**: 249.

Shaunann (1938) Uber die pathogenese des lupus erythematosus. *Acta Derm Venereol* **1**: 545.

Sicard A (1926) Traitement de la maladie de Dupuytren. *Gazette Hop* **99**: 418.

Sicard A (1930) A propos de la maladie de Dupuytren. *Presse Médicale* **38**: 1031.

Sicilano L (1906) Gli atteggiamenti viziati delle mani nei loro rapporti colla neuropatologia. *Rivista Critica Clin Med* **7**: 379.

Silva FL (1926) Malattia di Dupuytren: caso clinico della stessa. *Zentralorgan Chir* **23**: 75.

Simon (1937) Dupuytren'sche Fingerkontraktur. *Zentralbl Chir* **64**: 2597.

Skinner HL (1941) Dupuytren's contraction. Operative correction by use of tunnel skin graft. *Surgery* **10**: 313.

Sluys (1925) Traitement röntgenthérapique de la maladie de Dupuytren. *J Radiol Electrol* **9**: 476–77.

Smend H (1911) *Ueber einen Fal von Knochenbildung im menschlichen Penis, in Verbindung mit doppelseitiger Dupuytren'schen Kontraktur der III und IV Finger.* Inaugural dissertation, Leipzig.

Smith KD, Masters WE (1939) Dupuytren's contraction among upholsters. *J Ind Hygiene Toxicol* **21**: 97.

Smith N (1884) Dupuytren's contraction. *Lancet* **i**: 565.

Smith N (1885) Seventy cases of Dupuytren's contraction of the palmar fascia. *BMJ* **1258**: 275.

Smith N (1885) The treatment of Dupuytren's contraction of the palmar fascia. *BMJ* **1260**: 378.

Smith N (1885) The treatment of Dupuytren's contraction of the palmar fascia. *BMJ* **1268**: 781.

Smith N (1890) Treatment of Dupuytren's finger contraction. *BMJ* **1526**: 722.

Solomon J (1926) Maladie de Dupuytren. *Précis de Radiotherapie profonde*, 425, Masson, Paris.

Solomon J, Bisson, A, Gibert P (1925) Le traitement röntgenthérapique de la maladie de Dupuytren. *J Radiol Electrol* **9**: 476.

Sommer (1933) Die traumatische Aetiologie der Dupuytren'schen Kontraktur. *Arch orthopäd unfall – Chirurg* **32**: 651.

Sonntag (1921) Ueber induratio penis plastica nebst einen Bitrag zu ihrer operativen Behandlung. *Langenbeck's Arch klinisch Chirurg* **117**: 612.

Sonntag *Grundriss der gesamte Chirurgie* (cited by Scholle (1930)).

Southam FA (1882) Contraction of the palmar fascia. *BMJ* **1**: 86.

Souza, Leite (1886) Rétraction de l'aponéurose palmaire et de l'aponéurose plantaire. Rheumatisme articulaire. Afféction cardiaque. *Progrès Médical* **40**: 816.

Sovetow N (1932) La contrattura delle dita di Dupuytren e la sua dipendenza dal mestiere. *Zentralorg Chir* **59**: 390.

Spaak cited without bibliographical references in Sonntag.

Spandri P (1903) Sull'ulcera perforante della mano. *Rivista Veneta Scienze Med* **20**: 440.

Specklin P, Stoeber R (1922) Rétraction des aponévroses palmaires et plantaires avec névralgie:

guérison par les radiations. *Presse Médic* **30**: 743.

Spitzky H (1915) Behandlung von Hand – unf Fingerkontrakturen mit Künstlicher Fettumscheidung. *Zeitschr orthopäd Chirurg* **35**: 550.

Sprogis G (1926) Beitrag zur Lehre von der Vererbung der Dupuytren'schen Fingerkontraktur. *Deutsche Zeitschr Chirurg* **194**: 259.

Stackebrandt H (1932) *Die Heredität bei der Dupuytren'schen Kontraktur, dargestellt an 5 Stammbäumen.* Inaugural dissertation, Münster.

Stahnke E (1927) Zur Behandlung der Dupuytren'schen Fingerkontraktur. *Zentralbl Chir* **54**: 2438.

Stegemann (1933) Therapie der Dupuytren'schen Kontraktur. *Zentralbl Chir* **60**: 2216.

Stein RO (1909) Induratio penis plastica und Dupuytren'sche Kontraktur. *Wiener klinisch Wochenschr* **22**: 1821.

Steindl (1926) Behandlung der Dupuytren'schen Kontraktur. *Zentralbl Chir* **53**: 724.

Stejskal (1924) Dupuytren'sche Kontraktur: Proteintherapie. *Wiener klinisch Wochenschr* **37**: 605.

Stephenson SHA (1885) Hereditary transmission of Dupuytren's contraction. *BMJ* **1263**: 536.

Stetter (1880) Erfahrungen im Gebiete der praktischen Chirurgie. *Deutsche Zeitschr Chirurg* **14**: 50.

Stiber (1911) *Medizin Klinik* (edited by Mauclaire (1913, 1914)).

Stiefler G (1910) Dupuytren'sche Kontraktur. *Wiener klinisch Wochenschr* **32**: 1192.

Stiefler G (1911) Die Dupuytren'sche Kontraktur als trophische Störung im Symptomenbilde einer Tabes dorsalis. *Zeitschr orthopäd Chir* **28**: 606.

Stoppato U (1923) Fibroma della palma della mano. *Tumori* **9**: 31.

Strong cited without bibliographical references in Binda P.

Stuparich (1898) Symmetrische Dupuytren'sche Kontraktur am kleinen Finger. *Wiener med Presse* **2**.

Sultan G (1910) Contrattura delle dita di Dupuytren. *Atlante e compendio di Patologia Speciale Chirurgica*, Vol. 2, 394. Soc Editr Libraria Milano.

Sulzen L (1930) *Doppelsetige Dupuytren'sche Fingerkontraktur des Daumens.* Inaugural dissertation, Köln.

Suzuki (1931) *Acta Dermatologica* (edited by Policaro (1937)).

Sversen (1909) *Traumatische Entstehung der Dupuytren'schen Kontraktur.* Inaugural dissertation, München.

Taddei D (1924) Retrazione dell'aponevrosi palmare o malattia di Dupuytren. *Trattato di semeiologia e di diagnostica chirurgica*, Vol. 1, 727. UTET, Torino.

Tamplin RW cited without bibliographical references in Antonioli GM, Canestro C, Ebstein W and Neutra W.

Tamplin RW (1846) *Lectures on the Nature and Treatment of Deformities*, 256–67. Longman, London.

Tarnowsky (1887) *Ueber die Retraktion der Palmaraponeurose.* Inaugural dissertation, Erlangen.

Teissier (1835) *Bull Soc Anat* (edited by Lancereaux (1883, 1885)).

Teleky L (1939) Dupuytren's contraction as an occupational disease. *J Ind Hygiene Toxicol* **21**: 233.

Terillon (1888) Rétraction de l'aponévrose palmaire des deux mains; opération; redressement des doigts. *Bull Soc Chirurg* **14**: 265.

Termehr F (1924) *Ueber einem Fall von Fascienkontraktur am Unterarm.* Inaugural dissertation, Köln.

Terrier (1888) Rétraction de l'aponévrose palmaire. *Semaine Méd* **8**: 131.

Teschemacher (1904) Ueber das Vorkommen der Dupuytren'schen Fingerkontraktur bei Diabetes mellitus. *Deutsche Med Wochenschr* **30**: 604.

Testi A (1895) Contributo alla patogenesi della mallattia di Dupuytren. *Vol Lavori dei Congr Med Int*, 234. Roma.

Testi A (1902) La patogenesi della malattia di Dupuytren. *Archivio di Otopedia* **19**: 304.

Testi A (1902) Per l'anatomia patologica della malattia di Dupuytren. *Vol Lavori dei Congr Med Int*, 499. Roma.

Testi A (1905) Nuovo contributo alla patogenesi della malattia di Dupuytren. *Riforma Med* **21**: 820.

Testi A (1905) Sulla patogenesi della malattia di Dupuytren. *Faenza, Stabil Tipolotogr del Cav Montanari.*

Testi A (1905) Terzo contributo alla patogenesi della malattia di Dupuytren. *Vol Lavori dei Congr Med Int*, 231. Roma.

Testut L (1893) *Traité d'anatomie humaine.* Octave Doin, Paris.

Then Bergh H (1939) Konkordantes Vorkommen von Dupuytren'scher Fingerkontraktur bei 3 Zwillingspaaren. *Allgem Zeitschr Psychiatr* **112**: 327.

Thévenot (1903) Rétraction de l'aponévrose palmaire d'origine tuberculeuse. *Lyon Médical* **51**.

Thiem C (1910) Palmarfasciencontractur. *Handbuch der Unfalerkrankungen. Deutsche Chirurgie*, 2nd edn, Vol. 2, 156. Enke, Stuttgart.

Tichet H (1904) Rémarques sur la rétraction de l'aponévrose palmaire chez les paralytiques generaux. Thèse, Paris.

Tillaux P (1888) Rétraction de l'aponévrose palmaire. In: *Traité de Chirurgie Clinique*, 2nd edn. Vol. 1, 652. Asselin et Houzeau, Paris.

Tillmanns H Contrattura della dita secondo Dupuytren. In: *Trattato di Patologia generale e speciale Chirurgica*, 6th edn, Vol. 3, 586. Vallardi, Milano.

Tilmann (1931) Zur Behandlung der Dupuytren'schen Kontraktur. *Zentralbl Chir* **58**: 1533.

Tinel J (1916) Rétraction de l'aponévrose palmaire. *Les blessures des nerfs*, 161. Masson, Paris.

Tinel J (1937) Rétraction de l'aponévrose palmaire. *Les Système nerveux végétatif*, 494. Masson, Paris.

Tinel J, Borel (1925) Rétraction de l'aponévrose palmaire au cours d'une crise mélancolique. *Soc Psychiatr*, 19 novembre.

Tixier L (1922) Retrazione dell'aponevrosi palmare (morbo del Dupuytren). In: Bégouin, *Compendio di Patologia Chirurgica*, Vol. 4, 869. Vallardi, Milano.

Tobiásek (1930) Operazione di Tobiásek nella contrattura di Dupuytren. *Zentralorgan Chir* **50**: 634.

Todd AH (1927) Dupuytren's contracture in a girl of fifteen. *Proc Roy Soc Med, London* **21**: 10.

Tolosa A (1933) Retraçâo aponevrotica palmar de Dupuytren, de provavel origem medular. Co-existencia de perturbações sensitivas de tipo siringo-mielico. *Bol Soc Med Cir São Paulo (Brazil)* **16**: 158.

Tománek F (1935) Radioterapia della contrattura di Dupuytren. *Zentralorgan Chir* **72**: 585.

Topinard (1859–1863) Flexion permanente des doigts spontanée et héréditaire. *Soc Méd Paris.*

Touche (1902) Deux cas d'hémiatrophie faciale avec autopsie. *Revue Neurologique* **8**: 375.

Tranquilli E (1892) Due casi di retrazione dell'aponevrosi palmare (malattia di Dupuytren). *Boll Soc Lancisiana Ospedali di Roma* **12**: 162.

Tranquilli E (1904) Morbo di Dupuytren e diabete. *Malpighi: Gazz Med Roma* **30**: 645.

Trélat U (1887) De la rétraction de l'aponévrose palmaire et de son traitement. *Revue Soc Méd* **15**: 366.

Trélat U (1887) Rétraction de l'aponévrose palmaire (maladie de Dupuytren). *Gazette Hop* **4**: 27.

Trélat U (1891) De la rétraction de l'aponévrose palmaire. *Clinique Chirurgicale, Leçons publiées par M. Delbet*, Vol. 2, 66. Baillière, Paris.

Tricomi E (1903) Asportazione totale di ambedue le aponevrosi palmari per malattia del Dupuytren. *R Acad Sci dell'Istituto Bologna; Rendiconti* **7**: 125. Gamberini e Parmeggiani, Bologna.

Tricomi E (1907) Su tre asportazioni totali di

ambedue la aponevrosi palmair per malattia di Dupuytren. *Archiv Ortopedia* **24**: 1.

Trumper WA (1931) A case of Dupuytren's contraction. *Lancet* **ii**: 17.

Tubby AH (1901) The treatment of Dupuytren's contraction and other points in the surgery of the hand. *Lancet* **i**: 90.

Tubby AH (1904) *Trans Am Orthop Assoc* **13**: 152.

Tubby AH (1910) Dupuytren's contraction. *Med Press* 674.

Tubby AH (1913) Dupuytren's contraction successfully treated by open incision and (thiosinamin) fibrolysin. *BMJ* **2758**: 1203.

Tubby AH (1923) Dupuytren's contraction of the palmar fascia and some other deformities. *Practitioner* **110**: 214.

Tugler JA (1932) Sur un nouveau procédé de traitement chirurgical de la maladie de Dupuytren. Thèse, Paris.

Tùma V (1934) Ein Versuch der Züchtung des Gewebes aus der Dupuytren'chen Kontraktur des erwachsenen Menschen. *Arch experim Zellforsch* **15**: 173.

Tytgat E (1922) Un cas de maladie de Dupuytren traité et guéri par l'extirpation de l'aponévrose palmaire. *Le Scalpel* **75**: 569.

Uffreduzzi O (1937) Retrazione della fascia palmare (morbo di Dupuytren). In: *Trattato di Patologia Chirurgica generale e speciale*, 2nd edn, Vol. 1, 679. UTET, Torino.

Umber F (1909) Lehrbuch der Ernährungs – und Stoffwechselkrankheiten. *Berlin und Wien* 301.

Ungureanu V (1930) Un caso clinico di malattia di Dupuytren. *Zentralorgan Chir* **49**: 636.

Urechia CJ, Dragomir L (1935) Rétraction de l'aponévrose palmaire, maladie de Dupuytren, avec dissociation syringomyélique de la sensibilité. *Paris Médical* **25**: 274.

Valcarcel AG (1938) Einige Bemerkungen über die Dupuytren'sche Kontraktur und Verkürzung des Bindegewebes. *Zentralbl Chir* **65**: 2506.

Valentin (1930) Ueber Dupuytren'scher Fingerkontraktur. *Zentralbl Chir* **57**: 1103.

Van Braam, Houckgeest AQ (1924) La contrattura di Dupuytren. *Zentralorgan Chir* **25**: 139.

Variot cited without bibliographical references in Barison F, Mauclaire PL and Savarese E.

Vautrin cited without bibliographical references in Mauclaire PL.

Velpeau ALM (1835) Sur la rétraction des doigts. *Gazette Med Paris* **2–3**: 511.

Velpeau ALM (1841) Rétraction permanente des doigts. *Leçons orales de clinique chirurgicale, rec. et pub. par Jeanselme et Pavillon*, 574. Meline Cans et C, Bruxelles.

Velpeau ALM (1842) Rétraction des doigts. *Bull Acad Méd* **8**: 129.

Velpeau ALM (1848) Flexion permanente des doigts. *Gazette Hop* **23**.

Verdelli C (1896) Morbo di Dupuytren o retrazione dell'aponevrosi palmare. In: Charcot, Bouchard, Brissaud, *Trattato di medicina*, Vol. 6, 496. UTET

Vergely (1906) Maladie de Dupuytren et tuberculose. *J Méd Bordeaux* **51**.

Vernet cited without bibliographical references in Tichet H.

Verneuil (1857) Observations pour servir `a l'histoire de la flexion permanente des doigts. *Revue de Thérapeutique Médico-Chirurgicales* **5**: 225–30.

Verneuil A (1863) Affection singulaire et non décrite des doigts et des mains, par Miraultd'Angers; commentaires et discussion pour prouver que cette affection se rattache au rhumatisme. *Gazette hébdom méd chir* **113**, 131.

Vespa B (1896) Sulla malattia di Dupuytren. *Boll Soc Lancisìana Ospedali di Roma* **16**: 57.

Vidal (de Cassis) A (1832) – *Gazette méd Paris*, 27 juin.

Vidal (de Cassis) A (1861) Flexion permanente des doigts. *Traité de Pathologie externe et de Médecine opératoire*, 5th edn, Vol. 5, 673. Baillière, Paris.

Viger J (1883) De la rétraction de l'aponévrose palmaire chez les diabétiques. These no. 1883/57, Paris.

Vigoroux cited without bibliographical references in Tichet H.

Vizioli R (1886) Casi di contrattura ereditaria ripetentesi in tre generazioni. *Giornale Neuropatologia* **4**: 1.

Vogeler (1935) Dupuytren'sche Fingerkontraktur. *Münchener med Wochenschr* **82**: 276.

Vogt P (1868) Verkrummung und Steifigkeit der Finger. In: von Pitha, Billroth CAT eds, *Handbuch der allgemeine und speciellen Chirurgie*, Vol. 4, Part 2B, Section 10, 141–45. Enke, Stuttgart.

Vogt P (1881) Dupuytren'schen Fingercontractur. In: Billroth, Lücke, *Deutsche Chirurgie*, Vol. 64, 88. Stuttgart.

Von Albertini A (1929) Die sogenannte Dupuytren'sche Palmarkontraktur. In: Henke F, Lubarsch G, *Handbuch der spez. patholog. Anatomie und Histologie*. Vol. 1, 577. Springer, Berlin.

Von Bülow W (1926) Inaugural dissertation, Königsberg (cited by Stahnke (1927)).

Von Eiselsberg AF (1916) Dupuytren'sche Kontraktur des Daumens. *Wiener klinische Wochenschr* **29**: 436.

Von Eiselsberg AF (1922) *Arch klin Chir* **121**: 108.

Von Eiselsberg AF (1926) Behandlung der Dupuytren'schen Kontraktur. *Zentralbl Chir* **53**: 725.

Von Gaza (1922) *Arch klin Chirurg* **121**: 109.

Von Mosengeil (1876) Ueber Massage, deren Technik, Wirkung und Indicationen dazu, nebst experimentellen Untersuchungen darüber. *Langenbeck's Arch klinisch Chirurg* **19**: 428.

Von Preuschen (1888) Aetiologie der Dupuytren'schen Fingerkontraktur. *Deutsche med Wochenschr* **14**: 761.

Von Seemen H (1936) Zur Operation der Dupuytren'schen Fingerkontraktur. *Zentralbl Chir* **63**: 2192.

Von Seemen H (1936) Zur Operation der Palmarkontraktur (Dupuytren'sche Fingerkontraktur). *Deutsche Zeitschr Chirurg* **246**: 692.

Vulpian (1883) *Gazette Hop* (cited by Neutra 1901, 1903)).

Wagner E (1936) *Wesen und Operationserfolge der Dupuytren'schen Kontraktur.* Inaugural dissertation, Frankfurt.

Wagner W (1932) Ergebnisse der operativen Behandlung bei Dupuytren'scher Kontraktur. *Brun's Beiträge zur klinisch Chirurg* **155**: 271.

Wainwright L (1926) Dupuytren's contraction. *Practitioner* **117**: 263.

Walsham (1884) Dupuytren's contraction. *Lancet* **i**: 565.

Walter P (1920) *Zur Dupuytren'schen Fingerkontraktur.* Inaugural dissertation, Breslau.

Walzberg, Riedel (1881) Die chirurgische Klinik in Göttingen vom 1 oct. 1875 bis 1 oct. 1879. (Schrumpfung der Palmarfascie). *Deutsche Zeitschr Chirurg* **15**: 114.

Wan Chun Fen (1923) *Dupuytren'sche Fingerkontraktur und die Ergebnisse ihrer Behandlung.* Inaugural dissertation, Berlin.

Warner E (1884) A case of Dupuytren's contraction. *Boston Med Surg J* **111**: 345–46.

Weber FP (1938) A note on Dupuytren's contraction, camptodactylia and knuckle – pads. *Br J Dermatol Syphil* **50**: 26.

Wederhake (1918) Ueber die Verwendung des menschlichen Fettes in der Chirurgie. *Berliner klinisch Wochenschr* **55**: 47.

Weill F, Roger M (1934) Rétraction de l'aponévrose palmaire et sclérodermie. *Zentralorgan Chir* **68**: 363.

Weinlechner (1879) *Dupuytren'sche Fingercontractur an beiden Handen, vorwiegend linkerseits. Die von Prof. Busch empfohlene Trennung der Fascia palmaris nach Bildung eines dreieckigen Lappens hatte, weil an der Contractur die Sehnen selbst einen grossen Antheil nahmen, nur einen mässigen Erfolg,* 458–59. Bericht der KK Krankenalstalt Rudolph Stiflung in Wien in Jahr 1878.

Weinlechner (1880) *Dupuytren'sche Verkrümmung des kleinen und Ringfingers. Operirt nach Busch, der Lappen gangranescirt und Patient vor Heilung der Wunde an Tuberculose gestorben,* 473. Bericht der KK Krankenalstalt Rudolph Stiflung in Wien in Jahr 1879.

Weitbrecht J (1742) Syndesmologia sive Historia Ligamentorum Corporis Humani. Translated by EB Kaplan (1969). In: *Syndesmology.* WB Saunders, Philadelphia.

Wendenburg F (1913) *Die Dupuytren'schen Fingerkontraktur.* Inaugural dissertation, Berlin.

Wermel SS (1937) Patogenesi ed etiologia della contrattura di Dupuytren. *Zentralorg Chir* **85**: 251.

Wertheim, Salomonson JKA (1911) Dupuytren'sche Fascienkontraktur. In: Lewandowsky, *Handbuch der Neurologie,* Vol. 2, *Spezielle Neurologie,* 78. Springer, Berlin.

Wette W (1937) Dupuytren'sche Kontraktur und Unfall. *Monatschr Unfallheilk* **44**: 195.

Whelan B (1891) A case of Dupuytren's contraction. *Trans Michigan State Med Soc* **15**: 193–94.

Whitacre (1910) *New York Med J* **91**: 586.

Wiemers (1931) Zur Behandlung der Dupuytren'schen Kontraktur. *Zentralbl Chir* **58**: 1533.

Wienhold (1917) *Ueber die Behandlung der Dupuytren'schen Kontraktur.* Inaugural dissertation, Berlin.

Wigoder cited without bibliographical references in Savarese E.

Windsor J (1834) Permanent contraction of the fingers. *Lancet* **ii**: 501–502.

Wolf J (1936) Ueber Vorkommen und Bedeutung der Dupuytren'schen Kontraktur bei Nervenkrankheiten. *Zentralorgan Chirurg* **78**: 155.

Wyss O (1909) Akute posttraumatische Dupuytren'sche Fingerkontraktur. *Münchener med Wochenschr* **56**: 138.

Yovanovich BY (1936) Terapia chirurgica della malattia di Dupuytren. *Voino-sanitelski glasnik* **7**: 331.

Zahrtmann MK (1897) Om Patogenesen af Retractio

palmaris (Dupuytren). *Hospitalstidende, Kjøbenhaven* 4R **5**: 1037–47.

Zarwulanoff N (1907) *Zur Aetiologie der Dupuytren'schen Fingerkontraktur.* Inaugural dissertation, Würzburg.

Zimmermann (1898) Dupuytren'schen Krankheit. *Wiener klinisch Wochenschr* **11**: 224.

Ziveri A (1917) Sopra un caso di malatia di Dupuytren. *Rivista Patologia Nervosa Mentale* **22**: 377.

Zschau JL (1917) Ueber den Zusammenhang eines Leidens (Dupuytren'sche Verdickung der Sehnenhaut an der Hand) mit einem Unfall. *Monatschr Unfallheilk* **24**: 39.

Zur Verth (1926) Hypoplasie der Hypophysis. *Zentralbl Chir* **53**: 1284.

Zur Verth (1930) Ueber Dupuytren'scher Finger-kontraktur. *Zentralbl Chir* **57**: 1103.

Zur Verth, Scheele (1913) Induratio penis plastica. *Deutsche Zeitschr Chirurg* **121**: 298.

REFERENCES AFTER 1942

Alioto RJ, Rosier RN, Burton RI et al. (1994) Comparative effects of growth factors on fibroblasts of Dupuytren's tissue and normal plantar fascia. *J Hand Surg* **19A**: 442–52.

Allen RA, Woolner LB, Ghormley RK (1955) Soft tissue tumors of the sole – with special reference to plantar fibromatosis. *J Bone Joint Surg* **37A**: 14–26.

Allieu Y (1988) La 'paume ouverte' dans la traitement de la maladie de Dupuytren. Technique et indications. *Rev Chir Orthop* **74**: 46–49.

Allieu Y, Tessier J (1986) La technique de la 'paume ouverte' dans la traitement de la maladie de Dupuytren. In: Tubiana R, Hueston JT, eds, *La Maladie de Dupuytren. Monographies du GEM.* L'Expansion Scientifique Française, Paris: 160–64.

Alnot JY, Morane L (1986) Appréciation des facteurs de risque évolutif dans la maladie de Dupuytren. In: Tubiana R, Hueston JT, eds, *La Maladie de Dupuytren*, 3rd edn, 122–25. L'Expansion Scientifique Française, Paris.

An HS, Southworth SR, Jackson WT et al. (1988) Cigarette smoking and Dupuytren's contracture of the hand. *J Hand Surg* **13A**: 872–74.

Andrew JG (1987) Calcification in Dupuytren's disease: a report of two cases. *J Hand Surg* **12B**: 277–78.

Andrew JG (1991) Contracture of the proximal interphalangeal joint in Dupuytren's disease. *J Hand Surg* **16B**: 446–48.

Arafa L, Noble J, Royle SG et al. (1992) Dupuytren's and epilepsy revisited. *J Hand Surg* **17B**: 221–24.

Arieff AJ, Bell J (1956) Epilepsy and Dupuytren's contracture. *Neurology* **6**: 115–17.

Aron E (1968) Le traitement médical de la maladie de Dupuytren par agent cytostatique (methyl-hydrazine). *Presse Med* **76**: 1956–58.

Aron E (1977) Maladie de Dupuytren et alcoolisme chronique – recherche d'un lien pathogenique groupes HLA. *Sem Hop Paris* **53**: 139.

Attal N (1997) Algodystrophies. Aspects cliniques, physiopathogéniques et thérapeutiques. In: Evaluation et traitement de la douleur. Proceedings of the *39th Congrès National d'Anesthésie et de Réanimation*. Société Française d'anesthésie et de réanimation (SFAR), 73–92, Elsevier, Paris.

Attali P, Ink O, Pelletier G et al. (1987) Dupuytren's contracture, alcohol consumption, and chronic liver disease. *Arch Int Med* **147**: 1065–67.

Aviles E, Arlen E, Miller T (1971) Plantar fibromatosis. *Surgery* **69**: 117–20.

Badalamente MA, Hurst LC (1983) The pathogenesis of Dupuytren's contracture: contractile mechanisms of the myofibroblasts. *J Hand Surg* **8A**: 235–43.

Badalamente MA, Hurst LC (1996) Enzyme injection as a non-operative treatment for Dupuytren's disease. *J Drug Delivery* **3**: 35–40.

Badalamente MA, Hurst LC, Sampson SP (1988) Prostaglandins influence myofibroblast contractility in Dupuytren's disease. *J Hand Surg* **13A**: 867–71.

Badalamente MA, Hurst LC, Sampson SP (1992) Platelet derived growth factor in Dupuytren's disease. *J Hand Surg* **17A**: 317–23.

Badalamente MA, Sampson SP, Hurst LC (1996) The role of transforming growth factor beta in Dupuytren's disease. *J Hand Surg* **21A**: 210–15.

Badois FJ, Lermusiaux JL, Masse C, Kuntz D (1993) Traitement non chirurgical de la maladie de Dupuytren par aponévrotomie à l'aiguille. *Rev Rhum* **60**: 808–13.

Bailey AJ, Sims TJ, Gabbiani G et al. (1977) Collagen of Dupuytren's disease. *Clin Sci Mol Med* **53**: 499–502.

Bailey AJ, Tarlton JF, van der Stappen J et al. (1994) The continuous elongation technique for severe Dupuytren's disease: a biochemical mechanism. *J Hand Surg* **19B**: 522–27.

Baird KS, Crossan JF, Ralston SH (1993) Abnormal growth factor and cytokine expression in Dupuytren's contracture. *J Clin Pathol* **46**: 425–28.

Barclay TL (1958) Edema following operation for

Dupuytren contracture. *Plast Reconstr Surg* **23**: 348–60.

Barsky HK (1984) *Guillaume Dupuytren – A Surgeon in His Place and Time.* Vantage Press, New York.

Bassot J (1965) Traitement de la maladie de Dupuytren par exérèse pharmaco-dynamique isolée ou complétée par un temps plastique uniquement cutané. *Lille Chirurg* **20**: 1

Bassot J (1969) Traitement de la maladie de Dupuytren par exérèse pharmaco-dynamique: bases physio-biologiques; technique. *Gazette Hop* 557.

Baxter H, Schiller C, Johnson LH et al. (1952) Cortisone therapy in Dupuytren's contracture. *Plast Reconstr Surg* **9**: 261–73.

Bazin S, LeLous M, Duance VC (1980) Biochemistry and histology of the connective tissue of Dupuytren's disease lesions. *Eur J Clin Invest* **10**: 9–16.

Beard AJ, Trail IA (1996) The 'S' Quattro in severe Dupuytren's contracture. *J Hand Surg* **21B**: 795–96.

Bedeschi P (1990) Various views and techniques. Management of the skin. Honeycomb technique. In: McFarlane RM, McGrouther DA, Flint MH, eds, *Dupuytren's Disease: Biology and Treatment.* 311–14. Churchill Livingstone, Edinburgh.

Beltran JE, Jimeno-Urban F, Yunta A (1976) The open palm and digit technique in the treatment of Dupuytren's contracture. *Hand* **3**: 73–77.

Bergenudd H, Lindgarde F, Nilson BE (1993) Prevalence of Dupuytren's contracture and its correlation with degenerative changes of the hands and feet and with criteria of general health. *J Hand Surg* **18B**: 254–57.

Berndt A, Kosmehl H, Katenkamp D et al. (1994) Appearance of the myofibroblastic phenotype in Dupuytren's disease is associated with a fibronectin, laminin, collagen type IV and tenascin extracellular matrix. *Pathobiology* **62**: 55–58.

Bohannon RW (1982) Whirlpool versus whirlpool and rinse for removal of bacteria from a venous stasis ulcer. *Phys Ther* **62**: 304–308.

Bojsen-Moller F, Schmidt L (1974) The palmar aponeurosis and the central spaces of the hand. *J Anat* **117**: 55–68.

Bonnici A, Birjandi F, Spencer J et al. (1992) Chromosomal abnormalities in Dupuytren's contracture and carpal tunnel syndrome. *J Hand Surg* **17B**: 349–55.

Borden J (1974) The open finger treatment of Dupuytren's contracture. *Orthop Rev* **8**: 25–29.

Bower M, Nelson M, Gazzard BG (1990) Dupuytren's contracture in patients infected with HIV. *BMJ* **300**: 164–65.

Boyer MI, Gelberman RH (1999) Complications of the operative treatment of Dupuytren's disease. *Hand Clin* **15**: 161–46.

Boyes JH (1954) Dupuytren's contracture: notes on the age at onset and the relationship to handedness. *Am J Surg* **88**: 147–54.

Boyes JH, Jones FE (1968) Dupuytren's disease involving the volar aspect of the wrist. *Plast Reconstr Surg* **41**: 204–207.

Bradlow A, Mowat AG (1986) Dupuytren's contracture and alcohol. *Ann Rheum Dis* **45**: 304–307.

Brand PW (1985) *Clinical Mechanics of the Hand*, 180. Mosby, St Louis.

Brand PW, Hollister AM (1999) *Clinical Mechanics of the Hand*, 3rd edn, 253–54. Mosby, St Louis.

Brand PW, Wood H (1977) Hand Volumeter Instruction Sheet. US Public Health Service Hospital, Carville, LA.

Brandes G, Messina A, Reale E (1994) The palmar fascia after treatment by the continuous extension technique for Dupuytren's contracture. *J Hand Surg* **19B**: 528–33.

Bray E, Galeazzi M (1980) First results in the treatment of Dupuytren's disease. *Arthritis Rheum* **23**: 1408.

Breed CM, Smith PJ (1996) A comparison of methods of treatment of PIP joint contractures in Dupuytren's disease. *J Hand Surg* **21B**: 246–51.

Brenner P, Mailänder P, Berger A (1994) Epidemiology of Dupuytren's disease. In: Berger A, Delbrück A, Brenner P, Hinzmann R, eds, *Dupuytren's Disease*, 244–54. Springer Verlag, Berlin.

Brickley-Parsons D, Glimcher MJ, Smith RJ et al. (1981) Biochemical changes in the collagen of the palmar fascia in patients with Dupuytren's disease. *J Bone Joint Surg* **63A**: 787–97.

Bridge P (1994) *The Calculation of Genetic Risks.* Johns Hopkins Press, Baltimore.

Briedis J (1974) Dupuytren's contracture: lack of complications with the open palm technique. *Br J Plast Surg* **27**: 218–19.

Brouet JP (1986) Etude de 1000 dossiers de maladie de Dupuytren. In: Tubiana R, Hueston JT, eds, *La Maladie de Dupuytren*, 98–105. L'Expansion Scientifique Française, Paris.

Bruner JM (1949) The use of the dorsal skin flap for the coverage of palmar defects after aponeurectomy for Dupuytren's contracture. *Plast Reconstr Surg* **4**: 599.

Bruner JM (1951) Incisions for plastic and reconstructive (non-septic) surgery of the hand. *Br J Plast Surg* **4**: 48.

Bruner JM (1970) The dynamics of Dupuytren's disease. *Hand* **2**: 172–77.

Bruner JM (1974) Technique of selective aponeurectomy for Dupuytren's contracture. In: Hueston JT, Tubiana R, eds, *Dupuytren's Disease*, 93–94. Churchill Livingstone, Edinburgh.

Bryan AS, Ghorbal MS (1988) The long-term results of closed palmar fasciotomy in the management of Dupuytren's contracture. *J Hand Surg* **13B**: 254–56.

Bunnell S (1944) *Surgery of the Hand*. JB Lippincott, Philadelphia.

Burch PRJ (1966) Dupuytren's contracture: an autoimmune disease? *J Bone Joint Surg* **48B**: 312–19.

Burge P (1994) Fasciotomy and the open palm technique. In: Berger A, Delbrück A, Brenner P, Hinzmann R, eds, *Dupuytren's Disease: Pathobiochemistry and Clinical Management*, 264–66. Springer Verlag, Berlin.

Byron PM, Muntzer EM (1986) *Therapist's Management of the Mutilated Hand. Hand Clinics, Hand Rehabilitation*. WB Saunders, Philadelphia.

Caroli A, Marcuzzi A, Pasquali-Ronchetti I et al. (1992) Correlation between Dupuytren's disease and arcus cornealis senilis: is dyslipidaemia a common aetiopathogenic factor? *Ann Chir Main* **11**: 314–19 (in French, English summary).

Caughill KA, McFarlane RM, McGrouther DA *et al.* (1988) Developmental anatomy of the palmar aponeurosis and its relationship to the palmaris longus tendon. *J Hand Surg* **13A**: 485–93.

Chammas M, Bousquet P, Renard E et al. (1995) Dupuytren's disease, carpal tunnel syndrome, trigger finger, and diabetes mellitus. *J Hand Surg* **20**: 109–14.

Chiu HF, McFarlane RM (1978) Pathogenesis of Dupuytren's contracture: a correlative clinical–pathological study. *J Hand Surg* **3**: 1–10.

Chow SP, Luk KDK, Kung TM (1984) Dupuytren's contracture in Chinese. *J R Coll Surg Edin* **29**: 49–51.

Cimmino MA, Cutolo M, Beltrame F (1982) Local injections of tiopronin in Dupuytren's contracture. *Arthritis Rheum* **25**: 1505.

Citron N, Messina JC (1998) The use of skeletal traction in the treatment of severe primary Dupuytren's disease. *J Bone Joint Surg* **80B**: 126–29.

Clarkson P (1961) The aetiology of Dupuytren's disease. *Guy Hosp Rep* **110**: 52–62.

Clarkson P (1963) The radical fasciectomy operation for Dupuytren's disease. A condemnation. *Br J Plastic Surg* **16**: 273–79.

Classen DA, Hurst LN (1992) Plantar fibromatosis and bilateral flexion contractures: a review of the literature. *Ann Plast Surg* **28**: 475–78.

Cleland H, Morisson WA (1986) Dupuytren's disease in the thumb: two cases of a central cord. *J Hand Surg* **11B**: 68–70.

Coleman SS, Anson GJ (1961) Arterial patterns in the hand based upon a study of 650 specimens. *Surg Gynecol Obstet* **113**: 409.

Colville J (1983) Dupuytren's contracture. The role of fasciotomy. *Hand* **15**: 162–66.

Comtet JJ, Bourne-Branchu B (1986) La maladie de Dupuytren est-elle d'origine vasculaire? In: Tubiana R, Hueston JT, eds, *Monographies du groupe d'Etude de la Main*, 79–83. L'Expansion Scientifique Française, Paris.

Conolly WB (1974) Spontaneous healing and wound contraction of soft tissue wounds in the hand. *Hand* **6**: 26–32.

Constantinesco A, Brunot B, Demangeat JL et al. (1986) Apport de la scintigraphie osseuse en trois phases au diagnostic précoce de l'algoneurodystrophie de la main. *Ann Chir Main* **5**: 93–104.

Conway H, Stark RB (1954) Arterial vascularization of the soft tissues of the hand. *J Bone Joint Surg* **36A**: 1238–40.

Cooney WP (1997) Somatic versus sympathetic mediated chronic limb pain. *Hand Clinics* **13**: 355–61.

Critchley EMR, Vakil SD, Hayward HW, Owen VMH (1976) Dupuytren disease in epilepsy: result of prolonged administration of anticonvulsants. *J Neurol Neurosurg Psychiatr* **39**: 498.

Crombrugghe BD, Karsenty G, Maity S (1990) Transcriptional mechanisms controlling Types I and III collagen genes. *Ann N Y Acad Sci* **580**: 88–96.

Crowley B, Tonkin MA (1999) The proximal interphalangeal joint in Dupuytren's disease. *Hand Clin* **15**: 137–47.

Curtis RM (1974) Volar capsulectomy in the proximal interphalangeal joint in Dupuytren's contracture. In: Hueston JT, Tubiana R, eds, *Dupuytren's Disease*, 135. Churchill Livingstone, Edinburgh.

D'Arcangelo M, Maffulli N, Kolhe S (1995) Traumatic release of Dupuytren's contracture. *Acta Orthop Belg* **61**: 53–54.

De Frenne HA (1977) Les structures aponévrotiques au niveau de la première commissure. *Ann Chir* **31**: 1017–19.

De la Caffinière JY (1983) Travail manuel et maladie de Dupuytren. Résultat d'une enquête informatisée en milieu sidérurgique. *Ann Chir Main* **2**: 66–72.

De la Caffinière JY (1986) Travail manuel et maladie de Dupuytren. In: Tubiana R, Hueston JT, eds, *La Maladie de Dupuytren*, 3rd edn, 92–97. L'Expansion Scientifique Française, Paris.

De Seze S, Debeyre N (1957) Traitement de la maladie de Dupuytren par l'hydrocortisone locale associée aux manoeuvres de redressement (70 cas traités). *Rev Rhum* **24**: 540–50.

Debeyre N (1958) Traitement de la maladie de Dupuytren par l'hydrocortisone locale associée aux manoeuvres de redressement (135 cas traités). *Sem Hôp Paris (Thér)* **34**: 728–30.

Demers R, Blais JA (1960) Le caractère familial et héréditaire de la contracture de Dupuytren. *Union Med Can* **89**: 1238–49.

Desplas B (1951) A propos de la maladie de Dupuytren. *Mem Acad Chir* **77**: 425–28.

Dickie WR, Hughes NC (1967) Dupuytren's contracture: a review of the late results of radical fasciectomy. *Br J Plast Surg* **20**: 311–14.

Djermag Y (1983) *Contribution à l'étude de la maladie de Dupuytren: A propos de 104 cas revus.* Thèse Doctorat en Médecine, Université Paris VII.

Djermag Y (1999) *Traitement des formes sév`eres de la maladie de Dupuytren par distracteur articulaire progressif.* Communication à l'Académie Nationale de Chirurgie le 5 mai 1999.

Dolynchuk KN, Pettigrew NM (1991) Transglutaminase levels in Dupuytren's disease. *J Hand Surg* **16A**: 787–90.

Donato RR, Morrison WA (1996). Dupuytren's disease in the feet causing flexion contractures in the toes. *J Hand Surg* **21B**: 364–66.

Doury PCC (1997) Algodystrophy. *Hand Clinics* **13**: 327–37.

Early PF (1962) Population studies in Dupuytren's contracture. *J Bone Joint Surg* **44B**: 602–13.

Eaton RJ (1971) *Joint Injuries of the Hand.* Charles Thomas, Illinois.

Ebelin M, Divaris M, Leviet D, Vilain R (1987) Traitement des récidives dans la maladie de Dupuytren. *Chirurgie* **113**: 780–84.

Ebelin M, Leviet D, Auclair E et al. (1991) Traitement des récidives de la maladie de Dupuytren par incision scalaire et greffe 'coupe-feu'. *Ann Chir Plast Esthet* **36**: 26–30.

Egawa T, Senrui H, Horiki A, Egawa M (1990) Epidemiology of the oriental patient. In: McFarlane RM, McGrouther DA, Flint MH, eds, *Dupuytren's Disease*, 239–45. Churchill Livingstone, Edinburgh.

Eicher E, Moberg G (1970) Möglichkeiten zur Vermeidung von Amputationen bei schwerer Dupuytren'scher Kontraktur. *Handchirurgie* **2**: 56–60.

Elliot D (1988) The early history of the contracture of the palmar fascia. Part 1: The origin of the disease: the curse of the MacCrimmons: the hand of benediction: Cline's contracture. *J Hand Surg [Br]* **13**: 246–53.

Elliot D (1988) The early history of contracture of the palmar fascia. Part 2: The Revolution in Paris: Guillaume Dupuytren. *J Hand Surg [Br]* **13**: 372–78.

Elliot D (1999) The early history of Dupuytren's disease. *Hand Clin* **15**: 1–19.

Evans RB (1997) The source of our strength. *J Hand Ther* **10**: 18–19.

Fahmy NR (1990) The Stockport serpentine spring system for the treatment of displaced comminuted intra-articular phalangeal fractures. *J Hand Surg* **15A**: 303–11.

Fahrer M (1980) The proximal end of the palmar aponeurosis. *Hand* **12**: 33.

Fahrer M, Tubiana R (1976) Palmaris longus, anteductor of the thumb. An experimental study. *Hand* **8**: 287.

Fairfield L (1954) *Epilepsy.* Duckworth, London.

Falter E, Herndl E, Muhlbauer W (1991) Dupuytren's contracture. When operate? Conservative preliminary treatment? *Fortschr Med* **109**: 223–26.

Ferrarini M (1936) Morphogenesi della aponevrosi palmare. *Arch Ital Anat Embryol* **37**: 203–68.

Fietti VG Jr, Mackin EJ (1995) Open-palm technique in Dupuytren's disease. In: Hunter JM, Mackin EJ, Callahan AD, eds, *Rehabilitation of the Hand: Surgery and Therapy*, 4th edn, 981–94. CV Mosby, St Louis.

Finney R (1953) Dupuytren's contracture. A radiotherapeutic approach. *Lancet* **2**: 1064–66.

Fisk G (1974) The relationship of trauma to Dupuytren's contracture. In: Hueston JT, Tubiana R, eds, *Dupuytren's Disease*, 43–44. Churchill Livingstone, Edinburgh.

Fisk G (1985) The relationship of manual labour and specific injury to Dupuytren's disease. In: Hueston JT, Tubiana R, eds, *Dupuytren's Disease*, 2nd edn, 104–105. Churchill Livingstone, Edinburgh.

Flint M, McGrouther D (1990) Is Dupuytren's disease a connective tissue response? In: McFarlane R, McGrouther D, Flint M, eds, *Dupuytren's Disease. Biology and Treatment*, Vol. 5, 282–87. Churchill Livivingstone, Edinburgh.

Flowers KR (1985) String wrapping versus massage for reducing digital volume. *J Hand Surg* **10**: 583.

Fossati P, Romon M, Vennin Ph (1982) Maladie de Dupuytren et diabète sucré. *Ann Chir Main* **1**: 353–54.

Foucher G (1995) *L'Algodystrophie de la main.* Springer, Paris.

Foucher G (1998) Quoi de neuf dans la traitement de la maladie de Dupuytren? *Ann Chir Plast Esthet* **43**: 593–99.

Foucher G, Legaillard P (1996) Anterior tenoarthrolysis in flexion contracture of the fingers. A propos of 41 cases. *Rev Chir Orthop Rep App Mot* **82**: 529–34.

Foucher G, Schuind F, Lemarechal P et al. (1985) La technique de la paume ouverte pour le traitement de la maladie de Dupuytren. *Ann Chir Plast Esthet* **30**: 211–15.

Foucher G, Cornil C, Lenoble E (1992) Open palm technique for Dupuytren's disease: a five year follow-up. *Ann Chir Main* **11**: 362–66.

Fraser-Moodie A (1976) Dupuytren's contracture and cigarette smoking. *Br J Plast Surg* **29**: 214–15.

Freehafer A, Strong JM (1963) The treatment of Dupuytren's contracture by partial fasciectomy. *J Bone Joint Surg* **45A**: 1207–216.

French PD, Kitchen VS, Harris JRW (1990) Prevalence of Dupuytren's contracture in patients infected with HIV. *BMJ* **301**: 967.

Fröscher W, Hoffmann F (1983) Dupuytrensche Kontraktur und Phenobarbitaleinrahme bei Epilepsie-Patienten. *Nervenarzt* **54**: 413–19.

Furnas DW (1979) Dupuytren's contractures in a black patient in east Africa. *Plast Reconstr Surg* **64**: 250–51 (letter).

Gabbiani G, Majno G (1972) Dupuytren's contracture: fibroblast contraction? An ultrastructural study. *Am J Pathol* **66**: 131–46.

Gallizia F (1964) A collagen triad: la Peyronie's disease, Dupuytren's disease and fibrosis of the auricular cartilage. *J Urol Nephrol* **70**: 424.

Garrison FH (1966) *An Introduction to the History of Medicine*, 4th edn. WB Saunders, Philadelphia.

Gelberman RH, Amiel D, Rudolph RM et al. (1980) Dupuytren's contracture. An electron microscopic, biochemical, and clinical correlative study. *J Bone Joint Surg* **62A**: 425–32.

Gelberman RH, Panagis JS, Hergenroeder PT, Zakaib GS (1982) Wound complications in the surgical management of Dupuytren's contracture: a comparison of operative incisions. *Hand* **14**: 248–54.

Goetzee AE, Williams HO (1954–55) A case of Dupuytren's contracture involving the hand and foot in a child. *Br J Surg* **42**: 417–20.

Gonzalez RI (1971) Dupuytren's contracture of the fingers: a simplified approach to the surgical treatment. *Calif Med* **115**: 25–31.

Gonzalez RI (1971) Open fasciotomy and Wolfe graft for Dupuytren's contracture. In: Hueston JT, ed., *Transactions of the Fifth International Congress of Plastic and Reconstructive Surgery, Melbourne, 1971*, 630–31. Butterworth, Melbourne.

Gonzalez RI (1974) Open fasciotomy and full-thickness skin graft in the correction of digital flexion deformity. In: Hueston JT, Tubiana R, eds, *Dupuytren's Disease*, 123–28. Churchill Livingstone, Edinburgh.

Gonzalez AM, Buscaglia M, Fox R et al. (1992) Basic fibroblast growth factor in Dupuytren's contracture. *Am J Pathol* **141**: 661–71.

Gonzalez MH, Sobeski J, Grindel S et al. (1998) Dupuytren's disease in African-Americans. *J Hand Surg* **23B**: 306–307.

Gordon S (1948) Dupuytren's contracture. *Can Med Assoc J* **58**: 543.

Gordon S (1954) Dupuytren's contracture: the significance of various factors in its etiology. *Ann Surg* **140**: 683.

Gordon SD (1957) Dupuytren's contracture: recurrence and extension following surgical treatment. *Br J Plast Surg* **9**: 286–88.

Gordon S (1963) Dupuytren's contracture: the use of free skin grafts in treatment. *Transactions of the Third International Congress of Plastic Surgeons, Washington DC, 1963*, 963–67. Excerpta Medica, Amsterdam.

Gordon SD (1964) Dupuytren's contracture. The use of free skin grafts in treatment. *Transactions of the 3rd Congress of the International Society of Plastic Surgeons, Washington, 1963*, 963–67. Excerpta Medica, Amsterdam.

Gordon SD (1964) Dupuytren's contracture: plantar involvement. *Br J Plast Surg* **17**: 421–23.

Gosset J (1967) Maladie de Dupuytren et anatomie des aponévroses palmodigitales. *Ann Chir* **21**: 554–65.

Gosset J (1972) Anatomie des aponévroses palmo-digitales. In: Tubiana R, Hueston J, eds, *Maladie de Dupuytren*, 23–38. L'Expansion Scientifique, Paris.

Gosset J (1985) Dupuytren's disease and the anatomy of the palmodigital aponeuroses. In: Hueston JT, Tubiana R, eds, *Dupuytren's Disease*, 2nd edn, 13–26. Churchill Livingstone, London.

Goyrand G (1835) De la rétraction permanente des doigts. *Gazette Med Paris* **3**: 481–86.

Grace DL, McGrouther DA, Phillips H (1984)

Traumatic correction of Dupuytren's contracture. *J Hand Surg* **9B**: 59–60.

Graubard DJ (1954) *J Int Coll Surg* **21**: 15, cited in Hueston JT (1963) *Dupuytren's Contracture*, 15. Churchill Livingstone, Edinburgh.

Haedicke GJ, Sturim HS (1989) Plantar fibromatosis: an isolated disease. *Plast Reconstr Surg* **83**: 296–300.

Haeseker B (1981) Dupuytren's disease and the sickle-cell trait in a female black patient. *Br J Plast Surg* **34**: 438–40.

Haimovici N (1978) Die Alloarthroplastik. Therapicalternative bei der arthrogenen Beugekontracture der Finger bei Dupuytren'scher Krankheit. *Handchirurgie* **10**: 135–48.

Hakstian RW (1966) Long-term results of extensive fasciectomy. *Br J Plast Surg* **140**: 149.

Hakstian RW (1974) Late results of extensive fasciectomy. In: Hueston JT, Tubiana R, eds, *Dupuytren's Disease*, 79–84. Churchill Livingstone, Edinburgh.

Halliday N, Rayan G, Zardi L et al. (1994) Distribution of ED-A and ED-B containing fibronectin isoforms in Dupuytren's disease. *J Hand Surg* **19A**: 428–34.

Hamlin EJ (1952) Limited excision of Dupuytren's contracture. *Ann Surg* **135**: 94–97.

Heyse WE (1960) Dupuytren's contracture and its surgical treatment. Clinical study of a local resection method. *JAMA* **174**: 113–18.

Hillemand B, Joly JP, Huet P et al. (1975) Anomalies palmaires, maladie de Dupuytren et arc cornéen. *Sem Hop Paris* **51**: 2001–10.

Hodgkinson PD (1994) The use of skeletal traction to correct the flexed PIP joint in Dupuytren's disease: a pilot study to assess the use of the Pipster. *J Hand Surg* **19A**: 534–37.

Hoet F, Boxho J, Decoster E et al. (1983) Dupuytren's contracture – review of 326 operated patients. *Ann Chir Main* **7**: 251–55 (in French, English summary).

Holland AJ, McGrouther DA (1997) Dupuytren's disease and the relationship between the transverse and longitudinal fibers of the palmar fascia. A dissection study. *Clin Anat* **10**: 97–103.

Honner R, Lamb DW, James JIP (1971) Dupuytren's contracture: long term results after fasciectomy. *J Bone Joint Surg* **53**: 240–46.

Howard LD Jr (1959) Dupuytren's contracture. A guide for management. *Clin Orthop* **15**: 118.

Hueston J (1985) Overview of etiology and pathology. In: Hueston JT, Tubiana R, eds, *Dupuytren's Disease*, 2nd edn, 75–81. Churchill Livingstone, Edinburgh.

Hueston JT (1960) The incidence of Dupuytren's contracture. *Med J Aust* **2**: 999–1002.

Hueston JT (1961) Limited fasciectomy for Dupuytren's contracture. *Plast Reconstr Surg* **27**: 569–85.

Hueston JT (1962) Digital Wolfe grafts in recurrent Dupuytren's contracture. *Plast Reconstr Surg* **29**: 342–44.

Hueston JT (1962) Further studies on the incidence of Dupuytren's contracture. *Med J Aust* **1**: 586–88.

Hueston JT (1963) *Dupuytren's Contracture*. E & S Livingstone, Edinburgh.

Hueston JT (1963) The Dupuytren's diathesis. In: Hueston JT, ed., *Dupuytren's Contracture*, 51–63. E & S Livingstone, Edinburgh.

Hueston JT (1963) Recurrent Dupuytren's contracture. *Plast Reconstr Surg* **31**: 66–69.

Hueston JT (1965) Dupuytren's contracture: the trend to conservatism. *Ann Roy Coll Surg Engl* **36**: 134–51.

Hueston JT (1966) Local flap repair of fingertip injury. *Plast Reconstr Surg* **37**: 349–50.

Hueston JT (1968) Dupuytren's contracture and specific injury. *Med J Aust* **1**: 1084.

Hueston JT (1969) The control of recurrent Dupuytren's contracture by skin replacement. *Br J Plast Surg* **22**: 152–56.

Hueston JT (1971) Enzymatic fasciotomy. *Hand* **3**: 38–40.

Hueston JT (1973) Traumatic aneurysm of the digital artery: a complication of fasciectomy. *Hand* **5**: 232–34.

Hueston JT (1974) *Dupuytren's Disease*. Churchill Livingstone, Edinburgh.

Hueston JT (1974) The management of ectopic lesions in Dupuytren's contracture. In: Hueston JT, Tubiana R, (eds), *Dupuytren's Disease* 145–48. Churchill Livingstone, Edinburgh.

Hueston JT (1974) Prognosis as a guide to the timing and extent of surgery in Dupuytren's contracture. In: Hueston JT, Tubiana R, eds, *Dupuytren's Disease*, 1st edn, 61–62. Churchill Livingstone, Edinburgh.

Hueston JT (1974) Skin replacement in Dupuytren's contracture. In: Hueston JT, Tubiana R, eds, *Dupuytren's Disease*, 119–22. Churchill Livingstone, Edinburgh.

Hueston JT (1977) Dupuytren's contracture. In: Converse JM, ed., *Reconstructive Plastic Surgery*, Vol. 6, 2nd edn, 3403–27. WB Saunders, Philadelphia.

Hueston JT (1978) Review of Rank and Wakefield's series.

Hueston JT (1981) Historical Profiles. Archibald Hector McIndoe (1900–1960). In: Tubiana R, ed., *The Hand*, Vol. 1. WB Saunders, Philadelphia.

Hueston JT (1981) Historical profiles: Guillaume Dupuytren. In: Tubiana R, ed., *The Hand*, Vol. 1. WB Saunders, Philadelphia.

Hueston JT (1982) Dorsal Dupuytren's disease. *J Hand Surg* **7**: 384–87.

Hueston JT (1982) Dupuytren's contracture. In: Flynn JE, ed., *Hand Surgery*, 3rd edn, 797–822. Williams & Wilkins, Baltimore.

Hueston JT (1984) 'Firebreak' grafts in Dupuytren's contracture. *Aust N Z J Surg* **54**: 277–81.

Hueston JT (1984) Some observations on knuckle pads. *J Hand Surg* **9B**: 75–78.

Hueston JT (1985) Dermofasciectomy and skin replacement in Dupuytren's disease. In: Hueston JT, Tubiana R, eds, *Dupuytren's Disease*, 2nd edn, 149–53. Churchill Livingstone, Edinburgh.

Hueston JT (1985) The management of ectopic lesions in Dupuytren's disease. In: Hueston JT, Tubiana R, eds, *Dupuytren's Disease*, 2nd edn, 204–10. Churchill Livingstone, Edinburgh.

Hueston JT (1987) Dupuytren's contracture: medico-legal aspects. *Med J Aust* **147** (suppl): S1–S11.

Hueston JT (1988) Dupuytren's contracture. *Curr Orthop* **2**: 173–78.

Hueston JT (1990) Historical review-addendum. *Curr Orthop* **4**: 286.

Hueston JT (1991) Comment on 'Anatomy and pathogenesis of the digital cords and nodules'. *Hand Clin* **7**: 659–60.

Hueston JT (1991) Unsatisfactory results in Dupuytren's contracture. *Hand Clin* **7**: 759–63.

Hueston JT (1992) Regression of Dupuytren's contracture. *J Hand Surg* **17B**: 453–57.

Hueston JT (1998) Current views on etiology and pathogenesis. In: Tubiana R, ed., *The Hand*, Vol. 5. WB Saunders, Philadelphia.

Hueston JT, Seyfer AE (1991) Some medicolegal aspects of Dupuytren's contracture. *Hand Clin* **7**: 617–32.

Hueston JT, Tubiana R (1974) *Dupuytren's Disease*. Churchill Livingstone, Edinburgh.

Hueston JT, Tubiana R (1985) *Dupuytren's Disease*, 2nd edn. Churchill Livingstone, Edinburgh.

Hueston JT, Wilson WF (1973) Knuckle pads. *Aust N Z J Surg* **42**: 274.

Hurst LC (1996) Dupuytren's fasciectomy: zig-zag-plasty technique. In: Blair WF, ed., *Techniques in Hand Surgery*, 518–29. Williams and Wilkins, Baltimore.

Hurst LC, Badalamente M (1990) Associated diseases. In: McFarlane RM, McGrouther DA, Flint MH, eds,

Dupuytren's Disease, 253–60. Churchill Livingstone, Edinburgh.

Hurst LC, Badalamente MA (1999) Non-operative treatment of Dupuytren's disease. *Hand Clin* **15**: 97–107.

Hurst LC, Badalamente MA, Makowski J (1986) The pathobiology of Dupuytren's contracture: effects of prostaglandins on myofibroblasts. *J Hand Surg* **11A**: 18–23.

Iselin F, Cardenas-Baron L, Gouget-Audry I, Peze W (1988) La maladie de Dupuytren dorsale. *Ann Chir Main* **7**: 247–50.

Iselin M (1955) *Chirurgie de la Main*, Vol. 2. Livre de Chirurgien, Masson, Paris.

Jabaley ME (1999) Surgical treatment of Dupuytren's disease. *Hand Clin* **15**: 109–26.

James JIP (1974) The genetic pattern of Dupuytren's contracture and idiopathic epilepsy. In: Hueston JT, Tubiana R, eds, *Dupuytren's Disease*, 37–42. Churchill Livingstone, Edinburgh.

James JIP (1985) The genetic pattern of Dupuytren's disease and idiopathic epilepsy. In: Hueston JT, Tubiana R, eds, *Dupuytren's Disease*, 2nd edn, 94–99. Churchill Livingstone, Edinburgh.

James JIP, Tubiana R (1952) La maladie de Dupuytren. *Rev Chir Orthop* **38**: 352–406.

Jennings AM, Milner PC, Ward JD (1989) Hand abnormalities in Type II diabetes. *Diabet Med* **6**: 43–47.

Johnson HA (1980) The Hugh Johnson Sign of early Dupuytren's contracture. *Plast Reconstr Surg* **65**: 697.

Kaufhold N (1962) Die örtliche Behandlung mit 6-methyl-prednisolon (Urbason). *MMW* **104**: 2252–53.

Keilholz L, Seegenschmiedt M, Sauer R (1996) Radiotherapy for prevention of disease progression in early stage Dupuytren's contracture: initial and long-term results. *Int J Radiat Oncol Biol Phys* **36**: 891–97.

Kelly C, Varian J (1992) Dermofasciectomy – a long-term review. *Ann Hand Upper Limb Surg* **11**: 381–82.

Ketchum LD (1992) The use of full thickness skin graft in Dupuytren's contracture. *Hand Clin* **7**: 731–41.

Ketchum LD (1996) Dupuytren's contracture: triamcinolone injection. *Correspondence Newsletter, ASSH No. 131*.

Ketchum LD, Hixson FP (1987) Treatment of Dupuytren's contracture with dermofasciectomy and full thickness skin graft. *J Hand Surg* **12A**: 659–63.

King RA (1949) Vitamin E therapy in Dupuytren's contracture. *J Bone Joint Surg* **31B**: 43.

Kischer CW, Speer DP (1984) Microvascular changes in Dupuytren's contracture. *J Hand Surg* **9A**: 58–62.

Kline SC, Beach V, Holder LE (1993) Segmental reflex sympathetic dystrophy: clinical and scintigraphic criteria. *J Hand Surg* **18A**: 853–59.

Kloen P, Jenning CL, Gebhardt MC et al. (1995) TGF beta: possible roles in Dupuytren's contracture. *J Hand Surg* **20A**: 101–108.

Knowles HB (1981) Joint contractures, waxy skin, and control of diabetes. *N Engl J Med* **305**: 217.

Landsmeer JMF (1949) The anatomy of the dorsal aponeurosis of the human finger and its functional significance. *Anat Rec* **104**: 31–44.

Landsmeer JMF (1956) Les aponévroses dorsales de la main. *Compte Rendu de l'Association des Anatomistes* **43**: 443.

Landsmeer JMF (1976) *Atlas of Anatomy of the Hand.* Churchill Livingstone, Edinburgh.

Lane CS (1981) The treatment of Dupuytren's contracture with flexor tendon sheath involvement. The sliding volar flap. *Ann Plast Surg* **6**: 20–23.

Lankford LL (1988) Reflex sympathetic dystrophy. In: Green DP, ed., *Operative Hand Surgery*, 2nd edn, Vol. 1, 633–933. Churchill Livingstone, New York.

Lankford LL (1999) Reflex sympathetic dystrophy. In: Tubiana R, ed., *The Hand*, Vol. 5. WB Saunders, Philadelphia.

Lappi DA, Martineau D, Maher PA et al. (1992) Basic fibroblast growth factor in cells derived from Dupuytren's contracture: synthesis, presence, and implications for treatment of the disease. *J Hand Surg* **17**: 324–32.

Larkin JG, Frier BM (1986) Limited joint mobility and Dupuytren's contracture in diabetic, hypertensive, and normal population. *BMJ* **292**: 1494.

Larsen RD, Takagishi N, Posch JL (1960) The pathogenesis of Dupuytren's contracture. *J Bone Joint Surg* **42A**: 993–1007.

Latil F, Hueston JT (1992) JCB Goyrand (1802–1866): Chirurgien et Académicien Aixois. *Ann Chir Plast Esthet* **37**: 574–78.

Lawson PM, Maneschi F, Fohner EM (1983) The relationship of hand abnormalities to diabetes and diabetic retinopathy. *Diabetes Care* **6**: 140–43.

Le Chuiton M (1957) Traitement de la maladie de Dupuytren par téno-aponévrectomie antibrachiale du petit palmaire. *Mem Acad Chir* **83**: 29–30.

Le Gros Clark W (1958) *The Tissues of the Body*, 4th edn. Oxford University Press, London.

Le Roy Steinberg C (1951) Tocopherols in the treatment of primary fibrositis. *Arch Surg* **63**: 824–33.

Leclercq C, Tubiana R (1986) Résultats à long terme des aponévrectomies pour maladie de Dupuytren. *Chirurgie* **112**: 195.

Leclercq C, Tubiana R (1999) Recurrence in Dupuytren's contracture. In: Tubiana R, ed., *The Hand*, Vol. V, 484–92. Saunders, Philadelphia.

Lee GW, Weeks PM (1995) The role of bone scintigraphy in diagnosing reflex sympathetic dystrophy. *J Hand Surg* **20A**: 458–63.

Legge JWH, McFarlane RM (1980) Prediction of results of treatment of Dupuytren's disease. *J Hand Surg* **5**: 608–16.

Lennox I, Murali S, Porter R (1993) A study of the repeatability of the diagnosis of Dupuytren's contracture and its prevalence in the Grampian region. *J Hand Surg* **18B**: 258–61.

Leriche R (1945) La chirurgie à l'ordre de la vie, 153. Zeluck, Paris.

Lermusiaux JL, Debeyre N (1980) Le traitement médical de la maladie de Dupuytren. In: de Seze S, Rickewaert A, Kahn MF, Guerin C, eds, *L'Actualité Rhumatologique 1979*, 238–43. L'Expansion Scientifique Française, Paris.

Lettin A (1964) Dupuytren's diathesis. *J Bone Joint Surg* **46B**: 220–25.

Leviet D (1978) La translocation de l'auriculaire par ostéotomie intracarpienne (in French with English summary). *Ann Chir* **32**: 609–12.

Ling RSM (1963) The genetic factor in Dupuytren's disease. *J Bone Joint Surg* **45B**: 709–18.

Lister G (1977) *The Hand: Diagnosis and Indications.* Churchill Livingstone, Edinburgh.

Lister G (1978) Intraosseous wiring of the digital skeleton. *J Hand Surg* **3**: 427–35.

Littler JW (1974) Special points of technique in Dupuytren's contracture. In: Hueston JT, Tubiana R, eds, *Dupuytren's Disease*, 97–99. Churchill Livingstone, Edinburgh.

Liu Y, Chen WY (1991) Dupuytren's disease among the Chinese in Taiwan. *J Hand Surg* **16A**: 779–86.

Logan AM, Armstrong JR, Huerren J (1998) Dermofasciectomy in the management of Dupuytren's disease. Paper presented at the *7th Congress of the International Federation of Societies for Surgery of the Hand*, Vancouver.

Lubahn JD (1999) Open palm technique and soft-tissue coverage in Dupuytren's disease. *Hand Clin* **15**: 127–36.

Lubahn JD, Lister GD, Wolfe T (1984) Fasciectomy and Dupuytren's disease: a comparison between the open-palm technique and wound closure. *J Hand Surg* **9A**: 53–58.

Luck JV (1959) Dupuytren's contracture – a new concept of the pathogenesis correlated with surgical management. *J Bone Joint Surg* **41A**: 635–64.

Lyall H (1993) Dupuytren's disease in identical twins. *J Hand Surg* **18B**: 368–70.

MacCallum P, Hueston JT (1962) The pathology of Dupuytren's contracture. *Aust N Z J Surg* **31**: 241–53.

MacKenney RP (1983) A population study of Dupuytren's contracture. *Hand* **15**: 155–61.

Mackin EJ, Byron PM (1990) Postoperative management. In: McFarlane RM, McGrouther DA, Flint MH, eds, *Dupuytren's Disease*, 368–76. Churchill Livingstone, Edinburgh.

Mackinnon S, Holder LE (1984) The use of three-phase radionuclide bone scanning in the diagnosis of reflex sympathetic dystrophy. *J Hand Surg* **9A**: 556–63.

Madden J (1976) Chromosomal abnormalities in Dupuytren's disease. *Lancet* **1**: 207 (letter).

Maes J (1979) Dupuytren's contracture in an oriental patient. *Plast Reconstr Surg* **64**: 251 (letter).

Magro G, Colombatti A, Lanzafame S (1995) Immunohistochemical expression of Type VI collagen in superficial fibromatoses. *Pathol Res Pract* **191**: 1023–28.

Magro G, Lanzafame S, Micoli G (1995) Co-ordinate expression of alpha 5 beta 1 integrin and fibronectin in Dupuytren's disease. *Acta Histochem* **97**: 229–33.

Magro G, Fraggetta F, Colombatti A et al. (1997) Myofibroblasts and extracellular matric glycoproteins in palmar fibromatosis. *Gen Diagn Pathol* **142**: 185–90.

Makela EA, Jaroma H, Harju A et al. (1991) Dupuytren's contracture: the long-term results after day surgery. *J Hand Surg* **16B**: 272–74.

Mantero R, Ghigliazza GB, Bertolloti P et al. (1986) Les formes récidivantes de al maladie de Dupuytren (analyse d'une casuitique). In: Tubiana R, Hueston JT, eds, *La Maladie de Dupuytren*, 3rd edn, 208–209. Expansion Scientifique Française, Paris.

Matev I (1990) Dupuytren's contracture with associated changes in the plantar aponevroses and in the auricular conchae. *Ann Hand Surg* **9**: 379–80.

Matthews P (1979) Familial Dupuytren's contracture with predominantly female expression. *Br J Plast Surg* **32**: 120–23.

Mawhinney I, de Frenne H, Tubiana R (1999)

Historical, anatomical and clinical aspects of Dupuytren's disease. In: Tubiana R, ed., *The Hand*, 431–83, Vol. V. WB Saunders, Philadelphia.

McCarthy DM (1992) The long-term results of enzymatic fasciotomy. *J Hand Surg* **17B**: 356.

McCash CR (1964) The open palm technique in Dupuytren's contracture. *Br J Plastic Surg* **17**:271–80.

McCash CR (1974) The open palm technique in Dupuytren's contracture. In: Hueston JT, Tubiana R, eds, *Dupuytren's Disease*, 129–33. Churchill Livingstone, Edinburgh.

McFarlane R (1983) The current status of Dupuytren's disease. *J Hand Surg* **8A**: 703–708.

McFarlane R (1985) Some observations on the epidemiology of Dupuytren's disease. In: Hueston JT, Tubiana R, eds, *Dupuytren's Disease*, 122–28. Churchill Livingstone, Edinburgh.

McFarlane R, McGrouther D, Flint M (1990) *Dupuytren's Disease: Biology and Treatment.* Churchill Livingstone, Edinburgh.

McFarlane RM (1974) Pattern of the diseased fascia in the fingers in Dupuytren's contracture. *Plast Reconstruct Surg* **54**: 31.

McFarlane RM (1983) The current status of Dupuytren's disease. *J Hand Surg* **8A**: 703–8.

McFarlane RM (1985) The anatomy of Dupuytren's disease. In: Hueston JT, Tubiana R, eds, *Dupuytren's Disease*, 2nd edn. Churchill Livingstone, Edinburgh.

McFarlane RM (1985) Some observations on the epidemiology of Dupuytren's disease. In: Hueston JT, Tubiana R, eds, *Dupuytren's Disease*, 2nd edn, 122–28. Churchill Livingstone, London.

McFarlane RM (1986) Complications in Dupuytren's disease. In: Boswick JA, ed., *Complications in Hand Surgery*, 294–99. WB Saunders, Philadelphia.

McFarlane RM (1986) Epidemiologie de la maladie de Dupuytren. In: Tubiana R, Hueston, JT, eds, *La Maladie de Dupuytren*, 3rd edn. L'Expansion Scientifique Française, Paris.

McFarlane RM, McGrouther D, Flint M (1990) *Dupuytren's Disease. Biology and treatment.* Churchill Livingstone, Edinburgh.

McGregor IA (1967) The Z-plasty in hand surgery. *J Bone Joint Surg* **49B**: 448–57.

McGregor IA (1985) Fasciotomy and graft in the management of Dupuytren's contracture. In: Hueston JT, Tubiana R, eds, *Dupuytren's Disease*, 2nd edn, 164–71. Churchill Livingstone, Edinburgh.

McGregor IA (1986) Traitement de la maladie de Dupuytren par aponévrotomie et greffe. In: Tubiana R, Hueston JT, eds, *La Maladie de*

Dupuytren, 3rd edn, 165–71. L'Expansion Scientifique Française, Paris.

McGrouther D (1990) Is Dupuytren's disease an inherited disorder? In: McFarlane R, McGrouther D, Flint M, eds, *Dupuytren's Disease*, 280–81. Churchill Livingstone, Edinburgh.

McGrouther DA (1982) The microanatomy of Dupuytren's contracture. *Hand* **13**: 215–36.

McGrouther DA (1986) Anatomie microscopique de la maladie de Dupuytren. In: Tubiana R, Hueston JT, eds, *La Maladie de Dupuytren*, 3rd edn, 32–48. L'Expansion Scientifique Française, Paris.

McGrouther DA (1988) La maladie de Dupuytren. To incise or to excise? *J Hand Surg* **13B**: 368–70.

McGrouther DA (1998) Dupuytren's contracture. In: Green DP, Hotchkiss RN, Pederson WC, eds, *Green's Operative Hand Surgery*, Vol. 1, 4th edn, 563–91. Churchill Livingstone, New York.

McIndoe AH, Beare RLB (1958) The surgical management of Dupuytren's contracture. *Am J Surg* **95**: 197.

McKusick V (1983) *Mendelian Inheritance in Man.* Johns Hopkins University Press, Baltimore.

Medori C (1982) Résultats chirurgicaux de 80 mains atteintes de maladie de Dupuytren revues avec un recul moyen de 5 ans. Thesis, Paris.

Mennen U (1986) Dupuytren's contracture in the Negro. *J Hand Surg* **11B**: 61–64.

Mennen U, Gräbe RP (1979) Dupuytren's contracture in a Negro. A case report. *J Hand Surg* **4**: 451–53.

Menzel EJ, Piza H, Zielinski C et al. (1979) Collagen types and anticollagen antibodies in Dupuytren's disease. *Hand* **11**: 243–48.

Merle M, Merle S (1986) Maladie de Dupuytren et diabète. In: Tubiana R, Hueston JT, eds, *La Maladie de Dupuytren*, 3rd edn, 90–92. L'Expansion Scientifique Française, Paris.

Merle S (1970) Maladie de Dupuytren et diabète. Thesis, Nancy.

Messina A (1989) La TEC (Tecnica di estensione continua) nel morbo di Dupuytren grave. Dall'amputazione alla ricostruzione. *Riv Chir Mano* **26**: 253–56.

Messina A, Messina J (1991) The TEC treatment (continuous extension technique) for severe Dupuytren's contracture fingers. *Ann Chir Main Memb Super* **10**: 247–50.

Messina A, Messina J (1993) The continuous elongation treatment by the TEC device for severe Dupuytren's contracture of the fingers. *Plast Reconstr Surg* **7**: 84–90.

Michon J, Merle M (1986) Difficultés et complications dans la chirurgie de la maladie de Dupuytren. In: Tubiana R, Hueston JT, eds, *La Maladie de Dupuytren*, 3rd edn, 186. L'Expansion Scientifique Française, Paris.

Mikkelsen OA (1967) Dupuytren's disease and blood groups. *Scand J Plast Reconstr Surg* **1**: 148–49.

Mikkelsen O (1972) The prevalence of Dupuytren's disease in Norway. *Acta Chir Scand* **138**: 695–700.

Mikkelsen OA (1976) Dupuytren's disease – a study of the pattern of distribution and stage of contracture in the hand. *Hand* **8**: 265–71.

Mikkelsen OA (1977) Dupuytren's disease. Initial symptoms, age of onset, and spontaneous course. *Hand* **9**: 11–15.

Mikkelsen OA (1977) Knuckle pads in Dupuytren's disease. *Hand* **9**: 301–305.

Mikkelsen OA (1990) Epidemiology of a Norwegian population. In: McFarlane RM, McGrouther DA, Flint MH, eds, *Dupuytren's Disease*, 2nd edn, 191–200. Churchill Livingstone, Edinburgh.

Mikkelsen OA, Hoyeraal HM, Sandvik L (1999) Increased mortality in Dupuytren's disease. *J Hand Surg* **24B**: 515–18.

Milford L (1968) *Retaining Ligaments of the Digits of the Hand.* WB Saunders, Philadelphia.

Millesi H (1974) The clinical and morphological course of Dupuytren's disease. In: Hueston JT, Tubiana R, eds, *Dupuytren's Disease*, 49–60. Churchill Livingstone, Edinburgh.

Millesi H (1985) The clinical and morphological course of Dupuytren's disease. In: Hueston JT, Tubiana R, eds, *Dupuytren's Disease*, 2nd edn, 114–21. Churchill Livingstone, Edinburgh.

Millesi H (1986) Evolution clinique et morphologique de la maladie de Dupuytren. In: Tubiana R, Hueston JT, eds, *Maladie de Dupuytren*, 3rd edn, 115–21. L'Expansion Scientifique, Paris.

Mitra A, Goldstein RY (1994) Dupuytren's contracture in the black population: a review. *Ann Plast Surg* **32**: 619–22.

Moberg E (1973) Three useful ways to avoid amputation in advanced Dupuytren's contracture. *Orthop Clin North Am* **4**: 1001.

Moermans JP (1991) Segmental aponeurectomy in Dupuytren's disease. *J Hand Surg* **16B**: 243–54.

Mondor H (1945) *Dupuytren*, 2nd edn. Gallimard, Paris.

Montenero P, Colleti A, Fabri G (1965) *Maladie de Dupuytren et diabète.* Journées annuelles de Diabétologie de l'Hôtel-Dieu. 75–87. Flammarion, Paris.

Moorhead JJ (1953) Trauma and Dupuytren's contracture. *Am J Surg* **85**: 352–58.

Morane L (1983) Utilisation pronostique des facteurs de risque dans la maladie de Dupuytren. Thesis, Paris.

Morgan RJ, Pryor JP (1978) Porcarbazine (Natulan) in the treatment of Peyronie's disease. *Br J Urol* **50**: 111–13.

Muguti G, Appelt B (1993) Dupuytren's contracture in black Zimbabweans. *Central Afr J Med* **39**: 129–32.

Murrell GA (1991) The role of the fibroblast in Dupuytren's contracture. *Hand Clin* **7**: 669–80.

Murrell GAC, Hueston JT (1990) Aetiology of Dupuytren's contracture. *Aust N Z J Surg* **60**: 247–52.

Murrell GAC, Murrell TGC, Pilowski E (1987) A hypothesis for the resolution of Dupuytren's contracture with allopurinal. *Specul Sci Technol* **10**: 107–12.

Murrell TGC, Murrell GAC, Pilowski E (1986) Resolution of Dupuytren's contracture with allopurinol. *Proceedings of the 10th Fed Europ Connective Tissue Societies, Manchester,* July/August 1986.

Naylor IL, Coleman DJ, Coleman RA et al. (1994) Reactivity of nodular cells in vitro: a guide to the pharmacological treatment of Dupuytren's contracture. In: Berger A, Delbruck A, Brenner P, Hinzman R, eds, *Dupuytren's Disease*, 139–50. Springer Verlag, Berlin.

Neumuller J, Menzel J, Millesi H (1994) Prevalence of HLA-DR3 and autoantibodies to connective tissue components in Dupuytren's contracture. *Clin Immunol Immunopathol* **71**: 142–48.

Nezelof G, Tubiana R (1958) La maladie de Dupuytren: étude histologique. *Sem Hop Paris* **34**: 1102–10.

Niederhuber SS, Stribley RF, Koepke GH (1975) Reduction of skin bacterial load with use of therapeutic whirlpool. *Phys Ther* **55**: 482.

Noble J, Harrison DH (1976) Open palm technique for Dupuytren's contracture. *Hand* **8**: 272–78.

Noble J, Heathcote JG, Cohen H (1984) Diabetes mellitus in the aetiology of Dupuytren's disease. *J Bone Joint Surg* **66B**: 322–25.

Norotte G, Apoil A, Travers V (1988) A ten year follow-up of the results of surgery for Dupuytren's disease. A study of 58 cases (in French and English). *Ann Chir Main* **7**: 277–81.

Orlando JC, Smith JW, Goulian D (1974) Dupuytren's contracture: a review of 100 patients. *Br J Plast Surg* **27**: 211–17.

Parsons AR (1948) Dupuytren's contracture treatment by massive doses of vitamin E. *Ir J Med Sci* **270**: 272–75.

Pentland AP, Anderson TF (1985) Plantar fibromatosis responds to intralesional steroids. *J Am Acad Dermatol* **12**: 212–14.

Pickren JW, Smith AG, Stevenson TW, Stout AP (1951) Fibromatosis of the plantar fascia. *Cancer* **4**: 846–56.

Pittet B, Rubbia-Brandt L, Desmoulière A et al. (1994) Effect of gamma-interferon on the clinical and biologic evolution of hypertrophic scars and Dupuytren's disease: an open pilot study. *Plast Reconstr Surg* **93**: 1224–35.

Pittet-Cuenod B, Della Santa D, Chamay A (1991) Total anterior tenoarthrolysis to treat inveterate flexion contraction of the fingers: a series of 16 patients. *Ann Plast Surg* **26**: 358–64.

Piulachs P, Mir y Mir L (1952) Considerations sobre la enfermedad de Dupuytren. *Fol Clin Int* **II**: 415–16.

Plasse JS (1979) Dupuytren's contractures in a black patient. *Plast Reconstr Surg* **64**: 250 (letter).

Plewes L (1956) Sudeks's atrophy in the hand. *J Bone Joint Surg* **38B**: 195.

Pojer J, Jedlickova J (1970) Enzymatic pattern of liver injury in Dupuytren's contracture. *Acta Med Scand* **187**: 101–104.

Pojer J, Radivojevic M, William TF (1972) Dupuytren's disease – its association with abnormal liver function in alcoholism and epilepsy. *Arch Intern Med* **129**: 561–66.

Powell BW, McLean NR, Jeffs JV (1986) The incidence of a palmaris longus tendon in patients with Dupuytren's disease. *J Hand Surg* **11B**: 382–84.

Quintana GA (1988) Various epidemiologic aspects of Dupuytren's disease. *Ann Chir Main* **7**: 256–62.

Quintana Guitian A (1988) Epidemiological features of Dupuytren's disease. *Ann Chir Main* **7**: 256–62 (in French).

Rao GS, Luthra PK (1988) Dupuytren's disease of the foot in children: a report of three cases. *Br J Plast Surg* **41**: 313–15.

Rayan GM (1999) Palmar fascia complex. Anatomy and pathology in Dupuytren's disease. *Hand Clin* **15**: 73–86.

Rayan GM, Parizi M, Tomasek JJ (1996) Pharmacologic regulation of Dupuytren's fibroblast contraction in vitro. *J Hand Surg* **21B**: 1065–70.

Razemon J (1982) Le lambeau de rotation latéro digital dans les formes graves de la maladie de Dupuytren. A propos de 141 observations. *Ann Chir Main* **1**: 199.

Redfern AB (1986) Corresp newsl of *Am Soc Surg Hand* 71.

Reynolds JW, Bostram CF (1975) Plantar fibromatosis: an unusual location. *J Ann Podiatr Assoc* **65**: 154.

Richards HJ (1954) Dupuytren's contracture: surgical treatment. *J Bone Joint Surg* **36B**: 90–94.

Rives K, Gelberman R, Smith B, Carney K (1992) Severe contractures of the proximal interphalangeal joint in Dupuytren's disease. Results of a prospective trial of operative correction and dynamic extension splinting. *J Hand Surg* **17A**: 1153.

Robbins TH (1981) Dupuytren's contracture: the deferred Z-plasty. *Ann R Coll Surg Engl* **63**: 357–58.

Rodrigo JJ, Niebauer JJ, Brown RL, Doyle JR (1976) Treatment of Dupuytren's contracture: long-time results after fasciotomy and fascial excision. *J Bone Joint Surg* **58A**: 380–87.

Rombouts JJ, Noel H, Legrain Y, Munting E (1989) Prediction of recurrence in the treatment of Dupuytren's disease: evaluation of a histological classification. *J Hand Surg* **14A**: 644–52.

Rosenfeld N, Mavor E, Wise L (1983) Dupuytren's contracture in a black female child. *Hand* **15**: 82–84.

Rowe DW, Starman BJ, Fujimoto WY, Williams RH (1977) Abnormalities in proliferation and protein synthesis in fibroblast cultures from patients with diabetes mellitus. *Diabetes* **26**: 284.

Rowley DI, Couch M, Cheesney RB, Norris SH (1984) Assessment of percutaneous fasciotomy in the management of Dupuytren's contracture. *J Hand Surg* **9B**: 163–64.

Rudolph R, Guber S, Suzuki M, Woodward M (1977) The life cycle of the myofibroblast. *Surg Gynecol Obstet* **145**: 389–94.

Saez Aldana F, Gonzales del Pino J, Delgado A, Lovic A (1996) Epidemologia de la enfermedad de Dupuytren: analisis de 314 casos. *Rev Ortop Traum* **40**: 15–21.

Saffar Ph (1983) Total anterior teno-arthrolysis. Report of 72 cases. *Ann Chir Main* **2**: 345–50.

Saffar Ph (1988) Total anterior tenoarthrolysis. In: Tubiana R, ed., *The Hand*, Vol. III, 297–303. WB Saunders, Philadelphia.

Saffar Ph, Rengeval JP (1978) La ténoarthrolyse totale antérieure. Technique de traitement des doigts en crochet. *Ann Chir* **32**: 579–82.

Salamon A, Hamori J (1980) The role of myofibroblasts in the pathogenesis of Dupuytren's contracture. *Hand Chir* **12**: 113–17.

Salamon A, Hamori J (1980) Possible role of myofibroblasts in the pathology of Dupuytren's disease. *Acta Morphol Acad Sci Hung* **28**: 71–82.

Schneider LH (1964) Dupuytren's contracture in diabetes mellitus. Personal communication. Vth congress of International Diabetes Federation, Toronto, Canada.

Schneider LH (1991) The open palm technique. *Hand Clin* **7**: 723–28.

Schneider LH, Hankin FM, Eisenberg T (1986) Surgery of Dupuytren's disease: a review of the open palm method. *J Hand Surg* **11A**: 23–27.

Schuind F, Burny F (1997) Can algodystrophy be prevented after hand surgery? *Hand Clinics* **13**: 455–76.

Searle AE, Logan AM (1992) A mid-term review of the results of dermofasciectomy for Dupuytren's disease. *Ann Hand Upper Limb Surg* **11**: 376–80.

Sergovich F, Botz J, McFarlane R (1973) Nonrandom cytogenetic abnormalities in Dupuytren's disease. *N Engl J Med* **308**: 162–63.

Short WH, Watson HK (1982) Prediction of the spiral nerve in Dupuytren's contracture. *J Hand Surg* **7A**: 84–86.

Shum DT (1990) Histopathology. In: McFarlane RM, McGrouther DA, Flint MH, eds, *Dupuytren's Disease*, 25–30. Churchill Livingstone, New York.

Shum DT, McFarlane R (1988) Histogenesis of Dupuytren's disease: an immunohistochemical study of 30 cases. *J Hand Surg* **13A**: 61–67.

Simons AW, Srivastava S, Nancarrow JD (1996) Dupuytren's disease affecting the wrist. *J Hand Surg* **21B**: 367–68.

Siratokova H, Elliot D (1997) A historical record of traumatic rupture of Dupuytren's contracture. *J Hand Surg* **22B**: 198–200.

Skoog T (1948) Dupuytren's contraction with special reference to aetiology and improved surgical treatment. Its occurrence in epileptics – Note on knuckle pads. *Acta Chir Scand* **96** (suppl 139): 1.

Skoog T (1967) The superficial transverse fibers of the palmar aponeuroses and their significance in Dupuytren's contracture. *Surg Clin North Am* **47**: 443.

Skoog T (1985) Dupuytren's contracture: pathogenesis and surgical treatment. In: Hueston JT, Tubiana R, eds, *Dupuytren's Disease*, 184–92. Churchill Livingstone, Edinburgh.

Sladicka SJ, Benfanti P, Raab M, Becton J (1996) Dupuytren's contracture in the black population: a case report and review of the literature. *J Hand Surg* **21A**: 898–99.

Smith P, Breed C (1994) Central slip attenuation in

Dupuytren's contracture. A cause of persistent flexion of the proximal interphalangeal joint. *J Hand Surg* **19A**: 840.

Smith PJ, Ross DA (1994) The central slip tenodesis test for early diagnosis of potential boutonnière deformities. *J Hand Surg* **19B**: 88.

Spencer J, Walsh K (1984) Histocompatibility antigen patterns in Dupuytren's contracture. *J Hand Surg* **9B**: 276–78.

Srivastava S, Nancarrow JD, Cort DF (1989) Dupuytren's disease in patients from the Indian sub-continent. Report of ten cases. *J Hand Surg* **14B**: 32–34.

Stack HG (1971) The palmar fascia and the development of deformities and displacements in Dupuytren's contracture. *Ann R Coll Surg Engl* **48**: 230.

Stack HG (1973) *The Palmar Fascia.* Churchill Livingstone, Edinburgh.

Starkweather K, Lattuga S, Hurst LC et al. (1996) Collagenase in the treatment of Dupuytren's disease: an in vitro study. *J Hand Surg* **21A**: 490–95.

Stewart HD, Innes AR, Burke FD (1985) The hand complications of Colle's fracture. *J Hand Surg* **10B**: 103.

Stiles PJ (1966) Ultrasonic therapy in Dupuytren's contracture. *J Bone Joint Surg* **48B**: 452–54.

Strickland JW, Bassett RL (1985) The isolated digital cord in Dupuytren's contracture. Anatomy and clinical significance. *J Hand Surg* **10A**: 118–24.

Strickland JW, Leibovic SJ (1991) Anatomy and pathogenesis of the digital cords and nodules. *Hand Clin* **7**: 645–57.

Stuhler T, Stankovic P, Ritter G, Schmulde E (1977) Epilepsie und Dupuytren'sche Kontraktur. *Hand Chir Mikrochir Plast Chir* **9**: 219–23.

Sugden P, Andrew JG, Andrew SM (1993) Dermal dendrocytes in Dupuytren's disease: a link between skin and pathogenesis? *J Hand Surg* **18B**: 662–66.

Tait B, Mackay L (1982) HLA phenotypes in Dupuytren's contracture. *Tissue Antigens* **19**: 240–41.

Terek RM, Jiranek WA, Goldberg MJ (1995) The expression of platelet derived growth-factor gene in Dupuytren's contracture. *J Bone Joint Surg* **77A**: 1–9.

Thomine J-M (1964) Contribution à l'étude de la maladie de Dupuytren et son traitement chirurgical. Thèse, Paris.

Thomine J-M (1965) Conjonctif d'enveloppe des doigts et squelette fibreux des commissures interdigitales. *Ann Chirurg Plast* **3**: 194–203.

Thomson GR (1949) Treatment of Dupuytren's contracture with vitamin E. *BMJ* **17**: 1382–83.

Thurston AJ (1987) Conservative surgery for Dupuytren's contracture. *J Hand Surg* **12B**: 329–34.

Tomasek JJ, Haaksma CJ (1991) Fibronectin filaments and actin microfilaments are organized into a fibronexus in Dupuytren's diseased tissue. *Anat Rec* **230**: 175–82.

Tomasek JJ, Rayan GM (1995) Correlation of alpha-smooth muscle actin expression and contraction in Dupuytren's disease fibroblasts. *J Hand Surg* **20A**: 450–55.

Tomasek JJ, Schultz RJ, Episalla CW et al. (1986) The cytoskeleton and extracellular matrix of the Dupuytren's disease 'myofibroblast': an immunofluorescence study of a non-muscle cell type. *J Hand Surg* **11A**: 365–71.

Tomasek JJ, Schultz RJ, Haaksma CJ (1987) Extracellular matrix–cytoskeleton connections at the surface of the specialized contractile fibroblast (myofibroblast) in Dupuytren's disease. *J Bone Joint Surg* **69A**: 1400–407.

Tonkin MA, Burke FD, Varian JP (1984) Dupuytren's contracture: a comparative study of fasciectomy in one hundred patients. *J Hand Surg* **9B**: 156–62.

Tonkin MA, Burke FD, Varian JPW (1985) The proximal interphalangeal joint in Dupuytren's disease. *J Hand Surg* **10B**: 358–64.

Touraine A, Ruel H (1945) La polyfibromatose héréditaire. *Ann Dermatol Syphiligr* **5**: 1–5.

Tubiana R (1955) Prognosis and treatment of Dupuytren's contracture. *J Bone Joint Surg* **37A**: 1155–68.

Tubiana R (1963) Les temps cutanés dans le traitement chirurgical de la maladie de Dupuytren. *Ann Chirurg Plast* **8**: 157–68.

Tubiana R (1964) Le traitement sélectif de la maladie de Dupuytren. *Rev Chirurg Orthoped* **50**: 311–33.

Tubiana R (1964) Limited and extensive operations in Dupuytren's contracture. *Surg Clin N Am* **44**: 1071–80.

Tubiana R (1967) *Maladie de Dupuytren.* L'Expansion Scientifique Française, Paris.

Tubiana R (1974) Surgical treatment of Dupuytren's contracture: technique of fasciotomy and fasciectomy. In: Hueston JT and Tubiana R, eds, *Dupuytren's Disease*, 85–92. Churchill Livingstone, Edinburgh.

Tubiana R (1985) Overview on surgical treatment of Dupuytren's disease. In: Hueston JT, Tubiana R, eds, *Dupuytren's Disease*, 2nd edn, 129–30. Churchill Livingstone, Edinburgh.

Tubiana R (1986) Evaluation des déformations dans la

maladie de Dupuytren. In: Tubiana R, Hueston JT, eds, *La Maladie de Dupuytren*, 3rd edn, 111–14. L'Expansion Scientifique Française, Paris.

Tubiana R (1996) Evaluation des lésions dans la maladie de Dupuytren. *Main* **1**, 3–11.

Tubiana R (1998) Dupuytren's disease. Surgical treatment. In: Tubiana R, ed., *The Hand*, Vol. 5, 442–48. WB Saunders, Philadelphia.

Tubiana R (1999) Dupuytren's disease of the radial side of the hand. *Hand Clinics* **15**: 149–59.

Tubiana R, Hueston JT (1972) *La Maladie de Dupuytren*, 2nd edn. L'Expansion Scientifique Française, Paris.

Tubiana R, Hueston JT (1986) *La Maladie de Dupuytren*, 3rd edn. L'Expansion Scientifique Française, Paris.

Tubiana R, Leclercq C (1985) Recurrent Dupuytren's disease. In: Hueston JT, Tubiana R, eds, *Dupuytren's Disease*, 2nd edn, 200–203. Churchill Livingstone, Edinburgh.

Tubiana R, Leclercq C (1986) Tubiana R, Hueston JT, eds, *La Maladie de Dupuytren*, 3rd edn, 203–207. L'Expansion Scientifique Française, Paris.

Tubiana R, Michon J (1961) Classification de la maladie de Dupuytren. *Mem Acad Chir* **87**: 886–87.

Tubiana R, Thomine J-M, Brown S (1967) Complications in surgery of Dupuytren's contracture. *Plast Reconstr Surg* **39**: 603–12.

Tubiana R, Michon J, Thomine J-M (1968) Scheme for the assessment of deformities in Dupuytren's disease. *Surg Clin North Am* **48**, 979.

Tubiana R, Fahrer M, McCullough CJ (1981) Recurrence and other complications in surgery of Dupuytren's contracture. *Clin Plast Surg* **8**: 45.

Tubiana R, Simmons BP, de Frenne HAR (1982) Location of Dupuytren's disease on the radial aspect of the hand. *Clin Orthop Relat Res* **168**: 222–29.

Tubiana R, Thomine J-M, Mackin E (1996) *Examination of the Hand and Wrist*. Martin Dunitz, London.

Tyrkko J, Viljanto J (1975) Significance of histopathological findings in Dupuytren's contracture. *Ann Chir Gynaecol Fenniae* **64**: 288–91.

Urban M, Feldberg L, Janssen A et al. (1996) Dupuytren's disease in children. *J Hand Surg* **21B**: 112–16.

Vandeberg JS, Rudolph R, Gelberman R, Woodward MR (1982) Ultrastructural relationship of skin to nodule and cord in Dupuytren's contracture. *Plast Reconstr Surg* **69**: 835–44.

Vigroux JP, Valentin LP (1992) Natural history of Dupuytren's contracture treated by surgical fasciectomy: the influence of diathesis (76 hands reviewed at more than 10 years). *Ann Chir Main* **11**: 367–74.

Vilain R, Michon J (1977) *Chirurgie plastique cutanée de la main et de la pulpe*, 2nd edn. Masson, Paris.

Viljanto JA (1973) Dupuytren's contracture: a review. *Semin Arthritis Rheum* **3**: 155–76.

Von Borchardt B, Lanz U (1995) Die präoperative kontinuierliche Extensionsbehandlung hochgradiger Dupuytrenscher Kontrakturen. *Handchir Mikrochir Plast Chir* **27**: 269–71.

Von Paeslack (1962) Dupuytren's contracture and diabetes mellitus. *Schweiz Med Wochenschr* **92**: 349–53.

Von Speiser P, Millesi H (1964) Hereditary serologic structure in Dupuytren's disease. *Wien Med Wschr* **114**: 756–57 (in German).

Von Stapelmohr S (1947) Om 14 ars Dupuytren- operatiomer `a Norrköpings lasarett. *Svenska läk Tidning* **44**: 81 (cited by Skoog (1948) (in Swedish)).

Vorstman B, Grossman JA, Gilbert DA et al. (1986) Maladie de La Peyronie. In: Tubiana R, Hueston JT, eds, *La Maladie de Dupuytren*, 3rd edn, 221–25. L'Expansion Scientifique, Paris.

Vuopala LU, Kaipainen WJ (1971) DMSO in the treatment of Dupuytren's contracture – a therapeutic experiment. *Acta Rheum Scand* **17**: 61–62.

Wallace AF (1965) Dupuytren's contracture in women. *Br J Plast Surg* **13**: 385–86.

Walsh K, Spencer J (1990) Immunology and genetics. In: McFarlane R, McGrouther D, Flint M, eds, *Dupuytren's Disease*, 99–103. Churchill Livingstone, Edinburgh.

Walsh M (1984) Relationship of hand edema to upper extremity position and water temperature during whirlpool. *J Hand Surg* **9A**: 609.

Walsh MT (1984) Therapist's management of reflex sympathetic dystrophy. In: Hunter JM, Mackin EJ, Callahan AD, eds, *Rehabilitation of the Hand: Surgery and Therapy*, 4th edn, CV Mosby, St Louis.

Watson HK, Lovallo JL (1987) Salvage of severe recurrent Dupuytren's contracture of the ring and small fingers. *J Hand Surg* **12A**: 287.

Watson HK, Light TR, Johnston TR (1979) Checkrein resection for flexion contracture of the middle joint. *J Hand Surg* **4**: 67–71.

Watson JD (1984) Fasciotomy and Z-plasty in the management of Dupuytren's contracture. *Br J Plast Surg* **37**: 27–30.

Wegmann T (1966) Dupuytren's contracture, diabetes mellitus and chronic alcoholism. *Schweiz Med Wochenschr* **96**: 852–54.

Wehbe MA, Hunter JM (1985) Flexor tendon gliding in the hand. I: in vivo excursions. *J Hand Surg* **10A**: 575–74.

Wehbe MA, Hunter JM (1985) Flexor tendon gliding in the hand. II: differential gliding. *J Hand Surg* **10A**: 575–79.

Weinzierl G, Flugel M, Geldmacher J (1993) Lack of effectiveness of alternative nonsurgical treatment procedures of Dupuytren's contracture. *Chirurg* **64**: 492–94.

Weinzweig N, Culver JE, Fleegler EJ (1996) Severe contractures of the PIP joint in Dupuytren's disease: combined fasciectomy with capsuloligamentous release versus fasciectomy alone. *Plastic Reconstr Surg* **97**: 560–66.

Whaley DC, Elliot D (1993) Dupuytren's disease: a legacy to the North? *J Hand Surg* **18B**: 363–67.

Wheeler ES, Meals RA (1981) Dupuytren's diathesis: a broad-spectrum disease. *Plast Reconstr Surg* **68**: 781–83.

Wolfe SJ, Summerskill WHJ, Davidson CS (1956) Thickening and contraction of the palmar fascia (Dupuytren's contracture), associated with alcoholism and hepatic cirrhosis. *New Engl J Med* **255**: 559–63.

Wong GY, Wilson PR (1997) Classification of complex regional pain syndromes. *Hand Clinics* **13**: 319–25.

Wood Jones F (1942) *The Principles of Anatomy as Seen in the Hand*, 2nd edn. Williams and Wilkins, Baltimore.

Wroblewski BM (1973) Carpal tunnel decompression and Dupuytren's contracture. *Hand* **5**:69–70.

Wurster-Hill D, Brown F, Park J et al. (1988) Cytogenetic studies in Dupuytren's contracture. *Am J Hum Genet* **43**: 285–92.

Wylock P, Vansteenland H (1989) Infection associated with a palmar skin pit in recurrent Dupuytren's disease. *J Hand Surg* **14A**: 518–20.

Yost J, Winters T, Fett HC (1955) Dupuytren's contracture. A statistical study. *Am J Surg* **90**: 568–71.

Zachariae L (1971) Dupuytren's contracture. The aetiological role of trauma. *Scand J Plast Reconstr Surg Hand Surg* **5**: 116–19.

Zachariae L, Zachariae F (1955) Hydrocortisone acetate in the treatment of Dupuytren's contracture and allied conditions. *Acta Chir Scand* **109**: 421–31.

Zachariae L, Dahlerup JV, Olesen E (1970) The electroencephalogram in patients with Dupuytren's contracture. *Scand J Plast Reconstr Surg Hand Surg* **4**: 35–40.

Zancolli EA, Cozzi EP (1992) The retinaculum cutis of the hand. In: Zancolli EA, Cozzi EP, eds, *Atlas of Surgical Anatomy of the Hand*. Churchill Livingstone, New York.

Zaworski RE, Mann RJ (1979) Dupuytren's contractures in a black patient. *Plast Reconstr Surg* **63**: 122–24.

Zemel N (1991) Dupuytren's contracture in women. *Hand Clin* **7**: 707–12.

Zemel NP, Balcomb TV, Skark HH et al. (1987) Dupuytren's disease in women: evaluation of long-term results after operation. *J Hand Surg* **12A**: 1012–16.

Index

Note: page numbers in *italics* refer to figures and tables